T0341318

EXPERIENCING FOOD: DESIGNING SUSTAINABLE AND SOCIAL PRACTICES

PROCEEDINGS OF THE 2ND INTERNATIONAL CONFERENCE ON FOOD DESIGN AND FOOD STUDIES (EFOOD 2019), 28–30 NOVEMBER 2019, LISBON, PORTUGAL

# Experiencing Food: Designing Sustainable and Social Practices

*Editors*

Ricardo Bonacho
*CIAUD Research Centre for Architecture, Urbanism and Design, University of Lisbon, Lisbon, Portugal*
*Higher Institute for Tourism and Hotel Studies, Estoril, Portugal*

Maria José Pires
*Higher Institute for Tourism and Hotel Studies, Estoril, Portugal*

Elsa Cristina Carona de Sousa Lamy
*Institute for Mediterranean Agrarian and Environmental Sciences (ICAAM), University of Évora, Évora, Portugal*

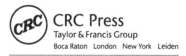

CRC Press
Taylor & Francis Group
Boca Raton London New York Leiden

CRC Press is an imprint of the
Taylor & Francis Group, an **informa** business

A BALKEMA BOOK

*CRC Press/Balkema is an imprint of the Taylor & Francis Group, an informa business*

© 2021 Taylor & Francis Group, London, UK

Typeset by MPS Limited, Chennai, India

*Library of Congress Cataloging-in-Publication Data*
Applied for

Published by:   CRC Press/Balkema
                Schipholweg 107C, 2316 XC Leiden, The Netherlands
                e-mail: Pub.NL@taylorandfrancis.com
                www.routledge.com – www.taylorandfrancis.com

ISBN: 978-0-367-49414-8 (Hbk)
ISBN: 978-1-003-04609-7 (eBook)
DOI: 10.1201/9781003046097
https://doi.org/10.1201/9781003046097

# Table of contents

# Preface

After the successful 1st International Food Design and Food Studies Conference in 2017 there was the challenge to follow the **Experiencing Food** motto. The then designed dialogues led to the discussion over **Designing Sustainable and Social Practices** and a growing search for solutions when designing food systems opened two main debates concerning sustainability: the social practices with food and creativity in food systems.

As for the former, the complexity of a food system triggers political, economic and industrial arguments, along with social issues and health choices. Clearly, these cannot avoid considering the relevance of the diversity of cultural factors, educational approaches and historic moments to be addressed, always bearing in mind lifestyles and learnings, social sustainability, accompanied by a growing concern over food security. Additionally, this debate also portrays situations from the urban scenario and foodscapes to the designing of menus in order to shape consumer perceptions of diverse cuisines and cross-cultural rituals. Such concerns bring about issues regarding the design of food items and the questioning of better forms of dealing with the natural resources to maintain an ecological balance in a near horizon. Therefore, there is a focus on the simultaneous awareness of the diversity in terms of developing gastronomic potential alternatives and of approaches in food production, preparation and management, as the food supply chain.

Reinventing solutions has led to working on sustainability and creativity in food systems: from alternatives in terms of production – product-development – to post-consumption, not forgetting the nutritional issues to food experience and eating behaviours and patterns. This equally portrays the presentation of different concepts when it comes to tableware and interactivity, ranging from everyday situations to fine dining experiences. Accordingly, food representations and transformative food experiences in creative processes from chefs, catering industries and designers reveal multiple connections and practices.

Questioning and understanding beyond both the tangible and intangible has brought to the table issues of how pleasure, creativity, bewilderment and innovation come together and allow us to envision trans-disciplinary collaborations that will help to better shape new sustainable connections and changes.

Maria José Pires
*Member of the Executive and Organizing Committees*
*Estoril Higher Institute for Tourism and Hotel Studies, Portugal*

*Experiencing Food: Designing Sustainable and Social Practices – Bonacho, Pires & Lamy (Eds)*
*© 2021 Taylor & Francis Group, London, ISBN 978-0-367-49414-8*

# Committee members

**CONFERENCE CHAIRS**
Ricardo Bonacho
*CIAUD – Lisbon School of Architecture, Universidade de Lisboa, Portugal*
*ESHTE, Estoril Higher Institute for Tourism and Hotel Studies, Portugal*

Maria José Pires
*ESHTE, Estoril Higher Institute for Tourism and Hotel Studies, Portugal*

Elsa Lamy
*ICAAM – Institute of Mediterranean Agricultural and Environmental Sciences, University of Évora, Portugal*

**ORGANIZING COMMITTEE**
Ricardo Bonacho
*CIAUD – Lisbon School of Architecture, Universidade de Lisboa, Portugal*
*Estoril Higher Institute for Tourism and Hotel Studies, Portugal*

Filipa Nogueira
*CIAUD, Lisbon School of Architecture, Universidade de Lisboa, Portugal*

João Paulo Martins
*CIAUD, Lisbon School of Architecture, Universidade de Lisboa, Portugal*

Maria José Pires
*ESHTE, Estoril Higher Institute for Tourism and Hotel Studies, Portugal*

Miguel Rafael
*CIAUD, Lisbon School of Architecture, Universidade de Lisboa, Portugal*

Luis Ginja
*CIAUD, Lisbon School of Architecture, Universidade de Lisboa, Portugal*

Elsa Lamy
*ICAAM – Institute of Mediterranean Agricultural and Environmental Sciences, University of Évora, Portugal*

**KEYNOTE SPEAKERS**
Carolien Niebling, *Designer*
Marije Vogelzang, *Dutch Institute of Food and Design*
Sonia Massari, *Gustolab International, Scuola Politecnica di Design, ISIA Design School*
Artur Gregório, *In Loco*

**INTERNATIONAL SCIENTIFIC COMMITTEE**
Adrian Woodhouse (Institute of Food Design, Otago Polytechnic, New Zealand)
Ana Cristina Dias (CIAUD – FA.ULisboa)
Ana Inácio (ESHTE)
Anabela Clemente Almeida (ESTM – IPL)
Cândida Cadavez (IHC – UNL / ESHTE)
Catarina Moura (LABCOM.IFP – UBI)
Catarina Prista (ISA – UL)
Cláudia Viegas (ESHTE)
Catarina Moura (LABCOM.IFP – UBI)
Cláudia Viegas (ESHTE)
Elisabete Rôlo (FA.ULisboa – CIAUD)
Elsa Lamy (ICAAM – UE)

Fabio Parasecoli (New School, New York)
Gonçalo Falcão (CIAUD – FA.ULisboa)
João Paulo do Rosário Martins (FA.ULisboa – CIAUD)
Manuela Guerra (ESHTE)
Maria José Pires (ESHTE)
Maria Teresa Pinto Correia (ICAAM)
Paulina Mata (FCT – UNL)
Pedro Moreira (FCNA – UP)
Raquel Lucas (CEFAGE)
Ricardo Bonacho (CIAUD – ESHTE)
Richard Mitchell (Otago Polytechnic Food Design Institute)
Sara Velez Estêvão (LABCOM.IFP – UBI)
Sonia Massari (Gustolab International, Scuola Politecnica di Design, ISIA Design School)
Teresa Cabral (CIAUD – FA.ULisboa)
Vera Barradas (C3i – IPP)

# Food design methods to inspire the new decade. Agency-centered design. Toward 2030

Sonia Massari

*ISIA Design School – Rome, Scuola Politecnica Design Milan, Roma Tre University, Rome, Italy*

ABSTRACT: Relationship between human beings and food, food experience and eating behaviors, and food supply chain and post-consumption activities, respond to a complex system of situational factors and choices that individuals make, often based on patterns that are intangible or not easily predictable. Public concern about food access and food security issues is increasing, everywhere in the world.

Food in its complexity must be studied and managed in a systemic and trans-disciplinary manner. Thus, understanding the role of design in the agri-food sector becomes fundamental. We need to design for more sustainable diets if we want to save the planet.

But there is a positive side to this story and that is there are several professions based on creativity that can make a difference. The professions of sustainability, where humanity is synonymous with a solution, and where food goes hand in hand with innovative systems. Among these, the food designer seems to be a promising career for future professionals who want to apply their skills beyond the food sector, such as the cross-cutting sectors suggested by the UN Agenda 2030 through the 17 Sustainable Development Goals (SDGs).

For this brief contribution, I decided to start from the conclusion of my keynote speech recently given at the 2nd International Food Design and Food Studies Conference entitled "Experiencing FOOD: Designing Sustainable and Social Practices", in Lisbon[1].

The conclusion of my speech was a call to action addressed to everybody, and particularly to designers and innovators who deal with the agri-food sector:

*"we have to design and propose visionary scenarios. We should inspire the humans. Maybe we should shock them. Or only hardly touch them. But only through our futuristic design projects and ideas will we be able to teach today's generations that a different world is possible. We could show them that a sustainable world is not only imaginable, but also achievable. We need to design our revolutionary future world from today. We need to envision sustainable scenarios. We must inspire the contemporary humanities on what the potential values of sustainability could be. More than before, today change makers need to be inspired by the future".*

Sustainability must become a human value soon.

## 1 DESIGN AND CREATIVITY FOR A MORE SUSTAINABLE WORLD

### 1.1 *Humans needs to be inspired to be more sustainable*

Sustainability must become a human value, but unfortunately, we are still far from this scenario. Food activities are always culturally mediated. There is no existing food activity or practice in the world that isn't culture-mediated. And the mediations are driven by human values.

Here is a simple example. I have breakfast everyday with coffee and brioche. Coffee and brioche are my final purpose, they are my food objects. The cultural mediation is in the ritual of breakfast itself. It is in its gestures and practices. I make my coffee every morning for breakfast, learned how to when I was young and have been doing since then. But that coffee and that brioche are also my mediation with the day that is about to start. My day won't be the same without coffee. Not being able to have breakfast the way I've been used to for years will probably affect me positively or negatively. It will have an impact. And where did I learn to have breakfast this way? Maybe from my family, maybe when I was a kid. Behind that breakfast there's much more than a simple act of nutrition. There is an experience, a food experience. There is my personal food experience. There is my story. My past, present and future. An experience that might have changed through the interaction with external factors. A disease for example, or a journey, or a relocation in

---

[1] http://efood.fa.ulisboa.pt/

a place where it might be hard to get a good coffee. Under these conditions, my breakfast will lighten, will change or will conform to the place where I live and to the people around me. For example, the presence of my daughter affects the dynamic of our breakfast for two, and temporarily changes the breakfast I've described above. Therefore, food is the subject of our cultural mediations.

This means that food is both the subject and means of our mediated activities. Mediations include not only the meaning, which is the reason why one does specific actions and activities. But they also include those deeper values of the human being, such as those cognitive acts that we struggle to change.

What does this mean? This means that if mediation does not reflect the subject, the action will be impossible and human values will disintegrate. This concept is very important when we talk about sustainability. Sustainability is that mediation that is still looking for its way in our cognition and in our culture. It is trying to become an important value for humans. And it is still not.

In fact, the word *sustainability* is a very overused term that suggests the possibility of maintaining the economic system in balance with the environment and overcoming the social imbalance. And, in order to work, sustainability has to be long-lasting both through years and generations (in French the word sustainability is translated with *"durable"* – long-lasting), and has to be shared by different communities so as to become a serious global change.

If our future and future generations depend on sustainability,
why can't we deal seriously with the issues connected to it?

The first reason is in the dominant model taught in most university departments and business schools and based on nineteenth-century assumptions. For example, we are still told that natural resources are limitless or limitlessly replaceable.

The second reason is because despite its great relevance, sustainability today is first and foremost a cultural issue which requires great educational changes that need to be tackled. In order to connect the big environmental and social issues such as climate change and deteriorating status of seas, biodiversity loss and mass migrations, all of them being global, interconnected and multidisciplinary, we need to be able to not only communicate beyond borders, but to play and design beyond cultural borders (rather that "design out of the box", we could start using "design out of the borders"). When we say borders, we mean geographical and disciplinary ones. But also, those between private and public sectors; scientific community and civil society, and different languages and disciplines.

It seems necessary to invest on design: an educational tool that can lead to a new cultural change. Design could be the most effective, powerful and inspiring way of teaching and inspiring the students of

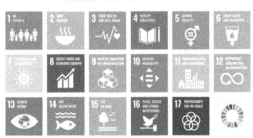

Picture 1. https://sustainabledevelopment.un.org/?menu=1300

the future. Collaboration and trans-disciplinarity are two of the necessary requirements seriously tackle the issue of sustainability. Additionally, the Sustainable Development Goals (SDGs) are helping us all to go in the same (and correct) direction.

## 2  TO ACHIEVE THE SDGS

### 2.1  *Education and innovation in the agri-food sector*

The Sustainable Development Goals (SDGs) are the 17 global goals (Picture 1) that are part of the *"2030 Agenda for a sustainable development"*.

Approved by the UN Assembly on September 2015, the Agenda 2030 is based on 169 targets along with over 240 indicators. "Common goals" means that they concern all countries and people: nobody is excluded, nor should be left behind on the long way that is necessary to take the world to sustainability.

It isn't just an agenda of government intervention. It is first and foremost an agenda of collaboration between "borders" of different natures, that through their work give origin to original collaborations and innovative partnerships.

A kind of common "language", an index and a standardized way that let us "measure our creative and innovative actions" to achieve and design a more sustainable world. Therefore, Agenda 2030 is an agenda of change and innovation. In fact, a revolution is necessary to implement it. A creative revolution that crosses and overlaps with the other great revolution in progress, the digital revolution. Both revolutions are now emerging and maybe are the only ones able to transform the world at the speed required by the SDGs.

A very important concept is the one concerning the role of food to achieve the SDGs.

As a point of reference, we can take "the wedding cake" model theorized by Rockström and Sukhdev in 2016 (keynote speakers at https://eatforum.org/), a conceptualization that shows the wide spectrum of possible goals that can be achieved regarding the biosphere, society, and economy, through actions connected to food (Picture 2).

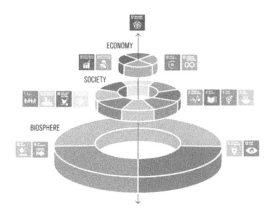

Picture 2. Sustainable Development Goals 2030 (SDGs) wedding cake from Azote Images for Stockholm Resilience Centre, 2016. https://eatforum.org/

The image of the "wedding cake" offered by Rockström and Sukhdev shows how food can contribute directly and indirectly to the achievement of all 17 Goals established by the 2030 Agenda, consistently with the evolution of a sustainability model that goes from being anthropocentric to being systemic-centric (or eco-centric). It recognizes, at the base of the cake, that the biosphere dimension is what contains and supports any social and economic plan.

This model changes our paradigm for development, moving away from the current sector-based approach in which social, economic and ecological developments have been considered as separate parts. Now we need to move to a global logic in which economy can be at the service of society so that it can evolve to save the planet.

Therefore, a series of relationships connect the different SDGs through food. Some are more evident: the aim of Goal 12, for example, is sustainable production and consumption and is directly linked to the creation of a new relationship between producer and consumer (SDG 17), to the reduction of world hunger (SDG 2), to health and welfare (SDG 3), which are in turn influenced by the achievement of goals related to natural capital (SDGs 15, 14, 6, and 13).

Moving from this conceptual frame, the important role of food design is clear, and not only in the agri-food sector. Sustainable innovation in food means to produce a positive impact on all the other 17 goals.

Ideas and solutions created by food designers will last much longer than any given deadline, so they will have reach beyond 2030. They will continue influencing and changing our world, its systems and the people in the years and generations to come. Therefore, the role of food design is so important not only to envision and to inspire, but also to act. The decisions of design will have the power not only to help us achieve the SDGs, but also guide us and educate us toward a sustainable future beyond them (http://oslomanifesto.org/sdgs/).

## 3 DESIGNING FOR THE NEW DECADE. THE LAST 10 YEARS AND THE NEXT 10 YEARS

### 3.1 *My experience at Gustolab International*

I like to think of these last 10 years, of cultural, economic, social, ethical, digital and environmental transformations through a professional and personal story. At the beginning of the new millennium, I was an adjunct professor in design at a university in the United States. Never would I have thought to deal with education regarding food and innovation in food systems. When you study (and then you teach) design methods, the first thing you are told is that you will have to be able to apply it to any sector. You will never be expert in a specific sector because design is a transdisciplinary research method.

I was focusing my PhD research on new ways of teaching and learning, when in 2008, back in Europe, I was asked to design the foundations of a new and pioneering institute in Rome (Italy), called *Gustolab*: a food-related center of studies geared towards foreign students during their period of study abroad. The initial name given to the center was quite indicative: *Gustolab* ("laboratory of taste"), Center for Food and Culture. Subtitle." Training your taste". Its main aim was to educate foreign students about food and its relation to culture. Or better, to explain that food is always a product of culture and the study of food requires a full immersion in its culture.

Food culture was my key concept.

In fact, food is the great unifier that connects us across cultures and generations. Food can quite literally propel you to another time, country or culture without ever leaving your dinner table, which is why food culture is such an important way that allows people to connect and relate to one another. Food-culture refers to the practices, attitudes, and beliefs as well as the networks and institutions surrounding the production, distribution, and consumption of food. Food culture is the connection, beliefs, and experience we have with food and our food system. It incorporates our cultural heritage and ethnicity, but is not limited to it. It is about our environmental culture and the way our surrounding impact the foods we eat and the way we experience them. This was my arduous goal for a few years: to explain to my students the meaning of food culture, the importance of history and culture in the evolution of the production of ingredients, in cooking, in nutrition and in social dynamics. At the beginning, the debate on climate change was limited, and even less about the waste of resources. Most of the analyses and studies were on the social role of food.

Food was in search of a discipline

By the end of the first decade of 2000, many U.S. universities decided to open Food Studies academic programs with the purpose of training future professionals with transversal skills in food and science, communication and food business management. The education promoted by food studies had the purpose of involving different stakeholders such as researchers, those working in the agriculture, producers and consumers. It also had the purpose of helping the exchange of skills and knowledge between industries and universities in order to enhance food competences and resources. In 2004, the anthropologist Guigoni defined Food Studies as a set of studies about the anthropological, historical, sociological and psychological aspects of nutrition. "This macro-discipline intersects (and sometimes blends) with *consumption studies*, that are studies aimed at analyzing trends, myths and representations of consumption practices and the value and meaning of commodities in the different social groups." (Guigoni, 2004).

Food Studies have had a quick growth as a discipline and today, does not just study historical and sociological aspects of food, but also deals with the sphere of production, distribution, consumption and post-consumption (waste, education, communication, etc.) of food; moreover, the subject of Food Studies has moved to issues in agriculture and to new methods of micro-production (i.e: vertical, social, urban farming), to the analysis and study of innovative models for a sustainable production and distribution and to communication systems aimed at supporting education, training and innovation in the agri-food sector.

As director of *Gustolab*, my job was to design innovative curricula for Food Studies oriented courses abroad since the beginning. As a designer, I went into a domain I had never had before, a real scientific field by proposing a way of seeing food in a more general and less specific manner and thus a great challenge in teaching and learning. Through design I tried to connect topics that had never come across one another, integrate future studies and knowledge that had always been considered far from formal education and associated only to agricultural or artisan cultural transmission. *Gustolab* was the very first experiment of an institute totally dedicated to hybrid, experiential, transformative and systemic education applied to food. Designing it meant not only creating the concept and testing the prototype, but also understanding in a visionary way the educational impact of this initiative on the final target: not only a larger group of students, but potential adults and citizens of the new millennium.

Design is an experiential method of research

Since the beginning, I applied design methods to *Gustolab* to develop most of the experiential learning academic activities. I have always defined the power of design as "metabolic": design allows you to immerse yourself in a culture, understand it, and see the world with different eyes. This was my primary goal in all the courses I've designed and coordinated. I was continually looking to producers, breeders, farmers, artisans, to find their identities and values.

It was 2015 and we had to imagine an evolution of our hybrid teaching methods: a new way to experience a foreign food culture. The objective of using design for pedagogical purposes in the agri-food sector became so predominant that it also impacted on the development of the goals of the study center. *Gustolab* changed its name to "Gustolab, Institute for Food Studies" and became more of a center dedicated to food studies scholars and students. It was an attempt into the field, notions and associate them immediately to issues on the field. I designed more teaching models based on ethnographic research applied to video storytelling with the engagement of local community in shared research projects. It meant involving the students from the very beginning in activities of collaborative and co-constructive learning and helping them to produce a new way of education themselves. I started designing curricula for new careers in sustainability. The title of our programs always included the word "critical": critical studies on food and culture, critical studies on food and media, etc to make it clear that food was complex and must be analyzed with a critical and not only cultural approach. But also, to make sure our students understood that analytics and scientific data are important to analyze food systems, but to solve them we need to improve our intercultural awareness and critical creativity.

Food is complex. We need critical creativity

Almost at the end of this decade (2018), the borders of academic education for sustainability and food studies have broadened and the divide between qualitative and quantitative has started to narrow. Today we talk about proximity, connections and construction of systems in which human beings are not at the center, but become an integral part of the food ecosystem. To the critical approach, we added the creative and systemic approaches. It was time to think about systems and their impact on our lives. The aim was now to give students more tools of analysis to study food in from the point of view of human values. Students should be able to understand food from different perspectives. The idea for me has been designing sustainability and food systems curricula that aren't ideological and politically-oriented, and to train students to create their visions critically. Analyzing the systems wasn't enough anymore: it was necessary to try and solve them. Only an evolving study of diversities can sustain a process of sustainable change. The design I've applied over the last 10 years in my work has helped make the food studies paths more participatory and engaging. In the learning process, the territory and the community were no longer omitted. Migration had changed the urban and peri-urban substratum of our cities. Food security was not only a problem for "others", but it was starting to become "our problem". The concept of authenticity changed its meanings. So *Gustolab* changed its name again in order to adapt to the globalized and multifaceted society, becoming *"Gustolab International, Food Systems and Sustainability"*.

The word sustainability could no longer be separated from food

But where are we going now? What awaits us over the next 10 years? How will the SDGs guide us towards 2030? Today's process of scientific collaboration required by the SDGs must be more similar to a co-construction of knowledge, rather than to an exchange of notions and methods. We need to be more pioneering in order to convince people to be innovators and show them that a sustainable world is possible. By using creativity, testing new models, inventing new paradigms and solutions, but most of all by thinking out of the box, it is necessary to proceed toward an education for sustainability which is both creative and critical.

We must design a world for sustainable natives, those who do not have issues with the language of sustainability and demonstrate sustainable behavior effortlessly, like digital natives that do not have any issues with learning and using digital tools and devices. That's why it is necessary to design food products, services, systems and create behavioral models to support people's abilities and knowledge in relation to their social and cultural context. It is time to create new and more sustainable food cultures.

I think I have one of the best jobs in the world because I get to work with people who are happy, energetic, full of joy, creatively positive and insightful: students. I love inspiring students because they will be the adults of the future, as much as I love inspiring design students, because they will be the makers of the future.

20 years of teaching experience in the food and design studies have taught me that three things are needed to teach sustainability:

- experiential-based teaching techniques,
- 50% creative and 50% critical thinking learning approaches
- student agency for 2030.

In a word, we could almost summarize these three things in the concept of "design methods ". Agri-food education needs more design methods.

Let's start from the experiential-based teaching techniques. When I started doing this job and designing Gustolab Center, it was very innovative: it was an open field, where it was possible to experiment, make a mistake, start again, win and commit to it. There was very little scientific literature on formal, non-formal and informal food studies education. Today there are quite a lot of scholars dealing with this subject, in particular experiential learning has become a common practice in food and sustainability studies. Experiential learning has evolved also thanks to the application of design thinking to different disciplines.

| 6Cs | 1. COLLABORATION<br>2. COMUNICATION | EXPERIENTIAL TEACHING APPROACHES | AGENCY–CENTERED DESIGN | DESIGN METHODS FOR AGRI-FOOD EDUCATION |
|---|---|---|---|---|
| | 3. CRITICAL THINKING<br>4. CREATIVE THINKING | EXPERIENTIAL LEARNING APPROACHES | | |
| | 5. CHOICE<br>6. CHANGE | MENTORSHIP And STUDENT AGENCY | | |

Picture 3.

At the same time, the debate on the importance of creativity in classroom (Massari, 2017) has become more interesting as a research focus. Especially in terms of critical skills and knowledge that are needed to understand the controversial issues linked to social, economic and environmental sustainability.

Over ten years ago, the U.S. National Education Association (NEA, 2010) identified four Cs as essential 21st century skills that students should learn:

1. COLLABORATION
2. COMMUNICATION
3. CRITICAL THINKING
4. CREATIVITY

I could say that collaboration (team-work) and communication (debate and sharing) are at the basis of all the experiential teaching methods. Critical thinking and creativity are the necessary skills to activate all the processes of awareness and conscious learning and they are paramount in food and sustainability studies.

I want to add CHOICE and CHANGE to this list not only as two important skills for students to learn, but as the main goals of each of my courses. When many learning activities and methods are available to students, students love it as much as they love choices and changes in their life. This is what mentorship means to me (Picture 3).

Choice and change are fundamental in agency. The concept of student agency is rooted in the principle that students have the ability and the will to positively influence their own lives and the world around them. Student agency is thus defined as the capacity to set a goal, reflect and act responsibly to effect change. It is about acting rather than being acted upon; shaping rather than being shaped; and making responsible decisions and choices rather than accepting those determined by others[2].

So, I believe design methods applied to food and sustainability education are wired for the 6 Cs. And since they're wired for the 6 Cs, revolutionary learning will happen and students will be inspired to create a better future. When students are allowed to engage in the 6 Cs, students will learn to enjoy and engage with their futures. They will be able to design and reset it. This requires that the professor to remove themselves from the front and center, becoming more of a guide on the side rather than a sage on the stage. This opens opportunities to not merely teach, but to coach, mentor, nurture and inspire, and that's why I love it so much.

[2] www.oecd.org/education/2030-project

# 4 CONCLUSIONS

## 4.1 *Envisioning sustainability through agency-centered design*

We need to design solutions that allow our different sustainable food experiences to create systems that can truly make a difference.

> There is no more time.
> We no longer have resources.
> The world is burning.
> Food is changing.

We must change too. Otherwise the consequences will be devastating.

My statements for the next 10 years are:

- We must increase education for creating more sustainable food systems,
- We must envision new creativities,
- We must improve humans-agency skills

Human values-centered design (or, people-centered design) in the last 10 years has characterized our way of designing. In my opinion, we are in search of a new way of designing.

> Humanity needs more than inspiration

This is important and we must understand what this means. We need to work on agency-centered design. Let me try to explain this better.

Do you remember that very popular video on YouTube[3] in which a three-year-old child argues whether or not he should eat the octopus his mother cooked for him? A very smart kid because from that situation he managed to conclude that all the animals that we eat are going to die and that he didn't particularly like the idea that they were supposed to die to satisfy someone's appetite, especially his. His mother, moved, listens to him and accepts his request. A situation of great value starts to circulate. She is moved and takes her son's request very seriously; the kid understood that he acted for the environment causing his mother's emotion. This emotion doesn't get lost, but it was useful for the child to understand that he had done something beautiful.

A single episode is probably not enough to establish agency, but surely this mother will have been able to repeat this beautiful dyadic interaction in other situations.

The concept of agency is different from that of self-confidence. Self-confidence is a way of feeling connected to an internal principle. Agency is more of an awareness of efficiently being able to affect the surrounding environment; from an individual principle to a global and the ability to affect external environment materializes more or less consciously.

People with agency can take advantage of institutional links of structure itself, exploit the resources

given by the system and are less exposed to discouragement imposed by it. Their choices are influenced by the degree of effectiveness in handling the events; perseverance and resilience increase and the quality of performance gets better. If I feel adequate and if I feel that the environment is supporting me, my performance will get better. Agency is the ability to make things happen by intervening on reality and exercising a casual power. Agency isn't simply a trait or an activity of the single individual, but rather a way of living in the world.

Just imagine what it could mean in terms of becoming "sustainable agents".

In this new decade food designers have a critical role more than ever, not only because they have to design the sustainability messages to transmit, but because they have to design spaces where these messages can evolve. Surely the innovations for more sustainable agri-food systems will come to end (exactly like they started) but in their daily enaction they will move more and more on a *continuum*.

While designing these systems, we cannot anticipate what cannot be designed, but we should create a framework of what is unexpected. The task and job of the food designer is not to grant the same vision for everybody, but to establish the conditions for different visions that can interact and lead to sustainable solutions. If in the last decade we've worked to explain how to design the best food experiences and focused on the systemic approach in the food world, today more than ever we need to unify this knowledge into a common project: designing more sustainable food systems.

This process can be developed on different levels, from the moment input is given to user to the moment when the system allows the user to produce output, but most of all during the communication that the continuous repetition produces for all the life cycle of experience (Antonelli, 2008).

It is now clear to everybody how in the last 10 years, first the digital transformation and then the SDGs, have changed our way of looking at things.

Furthermore, the values we give to short-lived consumption are essentially in growing contrast with the political and economic climate of today's western societies. People are worried about the future and think about sustainability. Our end-user has changed their minds in the past 10 years: they are no longer disoriented in the many chosen, as described in our design manuals (led by digital and post-modern marketing).

> Today's consumption is more mature.

We have reached that stage of human evolution in which we must begin to solve problems that affect the relationship between us and our planet. The problem that most worries our western countries is not understanding the quantity of products and objects that we can still design or how to produce and consume in a sustainable way. The real question, on the other hand, is what we should design, produce and consume that increases the people agency. What we need to understand as a designer is the type of relationship

---

[3] https://www.youtube.com/watch?v=tQIMJ648qgg

that exists between us and the quality of life we want to have. But above all the quality of sustainable life that we can design.

A part of this transformation has to be understood as a form of constant change and this is the reason why the job of the food designer is never static, but changes continuously:

> *The designer's challenge is to create a framework for the user to engage in conversation, but the designer is also now charged with engaging the user in conversation through the framework itself. Design solutions can no longer be concluded; they're now works in progress, objects that continually evolve and are continually reinvented. (Antonelli, p. 131)*

We need to design our visionary futures to inspire contemporary humanities and create more sustainable worlds. And … we should start now.

## REFERENCES

Antonelli, P. (2008). *Design and the plastic mind.* New York: The Museum of Modern Art.

Guigoni, A. (editedby) (2004). Foodscapes. Stili, mode e culture del cibo oggi. Polimetrica, Milano.

NEA (2010). Preparing 21st Century Students for a Global Society: An Educator's Guide to 'The Four Cs'. Washington DC, National Education Association. www.nea.org/tools/52217.htm.

Massari, S. (2017). 'Food design and food studies: Discussing creative and critical thinking in food system education and research', *International Journal of Food Design*, 2: 1, pp. 117–133.

## WEBSITES

http://efood.fa.ulisboa.pt/
http://oslomanifesto.org/sdgs/
https://sustainabledevelopment.un.org/
https://eatforum.org/
www.oecd.org/education/2030-project
https://www.youtube.com/watch?v=tQIMJ648qgg

# Designing with a fork: Lessons from past urban foodscapes for the future

M. Sanchez Salvador

*DINÂMIA'CET-IUL, ISCTE-IUL, Lisbon, Portugal*

ABSTRACT: Unlike other basic needs, food has been virtually absent from today's urban design and planning. Historically, however, food matters were key factors underlying the location of pre-industrial cities, the size attained, the organization and land use of their hinterlands. Food production was present around and within the city; distribution routes defined its roads and streets; food activities were remembered in place-names; markets were the beating hearts of urban life. Cities and food were interconnected.

Nowadays, apart from food consumption, food became almost invisible in the city, being relegated to distant places, private spaces and off-hours. This distance conveys severe environmental and cultural consequences, jeopardizing urban sustainable development. Food, however, might contribute to designing more sustainable cities for the future. Architects and urban designers have proposed creative solutions — edible buildings, productive continuous landscapes — which might be crucial in this context. These realities will be explored, for a more balanced future.

## 1 INTRODUCTION

Cities might be defined as "groups of populations that do not produce their own means of subsistence", implying a technical, social and spatial division of production, and exchanges between those who produce subsistence goods and those who produce manufactured goods, symbolic goods, power and protection (Ascher, 2010: 21). This does not mean, however, that cities have developed *regardless* of their food supplies.

In fact, the very origin of cities is intrinsically linked to a more constant and abundant food supply made possible by *agriculture*. Until then, almost the entire community had to be channelled to ensure food supply through harvesting, hunting, fishing or pastoralism. With agriculture, it became possible to sustain individuals engaged in different professions and crafts. Social classes, monumental architecture, writing and numerical systems, exact sciences, art, state and politics, taxes, commerce, etc. — civilization — have since arisen. Childe (1950) termed it *urban revolution*.

Therefore, cities can be characterized by not producing their own means of subsistence, not because food production is absent from urban space or the daily activities of its inhabitants, but rather because a set of other characteristics and activities overlap them. In the physical design of cities, however, this food dimension was very much present.

## 2 PRE-INDUSTRIAL URBAN FOODSCAPES

### 2.1 *The location of cities*

Several factors determined the location of pre-industrial cities: defence, policy, religion and symbolism, climatic and health issues, proximity to water resources, among others. However, throughout history, one factor was key: *transportation*. Since, for centuries, land transportation was difficult, conditioning the movement of products and raw materials, physical proximity to (food) resources was central. Inner cities were, therefore, dependent on the agricultural resources available in their immediate hinterland.

> "As soil can hardly be built, the general principle is to organise the entire community according to the best soils and, within possible, never occupy them with land uses other than food production." (Pereira dos Santos, 2010: 18–19)

For a community to be established in a place, the existence of a set of favourable conditions had to be identified — topography, water, soil fertility, temperature, rain cycles. Conditions, that is, which allowed it to survive and thrive. The location of cities could be the reason of their prosperity or the cause of their collapse, which translated into an aura of symbolism around the foundation of a city. For this very reason, in the Roman Empire, the sites were chosen by *augurs* who made careful observations of the natural phenomena before defining the location of the *mundus*, the well that marked the city centre and was its symbolic connection to the place and to land gods (Steel, 2013: 15). Vitruvius highlighted this importance in his *Ten Books of Architecture* (2006), describing a dialogue between Alexander the Great and Dinocrates, the architect who proposed him to build a new magnanimous city. Alexander liked the proposal, but inquired the architect about the existence of surrounding fields to supply the city with grain. When Dinocrates answered negatively, Alexander would have replied:

> "Just as a new-born child cannot feed himself or continue to grow into life without the milk of a nurse, so a city without fields and without fruit that comes into its walls cannot grow, since it cannot develop without the abundance of food, nor can it sustain its population if it has no resources." (Alexander the Great quoted by Vitruvius, 2006: 69–70)

Alexander reproved the chosen site, and Alexandria was later founded in a place where it could thrive. This episode reflects a fundamental reality: in the absence of fast connections to distant territories, pre-industrial cities depended predominantly on local *foodsheds* — the area from which a community extracts their food (Hedden, 1929: 17).

But it was not only fertility that was important in defining soil quality: in a context of rudimentary agriculture, it was important that the land was easy to work, resistant to erosion and easy to protect (Raison, 1986: 324). Thus, cities would settle as close as possible to the most fertile and workable soils, being often completely surrounded by cultivated soils.

The only exception, in this pre-industrial context, was granted by navigable rivers or seas: privileged communication routes, uniting different and distant peoples. Rivers and seas allowed the fast transportation of food products since Antiquity, at a cost rate up to 42 times cheaper than land transportation (Steel, 2013: 73), giving riverside and seaside cities an unequalled advantage over inner cities.

## 2.2 Size and distribution of pre-industrial cities

Food supply also conditioned the size — in both population and physical terms — that a city could attain, a condition which parallels biology's notion of *carrying capacity*, which defines the relationship between an ecosystem and the number of individuals it can sustain in terms of food, water and habitat (Brun et al., 1986: 24). In a pre-industrial context, the *maximum population* of a city depended directly on the productive capacity of its soils and complementary food resources (Mumford, 1970: 316).

> "[These cities] were still in essence agricultural towns: the main source of their food supply was in the land around them; [...] they could not grow beyond the limit of their local water supply and their local food sources." (Mumford, 1956)

During the Medieval Ages, European cities remained within a few thousands of inhabitants (Morris, 1995: 119), and respected a certain proportion of urban to rural populations to insure food supply.

The *physical size* cities could attain was connected to the fact that food products could hardly travel more than one day before spoiling, especially vegetables, meat and milk. This limited the distance of their provenance to about 30 km if travelled on foot, or a bit larger if wagons or animals were used, fixating a practical limit to the city's productive belt. Thus, there was a maximum area an urban settlement could attain before occupying its production lands and reducing them to an insufficient size:

> "A day's journey by cart, a distance of around 20 miles [32 km], was the practical limit for bringing in grain overland, which limited the width of the city's arable belt. The simple laws of geometry meant that the larger the city grew, the smaller the relative size of its rural hinterland became, until the latter could no longer feed the former." (Steel, 2013: 70–71)

For Braudel (1992a: 99), it was advisable for a city to be fed on what it possessed within its reach, and limiting this supply to a circle of 20 to 30 km would avoid expensive transportation and imports. These limitations to growth led to an urban expansion model through new satellite cities, which maintained a certain autonomy.

The distribution of urban settlements in the territory was also relatively homogeneous. According to Élisée Reclus, European cities tended to distribute equally as much as topography allowed, maintaining a distance of a day's travel on foot between them (Mumford, 1970: 59). Thomas More, in his *Utopia* (1973: 63), also advocated a similar model, with cities being about 24 miles apart, and never more than a day on foot. Likewise, each city should have 20 miles (about 32 km) of arable land around, "and sometimes more if, from either side, the distance between one city and another is greater".

## 2.3 The hinterland of pre-industrial cities

Food supply was so crucial that it constrained the hinterland's land use and type of crops. Throughout time, we can witness a particular organisation: the *aureolar models*. Von Thünen, in *The Isolated State* of 1826, conceived a pioneering model, based on an idealised situation for a city located at a fertile plain, with no topographic constraints (relief, watercourses) and a constant climate, where farmers made rational decisions to maximize profits.

> "Imagine a very large town, at the centre of a fertile plain [...] the soil is capable of cultivation and of the same fertility. Far from the town, the plain turns into an uncultivated wilderness which cuts off all communication between this State and the outside world. [...] The central town must therefore supply the rural areas with all manufactured products, and in return it will obtain all its provisions from the surrounding countryside." (Von Thünen, quoted by Björklund, 2010: 49)

The main factor defining land uses would thus be transportation and its costs, directly related to the distance travelled (Steel, 2013: 71). Under these conditions, the tendency would be for food production to be organized in concentric rings around the town. The first ring was devoted to more perishable fruit, vegetables and dairy products, to which closeness was crucial. Being more expensive, they could bear the higher land rents, while benefitting the most from urban wastes, used as manure. The second ring was an area of forest, supplying the city with timber and firewood. Proximity was necessary because wood is heavy and difficult to transport. The third ring consisted of grain fields which, being lighter, had cheaper transportation costs and deteriorated less. The fourth and last ring was devoted to pastures. Although located far from the town, cattle were able to walk and be slaughtered near its place of consumption. Beyond these rings, there was only wilderness, too distant to be useful for the city supply, since transport made these goods too expensive.

Ribeiro Telles (2016) also referred a similar territorial model, organized into four strips. The first strip (F1) was the urban settlement itself, while the second strip (F2) was for orchards, vegetable gardens and small cattle breeding, being women's role in the high productivity achieved highlighted. The third strip (F3) had extensive agriculture and rain-fed areas, intended for cattle breeding in the winter and growing grain in the spring/summer. It would have the greatest extension and the most determinant in the size attained by the community, being the responsibility of men. The fourth strip (F4) was polyvalent, consisting of bushes, eventually vineyards, wild berries and nuts. Its functions transcended food supply and included defence, livestock and manure.

Other concentric-ring models were composed of two or three zones, with different agri-pastoral functions. Ring limits were directly related to labour: intensive cultivation was closer to dwellings because it required greater work by a larger part of the population and allowed transporting manure in a shorter time. A smaller number of producers were mobilized for livestock breeding, so this area could be located further away (Lemonnier, 1986: 82). Examples occurred more significantly in the Middle Ages in the Western and Central Europe (Lemonnier, 1986: 81), and could be found in London, Caen, Paris, Frankfurt-am-Main, Worms, Basel and Munich, among others (Braudel, 1992a: 428; 1992b: 25–161). In London, intensive agricultural areas concentrated within 25–30 km of the city centre, in areas like Uxbridge, Brentford, Kingston, Hampstead, Hertford, Watford, St Albans, Croydon and Dartford (Braudel, 1992b: 26). There was, even, a subdivision of the first ring: closer to London's centre, vegetables but mainly delicate and exotic fruits were cultivated, requiring great care; beyond this area, less perishable vegetables were produced — peas, beans, onions, Brussels sprouts, broccoli and cauliflower — and, farther still, ordinary vegetables in rotation systems. A similar situation occurred for animal products:

> "[…] the whole country round London was easily separable into zones or annular belts […].

Milking, for the supply of the metropolis, was carried on within a circuit of six or eight miles, either by cow-keepers […] or by farmers who sent the milk in large upright tin cans by spring vans, to the retailers in town. Beyond, and surrounding this zone, was the veal and lamb suckling district, extending from ten to thirty miles; while still farther off was the fresh-butter district, whence heavy, broad-wheeled waggons brought the butter to London." (Dodd, 1856: 219–220)

Paris derived most food supply from an area roughly coincident with the Seine's watershed, protected by numerous regulations governing food production and trade (Braudel, 1992b: 24). London and Paris were also examples of an exception included by Von Thünen in his model: the presence of a river that allowed the fast movement of products at a lower cost. This variable changed the whole model configuration, turning the production rings into parallel stripes along the watercourse (Steel, 2013: 71).

Pre-industrial cities maintained a relationship of proximity and interdependence with their food production lands, at a local scale, and strongly rooted in the territory's potentialities and constraints. It was characterized by a *circular metabolism* of energy and matter flows between urban and rural. However, food systems also impacted the organisation and urban form within cities, with food land uses being intrinsically connected to the different elements of urban form: open spaces, streets and buildings.

### 2.4 *Food production within pre-industrial cities*

Food production has always been part of cities. Even when cities were enclosed by walls, there were cultivated spaces inside — orchards, vegetable gardens, even commons and pastures — shown in engravings and maps (Mumford, 2004: 285). *Urban* and *peri-urban agriculture* were ancient practices — *hortus conclusus* existed in Egypt, Persia, Greece, Rome, Pompeii and in Islamic Spain — and were present both in small and large European cities (Parham, 2015: 47–49; Mumford, 2004: 88–285).

> "[…] the town of the Middle Ages was not merely *in* the country but *of* the country; food was grown within the walls, as well as on the terraces, or in the orchards and fields, outside." (Mumford, 1970: 24)

The existence of agricultural and livestock areas within the walls ensured the city's *resilience* and even *survival*, in the event of war or prolonged siege (Björklund, 2010: 21; Mumford, 2004: 88; Braudel; 1992a: 435). The walls of Florence covered meadows and vegetable gardens, as in Paris, Toulouse, Poitiers, Prague, Barcelona and Milan (Morris, 1995: 106–218; Braudel, 1992a: 435). In the 17th and 18th centuries, nearby vegetable gardens played an important role in food security and innovation: vegetables, fruit and herbs represented a reservoir of food resources, but it was also here that one learned to cultivate delicate, little-known plants. In France, these were the first sites to welcome novelties: cabbages, cauliflowers, radishes, carrots, peas and, later, the potato (Roche, 1998: 252). The need for close food production even led to innovative solutions as the *hortillonnages* in Amiens: floating vegetable gardens covering around 300 hectares, which played an important role in the city's food supply.

Animals — such as pigs, chickens, rabbits, pigeons, etc. — were also raised in the city for meat, but mainly for milk. In New York, in 1840, milk supply came from 18 000 cows living in about 500 farms in the city and in Brooklyn, fed on grain waste of distilleries and breweries (Santlofer, 2017: 239). Atkins estimates urban milk production of 52% for Edinburgh (1921), 30% for Liverpool (1927) and 20% for Belfast (1929), while London will have declined from 80% in 1850 to 28% in 1880, and only 3% in 1910 (Atkins, 2003: 137). Often, raising animals was a practice complementary to agriculture, getting manure and because animals could be fed on waste or raised in plots unsuitable for crops, due to slopes or soil characteristics.

Working on agricultural land (owned or rented) and raising livestock were part of the daily lives of city dwellers, who possessed rear vegetables gardens and practiced these occupations within the city. Many bourgeois also possessed orchards, vineyards and olive groves in the outskirts (Mumford, 2004: 146–314). Cows and sheep grazed on commons and city dwellers still benefitted from municipal forest and fishing resources (Mumford, 2004: 314–315). The size of these lands could be significant: in Poland it reached an average of 8–10 ha/person; while some small towns in France controlled extensions up to 5 km away from the city (Björklund, 2010: 21). In Sweden, the area of orchards, arable land, meadows, grasslands and forests belonging to a city averaged 970 ha and could reach 2500 ha, in some cases (Björklund, 2010: 89–91).

"Living in such a city, there could be no doubt as to where your food came from: it was all around you, snorting and steaming and getting in the way." (Steel, 2013: 6)

## 2.5 Urban form: squares, streets and buildings in pre-industrial cities

Food systems covered virtually all dimensions of urban development, organising land and building uses, street layouts, squares, and other public spaces, allowing flows of people and products and the interaction of different professions and social classes. Food was a strong link between communities, cities and territories.

Food production spaces, livestock breeding and food processing coexisted with housing, services and other urban activities. Roads of food distribution later materialised into roads and streets. They were designed to accommodate these flows and, although their names

have changed over time, their layout has left indelible marks on the urban fabric (Martin-McAuliffe, 2015: 249). Fluvial ports also impacted the city and place-names. Squares received weekly, monthly and festive fairs. Specific buildings were designed to house food activities: barns, warehouses, markets, shops and restaurants. Attending food trade spaces was part of the daily routine and identity of these communities. City dwellers knew where and by whom food sold was produced, how and through where it was brought into the city. Food, in all its dimensions and activities, was part of the city.

"Look at the plan of any city built before the railways, and there you will be able to trace the influence of food. It is etched into the anatomy of every pre-industrial urban plan: all have markets at their heart, with roads leading to them like so many arteries carrying in the city's lifeblood." (Steel, 2013: 118)

Once established, food spatial uses — production, distribution, trade — tend to persist and, even if they fade, their memory still persists in place-names. For example, Oxford derives from the contraction of *oxen* with *ford*, emphasizing the importance of these animals in the area (Morris, 1995: 123). Other food-related place names can be found in several cities, as the case of *Olivais* ('olive groves') and *Laranjeiras* ('orange trees') in Lisbon, and streets referring to specific crops or vegetable gardens.

"There are a great many streets, neighbourhoods and even [...] towns that have their origin in the culture of food." (Martin-McAuliffe, 2015: 20)

According to Dodd — who devoted a full chapter of his *Food of London* to place names — the streets connecting Newgate and Aldgate ('gate' defining a 'unloading area by the Thames') all derived their names from food. *Cheapside* derives from the term *ceap*, 'to barter'. The bread market was located at Bread Street; corn was sold at *Cornhill* (Dodd, 1856: 31–75). The meat trade site, for over nine centuries, was Smithfield, literally a 'smooth' field. Turkeys and geese were traded at *Poultry*. Fish trade occurred on streets like Old Fish Street or Old Fish Street Hill, and Friday Street derives its name from a Friday fish market (Steel, 2013: 119–120; Dodd, 1856: 29). In Amsterdam, there are also Groenstraat and a Warmoesstraat, literally 'vegetable' streets.

Dublin's place names offer several examples of food activities, such as Fishamble Street, Winetavern Street or Cook Street (Mac Con Iomaire, 2016: 73). Other examples included Blackberry Lane, Bull Alley Street, Bull Wall, Castle Market, Cornmarket, Cherryfield Road, Distillery Road, Goatstown, Haymarket, Milltown, Orchard Road, Pig Lane, Red Cow Lane, Watermill Road or Wheatfield, and others related to pork, due to its importance in the Irish diet (Mac Con Iomaire, 2016, 2014).

Markets were also one of the most basic functions the city performed for its surroundings, being unbeatable for freshness, low prices — due to the absence of intermediaries — and supervised exchanges. Held once or twice a week, markets were the focus of social life: here people met and talked, novelties and political affairs circulated. Incidents, agreements and business took place here. Despite the annual or festive fairs, regular markets had the biggest impact on local life (Roche, 1998: 59).

Markets could take on different urban forms, in an open square or covered bazaar — a *plaza*, *campo*, *piazza*, *grand-place* — in the centre of the city (often by the temple or church); in a ground on the outskirts, progressively absorbed into the urban fabric; in a wider part of the main street, or occupying streets with stalls or shops (Mumford, 2004: 85–234; Morris, 1995: 108–109). Markets were later formalized into market-halls, which often occupied the former sites of open-air markets. One key characteristic was, in fact, their longevity in the urban fabric. Once a site was taken, it tended to persist, despite urban transformations, and food trade occurred at the same place, or nearby. For instance, in Marseille, the Greek *agora* was occupied by the Roman *forum* and by the medieval market, while in Lucca the *forum* gave way to a medieval market that persisted until today (Parham, 2015: 74–75).

The medieval marketplaces had triangular, oval, or polygonal plans, but there were also cases of regular squares. A certain proportion between building dimensions and market area seems to have been relevant, contributing to its social use and ambience, according to a study by Camillo Sitte on *positive* and *negative* space (Parham, 2015: 73). When a certain ratio was exceeded, the space was perceived as too broad or too claustrophobic, a principle also applicable to the spatial structure of the market itself, in the layout and density of the stalls.

Pre-industrial markets were often located near the culmination of food land routes, unloading docks, etc. The case of London is illustrative: while a single bridge crossed the Thames, markets clustered naturally in the City. In Lisbon, Figueira Market was located at the junction of two major food routes, while Ribeira Market stayed by the river docks. The same principle applied to cattle and meat markets. Animals arrived through specific roads, converging to designated markets. In 19th-century London, weekly, thousands of animals got to Smithfield, on Thursdays and Sundays, for the Friday and Monday markets respectively. Cattle converged from all the surrounding streets, mainly through the Great North Road, which terminated at St. John's Street:

"The great stream that passed through St. Johan's street during the night was amazing, comprising thousands, or it might be tens of thousands, of fine well-fattened animals. [...] Nine, ten, eleven, midnight, the 'sma' hours' of the morning, all witnessed successive arrivals;

and the area of four or five acres, by the time the salesmen and butchers arrived, presented an extraordinary scene." (Dodd, 1856: 234–238)

The increase of trade, coupled with growing urban hygiene concerns during the 19th and 20th centuries, led to the construction of *halles* in Europe: covered, permanent and specialized markets, often still surrounded by the previously existent outdoor markets (Braudel, 1992b: 19), a typology that has in fact become iconic of European cities. Diverse types of buildings were developed, using iron and glass structures, to accommodate different types of goods with specific requirements, having numerous galleries and spacious complementary cellars. These became some of the most important built structures of urban foodscapes, complementing the existing network of food shops, in place since Antiquity.

Open spaces, streets and buildings were, thus, influenced by food activities, being shaped to accommodate and integrate them into the city's fabric.

## 3 CONTEMPORARY URBAN FOODSCAPES

### 3.1 *From local foodsheds to global foodsheds*

From mid- to late-19th century, covered market-halls, slaughterhouses, cooling systems and innovative food preservation methods, such as canning and freezing, changed the logics underlying food systems. Moreover, food systems were profoundly transformed by railways, which also disrupted the former rules governing the shape, size, location and organization of cities.

"Up until the nineteenth century, food, and the natural geography that provided it, had determined where cities were built, and how large they could grow. But railways made it possible to build cities just about anywhere, and just about any size." (Steel, 2013: 90–91)

Railways allowed the transport of large amounts of cargo quickly *by land*, for the first time, resembling 'man-made rivers'. Trains efficiently brought products to and from ports, from distant areas to city centres. This new reality profoundly changed urban diets: it was now possible to consume food from anywhere in the world. Food supply routes became longer; food systems became global.

However, if the distance food can travel increases linearly, its impact on the *foodshed* is not proportional. That is, if these production circles were determined by their radius (r), then the area covered ($\pi r^2$) increases in proportion to its square. Thus, an improvement in transport that allows reaching twice the distance in the same time translates into a supply area increase to its quadruple, or to nine-fold, when the distance is tripled, and so on. The introduction of railways — and later trucking systems, cars and airplanes — thus represented a very significant increase in the *foodshed*

12

accessible by urban markets, extending them to the whole planet.

> "Most cities today do precisely that, having long outgrown their local farm belts. London [...] is fed by a global hinterland [...] more than a hundred times larger than itself — roughly equivalent in size to all the productive farmland in the UK." (Steel, 2013: 7)

For cities, this change carried an obvious consequence: if distribution issues come to prevail over the ancestral issues of proximity, then their relation towards their surrounding hinterlands changes. Agricultural soil loses importance and value, given the need of space for housing, industry, public buildings, infrastructures, etc. (Pereira dos Santos, 2010: 19). Built-up fabric spreads "like oil over a glass surface" over the surroundings (Telles, 2016: 82).

> "This means that one of the chief determinants of large-scale urbanization has been nearness to fertile agricultural land; yet, paradoxically, the growth of most cities has been achieved by covering over and removing from cultivation the very land (often, indeed, the richest alluvial soils) whose existence at the beginning made their growth possible." (Mumford, 1956)

If pre-industrial cities could be measured in tens or hundreds of hectares, the new conurbations take thousands of square kilometres. Western economy has shifted from rural, with some large cities and thousands of villages, to metropolitan (Mumford, 1956). The shape of concentric expansions is replaced by a tentacle-like form (Raison, 1986: 336). Urban areas are expanding faster than their populations. This threat becomes more significant when considered that most cities are located in close proximity of soils on average 1.77 times more fertile than the rest (Bren d'Amour et al., 2017: 8939).

Cities pose yet other challenges to the sustainability of food systems, being a factor of diet transformation (*nutritional transition*), which changes food production and puts added pressure over natural resources (Smit, Nasr, & Ratta, 2001: 18). There's an increasing physical and mental distance between city dwellers and food systems. Far from production areas, urban consumers tend to ignore how, where or by whom food is produced or processed, seeming to pop up on supermarkets as if by magic. This ignorance fuels indifference regarding the conditions under which food items are produced, promoting socially and environmentally damaging decisions and behaviours (Paxton, 2005: 41), while exacerbating fears about the products consumed. At the same time, food — apart from consumption — has progressively become invisible in the city and public spaces, with food being produced and processed on distant lands, being handled and delivered at off-hours to numerous supermarkets scattered in the city, by *private* companies. Contemporary cities are, in fact, increasingly characterized by processes of *food privatopia* (Parham, 2015: 219).

## 3.2 Sustainable cities for a sustainable future

Cities face, today, pressing challenges regarding sustainable development, which will be exacerbated by climate change. Urban sprawl alters habitats, biochemistry, hydrology and energy flows (Bren d'Amour et al., 2017: 8939). It can affect drainage systems, water supply, increase temperature and environmental pollution, and food insecurity. Currently, around 60% to 80% of total energy consumption takes place in cities, as well as 40% to 70% of the anthropogenic emissions of GHG (UN-HABITAT, 2011: 33–52). Cities are responsible for about 60% of drinking water consumption (Drescher & Iaquinta, 2002: 34) and receive about three-quarters of everything that is collected and extracted from the soil (Smit, Nasr, & Ratta, 2001: 9). Each urban inhabitant generates 0.6 kg of solid waste per day (Zeeuw & Dubbeling, 2009: 9). Cities *ecological footprints* are several times larger than themselves. Food is a major component of this reality, being pointed by the Global Footprint Network as the single biggest component of urban ecological footprints. Ensuring the food security of a growing urban world population, while preserving the environment for future generations, is considered as one of the greatest challenges mankind will face in the coming years. In this context, the importance of pursuing a *circular metabolism* — where the outputs of a process act as inputs for another — has been highlighted (Smit, Nasr, & Ratta, 2001: 10–17). This cannot be attained without taking food systems into account, considering the amount of flows of matter and energy involved, towards and outwards the city, and the environmental impact (on land, water, biodiversity, climate change) food systems represent.

In fact, in most international declarations — such as *The Future We Want*, *Our Common Future* or the *Sustainable Development Goals* — there are references to the importance of food issues for reaching a sustainable development, mainly through improved sustainable agriculture and food security. However, it was the *New Urban Agenda* (Habitat III, 2016) that, for the first time, brought food systems to the scope of urban planning, in its several dimensions and stages, from production to waste, and in its various links to other urban systems and dimensions.

Reconnecting these realities by planning *City Region Food Systems* (CRFS) has been pointed as crucial to balancing urban matter and energy flows, while tackling the social, environmental and economic issues raised by the current models of cities and urban food systems (Dubbeling et al., 2016).

## 3.3 How urban design can take lessons from the past for more sustainable cities

To achieve an urban circular metabolism and an environmentally and socially sustainable future, bringing food back into the cities is crucial. Despite numerous initiatives and projects in cities worldwide, stemming from different motivations and through different strategies, the spatial dimension of food (system) planning has been largely overlooked, being food often taken as an 'add-on' to design:

"[…] food has too often been relegated to the margins of the design disciplines, as a taken-for-granted aspect of place, narrowly conceived as offering a surface gloss of vitality or applied as a kind of pleasant afterthought in spatial design terms." (Parham, 2015: 268)

For architects, changing this means rethinking the principles that govern urbanism, urban form and buildings themselves, in a permanent dialogue with all the stakeholders. This work should cover the whole food system — from production to waste — considering that all these activities occupy and transform specific spaces, shaping *foodscapes*, and intersect with the various scales present in a city. It will be required to think geographic proximity to nutritious foods, plan land uses, rethink zoning regulations, food infrastructures and the typologies of food establishments (Cabannes & Marocchino, 2018: 9). The location of new cities and the expansion of former ones should consider this balance and dependence of natural resources, and city planning and design should be an extension of these principles. That is, *food should be taken as an urban infrastructure*, with specific requirements and spaces.

One of the main strategies of urban design pointed, in this context, is the implementation of public spaces with a productive food dimension. These production areas can be integrated into (existing) green belts, corridors, and other types of biophysical (infra)structure of cities.

A famous proposal, in this context, is the *Continuous Productive Urban Landscape* (CPUL) developed by André Viljoen and Katrin Bohn, who proposed interconnected productive spaces in existing cities, creating a new urban infrastructure and redefining multi-functional uses of public space (Viljoen, Bohn, & Howe 2005). CPULs would be spatially continuous networks of open spaces, promoting connections between urban and peri-urban. They would include urban agriculture (mainly fruit and vegetables, but also small livestock), outdoor recreational and commercial spaces, natural habitats, ecological corridors and circulation routes, being environmentally, socially and economically productive (Viljoen, Bohn, & Howe 2005: xviii–15).

The final shape and extent of CPULs would vary from city to city, according to the site's characteristics, conditions and competing pressures. They could be materialized into parks (new or pre-existent), urban forests, green lungs, axis and corridors, spaces of reflection, cultural meeting and leisure. CPULs seek to work with pre-existent spaces, complementing and adding to them (Viljoen, Bohn, & Howe, 2005: 11–12). Knowing the city's history is, therefore, key for successful CPULs.

The productive landscapes could also extend beyond the ground floor and expand into edible buildings, occupying balconies, terraces, roofs, walls and façades …for a truly three-dimensional and complete productive landscape.

"Vertical space can be used effectively to grow food. Walls can hold cages for poultry and livestock as well as vines. Recent hydroponic techniques minimize space needs with plastic tubes that can be suspended on brick walls. Some city farmers attach long, narrow planters or boxes to their walls. Others hang plastic pots or halves of plastic soda bottles. Plants such as cucumber and melon can grow up a wall or fence if supported with sticks or twine. Residences have the potential to be three-dimensional places of agricultural production." (Smit, Nasr, & Ratta, 2001: 85)

Productive skyscrapers and even floating farms and food forests have been proposed. But other food activities should also be brought back into urban fabric — markets, food-hubs, food stores, cooperatives, and so on — reintegrating food in a variety of architectural programmes, as it did in the past.

*Foodscape planning and design* are, in this context, crucial, since the incorporation of food in cities and in architecture can help rebuild the lost connection of city dwellers with food systems, but also with nature as a whole — seasonality, climate, weather, topography and vegetation — reversing their alienation and reconnecting them with the natural cycles and with the planet. Towards this goal, some key principles could include: take *food as a design process* (vs a 'green wallpaper'), include *all activities of food systems*, be *site-specific and holistic*, be *multi-scale* and *multifunctional*, be *tridimensional*, keep it *dynamic* and *flexible* (open to urban changes), see the city's food potential through 'the eyes of the urban farmer', aim for a *circular urban metabolism* (matter, energy & water flows) and *learn from the past*.

## 4  CONCLUSION

Food has been an intrinsic part of cities since the beginning, being a key factor in their location, size attained, land use of their hinterlands and urban form. Food and cities were interdependent and their relationship bound to, and balanced by, natural resources and territorial conditions. In the last 150 years, mankind was able to largely transcend many of the constraints previously imposed, but not without severe environmental and social consequences.

Today, unsustainable urban development is no longer viable, and new solutions are demanded. Surprisingly, the key for a sustainable future may reside in the past, learning from this previous connection between food and city and the environmental and social benefits underlying it. The architect's role and responsibility are to (re)integrate food activities into urban design and architecture, in all of their scales, exploring innovative and historical solutions, in order to promote a more balanced global future for all.

## REFERENCES

Ascher, F. 2010. *Novos Princípios do Urbanismo; Novos Compromissos Urbanos*. Lisbon: Livros Horizonte.

Atkins, P. J. 2003. 'Is it urban? The relationship between food production and urban space in Britain, 1800–1950'. in Hietala, Marjatta e Vahtikari, Tanja. (eds.) *The Landscape of Food*. Helsinki: Finnish Literature Society. p. 133–144.

Björklund, A. 2010. *Historical Urban Agriculture: Food Production and Access to Land in Swedish Towns before 1900*. Acta Universitatis Stockholmiensis, no. 20. Stockholm: Stockholm University.

Braudel, F. 1992a. *Civilização material, economia e capitalismo, séculos XV-XVIII. Tomo I: As Estruturas do Quotidiano*. Lisbon: Editorial Teorema.

Braudel, F. 1992b. *Civilização material, economia e capitalismo, séculos XV-XVIII. Tomo II: Os Jogos das Trocas*. Lisbon: Editorial Teorema.

Bren d'amour, C.; Reitsma, F.; Baiocchi, G.; BartheL, S.; Güneralp, B.; Erb, K-H.; Haberl, H.; Creutzig, F. & Seto, K. C. 2017. 'Future urban land expansion and implications for global croplands'. *PNAS*, August 22nd 2017, vol. 114, no. 34. p. 8939–8944.

Brun, B.; Lemonnier, P.; Raison, J-P. & Roncayolo, M. 1986. 'Ambiente'. *Enciclopédia Einaudi 8: Região*. Lisbon: Imprensa Nacional – Casa da Moeda. p. 11–36.

Cabannes, Y. & Marocchino, C. (eds). 2018. *Integrating Food into Urban Planning*. London: UCL Press; Rome, FAO.

Childe, V. G. 1950. 'The Urban Revolution'. *The Town Planning Review 21 (1)*. April 1950. p. 3–17.

Dodd, G. 1856. *The Food of London: a sketch of the chief varieties, sources of supply, probable quantities, modes of arrival, processes of manufacture, suspected adulteration, and machinery of distribution, of the food for a community of two millions and a half*. London: Longman, Brown, Green, and Longmans.

Drescher, A. M & Iaquinta, D. L. 2002. 'Urbanization: Linking Development across the Changing Landscape'. *SOFA – Special Chapter on Urbanization*. January 2002. [online] http://www.fao.org/fileadmin/templates/FCIT/PDF/sofa.pdf

Dubbeling, M.; Bucatariu, C.; Santini, G.; Vogt, C. & Eisenbeiß, K. 2016. *City Region Food Systems and Food Waste Management*. Deutsche Gesellschaft für Internationale Zusammenarbeit.

Elliott, S. B. 2010. *Landscape, Kitchen, Table: Compressing the Food Axis to Serve a Food Desert*. Master Thesis in Architecture. University of Tennessee, Knoxville.

Habitat III – United Nations Conference on Housing and Sustainable Urban Development. 2016. *New Urban Agenda: Quito Declaration on Sustainable Cities and Human Settlements for All*. Quito, 17–20 October 2016. [online] https://www2.habitat3.org/bitcache/99d99fbd0824de502 14e99f864459d8081a9be00?vid=591155&disposition=in line&op=view

Hedden, W. P. 1929. *How great cities are fed*. New York: D. C. Health and Company.

Lemonnier, P. 1986. 'Solo'. *Enciclopédia Einaudi 8: Região*. Lisboa, Imprensa Nacional – Casa da Moeda. p. 59–96.

Mac Con Iomaire, M. 2016. 'The Gastro-Topography and Built Heritage of Dublin, Ireland'. in S. L. Martin-McAuliffe (ed.) (2016) *Food and Architecture at the table*. London: Bloomsbury Academic. p. 73–93.

Martin-Mcauliffe, S. 2015. 'Feeding Dublin: The City Fruit and Vegetable Market'. in M. McWilliams (ed.) *Food and Markets*. Prospect. p. 241–253.

More, T. 1973. *Utopia*. Mem Martins: Publicações Europa-América.

Morris, A. E. J. 1995. *Historia de la forma urbana: desde sus orígenes hasta la Revolución Industrial*. Barcelona: Ediciones Gustavo Gili.

Mumford, L. 2004. *A Cidade na História: suas origens, transformações e perspectivas*. São Paulo: Martins Fontes.

Mumford, L. 1970. *The Culture of Cities*. New York: Harcourt Brace Jovanovich.

Mumford, L. 1956. *The Natural History of Urbanization*. [online] http://habitat.aq.upm.es/boletin/n21/almum.en.html

Parham, S. 2015. *Food and Urbanism: The Convivial City and a Sustainable Future*. London: Bloomsbury.

Paxton, A. 2005. '5: Food Miles'. in A. Viljoen; K. Bohn & J. Howe. *Continuous Productive Urban Landscapes: Designing Urban Agriculture for Sustainable Cities*. Oxford: Architectural Press, Elsevier. p. 40–47.

Pereira dos Santos, H. 2010. *Do Tempo e da Paisagem: Manual para a leitura de Paisagens*. Parede: Principia.

Raison, J-P. 1986. 'Fixação'. *Enciclopédia Einaudi 8: Região*. Lisbon: Imprensa Nacional – Casa da Moeda. p. 312–340.

Roche, D. 1998. *História das Coisas Banais: Nascimento do Consumo nas Sociedades Tradicionais (Séculos XVII–XIX)*. Lisbon: Teorema.

Santlofer, J. 2017. *Food City: Four centuries of food-making in New York*. Now York: W. W. Norton & Company.

Smit, J.; Nasr, J. & Ratta, A. 2001. *Urban Agriculture: Food, Jobs and Sustainable Cities*. The Urban Agriculture Network, Inc.

Steel, C. 2013. *Hungry City: How Food Shapes our Lives*. London: Vintage Books.

Telles, G. R. 2016. *Gonçalo Ribeiro Telles: Textos Escolhidos*. Lisbon: Argumentum.

UN-HABITAT – United Nations Human Settlements Programme. 2011. *Cities and Climate Change: Global Report on Human Settlements 2011*. ISBN 978-92-1-132296-5.

Viljoen, A.; Bohn, K. & Howe, J. 2005. *Continuous Productive Urban Landscapes: Designing Urban Agriculture for Sustainable Cities*. Oxford, Architectural Press, Elsevier.

Vitruvius, M. 2006. *Tratado de Arquitectura*. Os Dez Livros de Arquitectura. Lisbon: IST Press.

Zeeuw, H. & Dubbeling, M. 2009. *Cities, Food and Agriculture: Challenges and the Way Forward*. RUAF Foundation.

# Feeding new alternatives: Reducing plastic in the take-away industry

B. Marques, E. Duarte & S. Parreira
*FBAUL, Faculty of Fine-Arts, Universidade de Lisboa, Lisbon, Portugal*

ABSTRACT: This paper focuses on the study of disposable plastics and their particular use in packaging in the food industry. Using common methodologies to product design and food design, a broader view to more sustainable practices in packaging was adopted considering different points of view, analyzed through an informal brief study (consumer/designer/producer). The containers for soups, broths and creams have been carefully observed in the take-away sector (a growing market in Portugal) on commercial areas such as supermarkets. The main purpose of this research was to understand the presence of disposable plastics in our day-to-day life, its impact on the environment and how materials like glass can be brought back to use as part of a sustainable strategy. This approach has allowed the acquisition of valuable information and tools that can be applied to new alternatives to the current models of consumerism.

## 1 INTRODUCTION

With the demographic, economic and technological development that we have endured over the years, the environment has undergone unprecedented changes.

In the twentieth century, due to World War II, the food industry experienced one of the biggest revolutions in its history. This was the period that marked the beginning of the processed food market: fast, efficient and inexpensive. This phenomenon has also happened in the plastic industry, because of its multifunctional, durable, resistant, weight and low-cost features. By the end of the twentieth century, various problems began to appear, mainly in terms of health issues. This period also marks the beginning of an ecological crisis. In order to harmonize ecology with prosperous economic growth, the theme of sustainability started to get discussed. Throughout the report *Our Common Future* (1987), the concept of sustainable development is defined as a "development that meets the needs of the present without compromising the ability of future generations to meet their own needs" (Brundtland, 1987). Currently, our consumption models are not in accordance with the principles of sustainability. It is essential to demand for a paradigm shift towards a more responsible economic, social and environmental behavior (Peneda, 2011).

Regarding the Design field, sustainability has become an important asset in the process of developing new projects, with the increasing interest of consumers on contemporary environmental and social issues. Therefore, the innovation process itself must focus progressively on a more ecological and social perspective, accompanied by technological growth (Gouveia, 2010). Design has a crucial role in the early stages of project development as decisions made at this point have huge impact on the sustainability of the final product (Murray, 2013).

Concerning the environmental impact, large retail, food and beverage companies have been the main targets of criticism for the amount of plastic garbage they produce. Through a study, it is estimated that only 9% of the plastic material generated by 2015 was recycled and that a majority of 79% of it remains accumulated in landfills (Geyer, Jambeck, & Law, 2017). It has also been noted that a majority of plastic packaging products are discarded in the same year they are manufactured, leaving behind an unparalleled environmental footprint.

In order to address the less sustainable aspects of the packaging industry, a project was designed to rethink the use of plastic material and its disposal aspect in take-away soups. Through the application of Product Design and Food Design methodologies, a proposal that seeks to create more value for the consumer, for the market, for the environment and for technology was developed.

## 2 A FRAMEWORK FOR SUSTAINABILITY

### 2.1 *Sustainable food design*

The concept of sustainable development first appears in 1979 after the First World Climate Conference. The main purpose was to allow for underdeveloped countries to evolve as richer countries do and assure basic welfare needs for the world's population. After the conference it became clear the need to consider ecological concerns for a sustainable development. Currently, the difficulties we are facing reveal an urgency to change standards and adapt our behavior to guarantee a similar life's quality for all living beings (Peneda, 2011).

Sustainability is based on three fundamental pillars: economic, environmental and social matters, all connected and depend on each other to maintain a balanced and prosperous sustainable development. After exploring these ideas from a product design point of view, there are several opportunities and subjects of intervention. For example, Sustainable Design represents the embodiment of a philosophy of sustainability in the design of objects, environments and/or services (Murray, 2013). It can also be referred as Ecodesign, Green Design or Environmental Design. Similarly, Sustainable Food Design aspires to bring these concepts to the food industry, as food products are part of an extremely complex system involving stages from production, processing and conservation, transportation, consumption and discarding (Barbero, 2015). This implies that all services associated with these products must be sustainable in the sense of waste, behavior, materials, supply and disposal (Zampollo, 2016).

It is up to the designers to outline alternative strategies for the development of new products and services that not only promote quality but also an ecological and social awareness without compromising consumer comfort. One way to adapt these concepts to current problems is to analyze the issues from the very beginning.

## 2.2 *The fate of disposable plastics*

It was after the outbreak of World War II (1939–1945) that the food industry endured one of the greatest changes in its history. With a growing shortage of labor in the factories, women eventually took the place of men while they served in the war. The lack of time and availability to perform household chores contributed to an increasing demand for cheap, easy to make and affordable food products. Companies quickly realized that to meet the population's new eating habits they also had to adapt. The same products that were distributed to soldiers inside plastic wrappers eventually reached the supermarkets, and pre-made, frozen and fast-food meals begin to appear (Recordati, 2015). The industrialization processes of manufacturing these foods ended up evolving without planning, which resulted in a detachment of the nutritional aspects and the quality of the products.

Alongside the industrialization of food, plastics industry has also undergone a troubled evolution. Thanks to its multifunctional, durable, lightweight and low-cost features, plastic has been instantaneously successful within the public. The plastic material that was once used as a container to transport the food to the soldiers was quickly adapted to the day-to-day life. Before it was usual for people to store food in glass jars and metal cans, which they carefully preserved for years. This habit changed with the search for new, cheaper, versatile and innovative products, fueling the appearance of brands such as Tupperware in the mid-1940s (Knight, 2014). Tupperware eventually

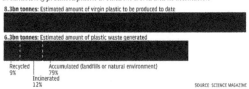

Billions of tonnes of plastic have accumulated in the environment
*Breakdown of produced plastic around the world and its destination*

**8.3bn tonnes:** Estimated amount of virgin plastic to be produced to date

**6.3bn tonnes:** Estimated amount of plastic waste generated

Recycled 9% | Accumulated (landfills or natural environment) 79%
Incinerated 12%

SOURCE SCIENCE MAGAZINE

Figure 1. Caption referring to the amount of accumulated and produced plastic until 2015 retrieved from The Telegraph (2018) based on Science Magazine article (2017).

reshaped the way people stored their meals at home and old habits fell into disuse (Gouveia, 2010).

In 2018, the pollution caused by disposable plastic materials was considered a worldwide calamity. Although the diversified characteristics of this material drove to the evolution of areas such as Design, the lack of planning turned out to be a bigger problem for sustainability. In the late twentieth century, the first signs of trouble began to appear. First in humans, where several toxic components were discovered in the bloodstream due to contact with plastic materials. Then in nature, as a result of a lack of planning in the way we produce, use and discard plastic (Freikel, 2018). It is estimated that over the last few years we have produced about 8.3 billion tons of plastic and that 6.3 billion tons of plastic garbage has been discarded by 2015 (Figure 1). From this waste, only 9% was recycled and approximately 12% was incinerated (Geyer et al., 2017). The very incineration of the material is a practice harmful to the environment by emitting carbon dioxide into the atmosphere (PAN, 2018).

The main targets of criticism regarding the disposal of plastics have been the retail, food and beverage companies. As we have seen so far, the current systems of production and treatment of this material have proved to be defective. There are products being retailed in supermarkets that are not designed to be recycled, such as adherent paper film, black take-away packaging, beverage labels and some colored plastics (Laville, n.d.). In order to address these problems, consumers, corporations and governments need to be mobilized into more sustainable paths. With customers' habits gradually changing it is up to retailers and governments to learn how to meet their needs. Private sectors should adopt innovative business models that reflect greater ecological and social responsibility for the impact of the products they promote, and governments should apply strict rules regarding the design, production and consumption of plastics. More than a pollution problem, we are facing a design dilemma (Solheim, 2018).

## 2.3 *Understanding the system*

As part of the research for this project, we proceed on observing some initiatives that have been taken in the scope of the reduction of disposable

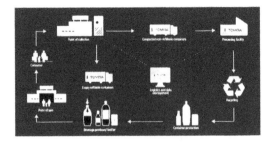

Figure 2. Caption of the process of recycling bottles and cans retrieved from TOMRA (2019).

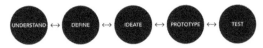

Figure 3. Caption of the design thinking methodology developed by André Gouveia (2017) based on the IDEO methodology (2008).

plastics, both in Portugal and abroad. Since change depends on a multidisciplinary task force that unites consumers, governors and entrepreneurs, it was considered relevant to unveil their roles in this process of transformation.

To better understand the consumer, an informal exploratory survey of consumerism habits was carried out. Throughout this experimental questionnaire, 150 consumers replied to key-questions related to the purchase of food products, focusing on the frequency of purchases, places of preference, importance of packaging and environmental awareness. In order to cross examine this results and complete the information, we also proceed on using methods like shadowing and experience sharing. In line with the literature review, consumers are gradually changing and there is more responsibility and information about ecological habits. As far as legislation is concerned, some initiatives have also been taken into consideration. Since 2003, resolution and law projects that warned for the reduction of plastic consumption and the awareness of recycling begun to appear (PEV, 2003). More recently, a resolution was approved in Portugal recommending that the government should terminate the use of disposable plastic dishes in catering services (PSD, 2018). In the case of supermarkets, they have already begun to adapt to the needs of consumers and are more available to reduce the use of plastics and to promote other alternatives (LIDL, 2018).

At the international standpoint, Germany has implemented a packaging deposit system introduced by the German government back in 2003. The *pfand* symbolizes an extra deposit that adds up to the value of the product at the time of purchase and can later be redeemed by the user after the seller retrieves the package. This process is facilitated through *Reverse Vending Machines* (RVM) (Oltermann, 2018).

Its operation is practical and intuitive. These machines have recycling or collecting preferences for reusing containers that are later collected by a particular company who transports the materials back to the factories (Figure 2).

To return a packet simply insert the empty container into the machine, wait for it to be processed by a computer through scanning, choose the most correct option in the digital interface and collect the refund

ticket from the deposit. These new systems allow for a renewal of old habits now facilitated by technology. Through a tax imposed on consumption and by encouraging sustainable initiatives, it becomes easier to control pollution (Walls, 2011).

## 3 CHANGING THE PARADIGM OF PACKAGING DESIGN

### 3.1 *Understanding*

In order to develop the final proposal, all the information collected during this work was taken into consideration. According to Tim Brown, renown designer and president of IDEO, Design projects must experience three phases: inspiration, ideation and implementation (Brown, 2008). During this process, Design methodologies were put into practice (Figure 3). These tools enable the end result to be user-centered, innovative, creative and meaningful.

The main focus was on the waste caused by disposable plastic materials, particularly within the food industry, in the take-away sector. Due to the ephemeral nature of this sort of packaging and the way it is designed, the environmental impact is quite substantial. This choice was based on the observation of the behavior of the consumers inside the supermarkets and the information collected during the literature review. Within the different areas in which plastic is used, the highest percentage concerns the use for packaging (Rodrigues, 2018). It was necessary to restrict the area of intervention, so only the soup containers example was considered, based on what was perceived. The challenge of the briefing was to develop a packaging design project for take-away soup containers that would allow the reuse of the product, preserving safety requirements and complying with the principles of sustainability. Other factors such as container portability and tightness, a fair and acceptable value for all, preservation of food and the reduction of waste produced by disposable packaging were also taken into consideration (Traitler, Coleman, & Hofmann, 2015).

### 3.2 *Defining consumers, competition and materials*

#### 3.2.1 *Consumers*
Being a user-centered project it was critical to define the target audience and understand it. Through design techniques such as face-to-face observation or shadowing, sharing of experiences and an informal survey of consumer habits, different types of users have been targeted. The focus group of consumers show

similarities regarding lack of time and dietary concerns. They can range from college students and young workers to families. Depending on the household these consumers can buy both individual and family soup packs. The quality of the products they purchase has been identified as one of the most important points when buying a food product, followed by the price and the ingredients. Most users are concerned about product packaging, favoring the material part over the aesthetic, albeit important. While product quality and trust in some brands are essential, when buying a different product consumers are more likely motivated by promotions and/or recommendations.

### 3.2.2 *Market study*

The next step was to understand the market and the competition with an evaluation of nearly fifty containers used for consumption of soups, broths and creams. This compilation was later split into two categories: lunchboxes and takeaway packages. For sustainable reasons lunchboxes were taken into consideration to this study, as it could provide an interesting overview of ecological features. The portable and sturdy characteristics of the lunchboxes make them reusable, on the other hand, takeaway packages have more versatility and a lower cost.

The lunchboxes are usually made of plastic, glass and stainless steel. They have a higher price due to the complexity of form, strength and reusability. Plastic packaging, similar to Tupperware style, is cheaper, lighter and more versatile. For the glass containers, they are also affordable, but more aesthetically limited. Amongst all the containers it was possible to perceive that there are negative points in the use of each one of them. Steel containers cannot be brought to the microwave; glass containers are heavier and can break; and plastic containers can eventually smell, gain color and even taste badly. Some plastics are also not designed for microwave use and may be harmful to health.

In the typology of take-away packaging there is much more variety. There are formats of cup, glass, sachet, bottle, mason jar, can and materials such as plastic, glass, cardboard mix and aluminum. The transversal features to these containers are the versatility and visual impact of the graphic element. As seen earlier, the worst attribute is its disposable component, which makes it difficult to reuse.

Through this compilation it was possible to define the product appeal of the final proposal and settle down for a compromise between the two typologies analyzed. More elements were taken into account before the materialization of the final product, like being 100% reusable, transparent, suitable for liquid consumption, resistant and part of a sustainable strategy.

### 3.2.3 *Materials*

To define the material for the project, a comparative brief study was carried out between the materials most used in the production of packaging in the food industry: glass, plastic and metal. Glass is produced from non-renewable sources such as sand, silica and limestone. So far, these raw materials exist in abundance on our planet and their collection is less harmful to the environment than other materials. However, the glass packaging manufacturing process requires too much energy (Spencer, 2012). The weight factor of the packaging also attributes less sustainable characteristics to the material. It requires additional precaution during transportation and storage due to its fragility. Regarding the disposal, glass can be 100% recycled, thus reducing the need to extract new raw material.

The most widely used plastic in the food industry is PET, a thermoplastic. This material is created from the extraction of petroleum, a non-renewable source extremely harmful to the environment. Plastic has a very low percentage of recycled material to date and only about 30% capacity to recycle (Spencer, 2012). About the transport aspect, plastic has a lower carbon footprint considering its weight.

The most used metal for packaging in the food industry is aluminum, due to its malleable characteristics. It is extracted from the mining of a material called bauxite and causes a significant environmental impact. Despite being an extremely lightweight material, easy to carry and 100% recyclable, the prerequisite of transparency restrains the use of this material.

We can conclude that each material has negative and positive aspects depending on the purpose for which they are designed. The material selected for the project was glass, for its transparency, reusability and recycling capabilities, but also because it is associated with better quality products (Balzarotti, Maviglia, Biassoni, & Ciceri, 2015). During the informal exploratory survey, when asked about choosing between a glass and a plastic packaging, a large majority of consumers revealed a preference for the glass material. Glass has been used satisfactorily over the years and continues to be considered one of the safest materials to protect food and drinks (Franco & Falqué, 2016). Although plastic also has some appealing characteristics, it has been previously demonstrated that this material has been responsible for polluting the environment and harming the health of humans and animals. Depending on the use of new raw material whenever this material is produced shows that disposable plastic for takeaway packaging is not part of a sustainable strategy.

### 3.3 *Sketching ideas*

This step represents the initial phase of product development and is characterized by elements such as creativity and quantity. At this stage, methods as brainstorming ideas and quick sketches allow a preview of the form and context for which the product will be designed. Drawing becomes a facilitating tool to preview some of the specifications of the product. The first ideas sketched were inspired by the traditional mason jar. Later on, this idea evolved into a hybrid between a bowl of soup and a jar, facilitating the use

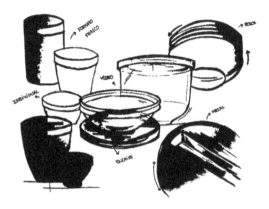

Figure 4. Caption of a composition of sketches made by the author (2018).

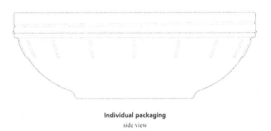

**Individual packaging**
side view

Figure 5. Caption of the individual package made by the author (2018).

of the product and maintaining the affective characteristics (Figure 4). The goal was for the consumer to immediately recognize the form and understand the action needed. The concept for the product comes from a familiar but appealing simplicity, which is committed to comfort and practicality.

### 3.4 Prototyping and testing

This stage is one of the most significant for the development of the project, since it allows to define technical specificities of the product. Through rough prototyping, we are able get a three-dimensional notion of the final product's appearance. The execution of quick prototypes gives a briefly perceive of the physical and technical constraints. For the execution of these prototypes materials such as gelatin sheet, roofmate, styrofoam and PLA, a biodegradable plastic, were used. Techniques like molding, sculpturing and 3D printing were also put into practice. The prototyping process was always accompanied by tests and the respective reformulation of the models along the way.

### 3.5 Project proposal

The final proposal aimed to reformulate the current take-away packaging based on the principle of re-use. For this purpose, two types of packaging were designed, one individual and another one family sized. Materials such as tempered glass and stainless steel

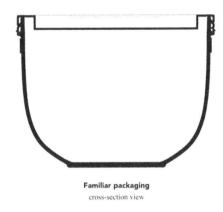

**Familiar packaging**
cross-section view

Figure 6. Caption of the familiar package cross section made by the author (2018).

were selected thanks to their resistance to temperatures and shocks. The individual packaging consists on a two-piece set, bowl and lid, fitted through a screw system reminiscent of mason jars (Figure 5). The general measures are 16 centimeters long and wide and 5.5 centimeters high.

The container has a circular base with a diameter of 8 centimeters to ensure more stability and the bowl has a thickness of 3 mm, reinforced in the areas of greater impact. Throughout the bowl, small protuberances have been designed to ease the opening act. At the top of the lid there is a circular shape that allows its use as a support for the base of the container. The individual package has a capacity of about 300 milliliters.

In order to create a uniform collection, the family sized package was designed based on the individual container (Figure 6).

The general measures are 16 by 16 centimeters and 12 centimeters in height. The package has a capacity of 1.2 liters. With the purpose of simplifying the production and standardization of the collection, the fitting and the lids are the same for the two containers.

Since the main resolution of this project was to encourage re-using habits and consumer awareness on this issue, it was contemplated the possibility to adapt the RVM systems to the final project proposal. Through the application of a deposit and reimbursement system, customers are encouraged to connect with a reusable strategy. The ultimate goal would be for the packaging project to be part of a closed-loop system, from production to disposal, thereby bringing added value to the environment, consumer and business. By applying this strategy, it becomes possible to minimize the most negative aspects of the extraction, production and transport of glass. Which means, through a re-use approach, the need to produce new material is eliminated and at least one stage of transport is reduced, for example, from the supermarket to the recycling factories. The strength, the look and the usability of the containers also allows the user to reuse the packaging at home as a lunchbox or container, according to their preference and necessities.

## 4 CONCLUSION

In conclusion, it is possible to perceive that there is still much capacity to exploit in the area of Food Design, mainly in Portugal. There is a latent need to adapt the concept of sustainable development to the current problems of society and the Food Industry itself. Throughout the study of historic events, we could analyze the problems associated with the excessive growth of food production and with a critical view prevent it from continuing to happen. The post-World War II industrial food revolution has brought more meaning to the role of the designer within this industry. Thanks to its creativity, innovative spirit and technological skills the designer has become a key player in the Food Industry.

Taking into account what was studied during this research and the requirements established for the development of this project, glass was considered the most suitable material for this type of object. The new reusability systems make it possible to reduce the negative aspects related to the use of glass, making this material a more sustainable choice.

We must use existing technologies and innovation as supplementary tools in the design process for a greener future. It is essential to learn how to reuse and reformulate products in an innovative and sustainable way socially, environmentally and economically. With a continuous cooperation between diverse scientific areas we can create more value within the Design field, the market and the industry, for the consumer and the world.

It is also valuable to understand consumer behavior and learn how to drive their choices towards more sustainable alternatives. New areas of interest such as trend analysis and forecasting should be explored. For future research it is advisable to conduct a detailed search of other alternative materials and a Life Cycle Assessment analysis of the process of a ready-to-eat or take-away product in a supermarket. From the design point of view, it is recommended to study product's shape, ergonomics and portability. For the implementation of the product in the market, it would be relevant to apply marketing strategies.

## REFERENCES

Balzarotti, S., Maviglia, B., Biassoni, F., & Ciceri, M. R. (2015). Glass vs. plastic: Affective judgments of food packages after visual and haptic exploration. *Procedia Manufacturing*, 3(Ahfe), 2251–2258.

Barbero, S. (2015). *Systemic Design for Sustainability. Sustainability Science.* Banff, Canada

Brown, T. (2008). Design thinking. *Harvard Business Review.*

Brundtland, G. (1987). *Report of the World Commission on Environment and Development: Our Common Future.* Genève, Switzerland.

Franco, I., & Falqué, E. (2016). Glass PACKAGING. *Reference Module in Food Science*, 10–11.

Freikel, S. (2018). Plastic: How it Changed the World. *BBC World Service.*

Geyer, R., Jambeck, J. R., & Law, K. L. (2017). Production, uses, and fate of all plastics ever made. *Science Advances*, 3(7), 5.

Gouveia, A. (2010). *Briefing innovation: Metodologia para a inovação de produto.* Fine-Arts Faculty.

Gouveia, A. (2017). *Da Ideia ao Produto.*

Knight, L. (2014). A brief history of plastics, natural and synthetic. *BBC News*, 1–8.

Laville, S. (n.d.). Quick guide: Plastics and our throwaway society.

LIDL. (2018). LIDL Portugal reduz o consumo de plástico em 20% até 2025.

Murray, B. (2013). Embedding environmental sustainability in product design, (may), 1–11.

Oltermann, P. (2018). Has Germany hit the jackpot of recycling? The jury's still out. *The Guardian*, 1–3.

PAN. (2018) Projecto-Lei n.º 752/XIII/3ª Determina a não utilização de louça descartável de plástico em determinados sectores da restauração.

Peneda, J. (2011). O paradigma da sustentabilidade. In *Arte & sociedade* (pp. 370–375). Lisbon.

PEV. (2003). Projeto de Lei n.º 342/IX Valorização de Resíduos.

PSD. (2018). Projeto de resolução n.º 1286/XIII/3.ª Recomenda ao Governo que promova estudos sobre as alternativas à utilização de louça descartável de plástico, realize campanhas de sensibilização para a redução do seu uso, e defina uma estratégia para a redução gradual da sua utilização.

Recordati, G. (2015). *The food industry: History, evolution and current trends.*

Rodrigues, R. J. (2018). Vai ser possível trocar plástico por senhas de supermercado. *Diário de Notícias.*

Solheim, E. (2018). The planet is on edge of a global plastic calamity. *The Guardian*, 1–3.

Spencer, C. (2012). *Disposable Drinking Bottles – Plastic vs. Glass vs. Aluminum.*

Traitler, H., Coleman, B., & Hofmann, K. (2015). Food Industry Design, Technology and Innovation. Hoboken, New Jersey: John Wiley & Sons, Inc.

Walls, M. (2011). Deposit-refund systems in practice and theory. *Resources for the Future Discussion Paper*, 15.

Wright, M., Kirk, A., Molloy, M., & Mills, E. (2018). The stark truth about how long your plastic footprint will last on the planet. *The Telegraph*, (January), 1–8.

Zampollo, F. (2016). *What is Food Design?*

# Food system photographic portraits: A necessary urban design agenda

T. Marat-Mendes, P. Bento d'Almeida & J. Cunha Borges
*ISCTE-IUL, Instituto Universitário de Lisboa, Lisbon, Portugal*

ABSTRACT: Research suggests that design solutions are an influential factor in the sustainability performance of food systems. Yet, such systems remain underexplored within architecture and urban design. We argue that some architectural surveys of the 20th century encapsulate urban form solutions which bear on food issues, and therefore deserve further consideration. Our findings point out that identifying food concerns within such surveys would promote proposals of urban form design solutions, which are necessary to integrate contemporary urban planning compendiums, but also to promote further dialogues among those concerned for food and urban design.

## 1 INTRODUCTION

### 1.1 *Food and the city*

The incorporation of food into urban planning is not a novel issue. Urban History provides a rich repository of examples, which testify the strong role of food on shaping a wide range of towns, villages, cities and territories, throughout all world continents and different periods.

Considering for example Nowdushan, located in Iran, a town of Persian origins conditioned by a rural system and irrigation ditches (Kostof 1991) or the case of Lisbon, the capital of Portugal, whose present public space derives from the need of the city to access water (Marat-Mendes et al. 2015; Marat-Mendes et al. 2016), one easily identifies how the main dietary elements (food and water) can shape urban areas throughout History. Furthermore if one considers the 14th century Abrogio Lorenzetti frescos of 'The Allegory of Bad and Good Government' painted in the Palazzo Pubblico in Siena, Italy, alongside the late 19th century Garden City theory by Ebenezer Howard, one will find these share a common proposition: a society and a governmental commitment towards the city and the territory in order to sustain in equilibrium, peace and public health, which implies the inclusion of the food system in urban environments. For instance, the Sienna agrarian and peasant way of life, determined specific urban form solutions, territorial arrangements outside the city walls and built structures inside them. As for the Garden City, specific housing arrangements and allotments, as well as areas for mass food production, including cereals, or fruits, flowers and vegetables, preferable for individual production, each determined particular urban form arrangements with implications on the food system.

The impact of food on urban form is indeed substantial, extending through several phases, including production, transportation, transformation, packaging, consumption and recycling (Steel 2013), but also several spheres and activities of human life. From the perspective of labour, major changes have occurred since the 1970s when agricultural labour started to decrease, to the point of near-disappearance (Fischer-Kowalski & Haas 2014). Such changes also influence the conviviality sphere, as previous common spaces shared by communitarian agrarian activities have meanwhile loss their use and meaning. Nevertheless, contemporary urbanism reclaims new convivial spaces, to which the food system can contribute to (Parham 2016).

The repository of urban elements, which cover all these dimensions of the food system and human activities, should be met with diversified and generous design solutions, responding to diverse socio-economic and environmental realities. It should include public space, rural systems, water elements like irrigation ditches, but also other elements, which have already been registered by Urban History and in contemporary urban forms, in use by society today, according to present needs.

This fascinating relationship between food, the city, the territory and society, suggests several research questions that have been gaining attention. Indeed, since the arrival of the new millennium, the time of publication of 'The Food System: a stranger to the planning field' by Pothukuchi and Kaufman (2000) that research literature in the field has gained greater momentum (Brinkley 2013; Marat-Mendes et al. 2018).

### 1.2 *The food system as an urban issue*

The spatial dimension of the food system, with its inherent urban forms, remains underexplored. A reduced and uninspired repository of morphological types has been found in urban food-production spaces in some municipalities of the Lisbon Region (Dias 2018; Marat-Mendes et al. 2018). Despite this lack of creativity and innovative design solutions, the production phase of the food system has received special attention from academic research, even though most authors would agree that the food system is a pattern or a holistic multi-level system.

A further opportunity for design is in assessing the role of food in the socio-metabolism of the territory, as this can inform designers on contributing to close loops of water, nutrients, energy and materials to improve sustainability (Kennedy et al. 2010). Infrastructures, and its associated urban form elements, are also determinative to improve the socio-metabolic functioning of cities, a relation in which the food system is strategic.

However, urban infrastructure has seldom been considered in this context. Such tendency as discussed by Pothukuchi and Kaufman (2000) points towards an 'estrangement' of the food system to urban planning. We would suggest however, that readings of the food system from the standpoint of infrastructure would allow for a greater 'spatial' reading of the food system and its design. Gandy (2004) has pointed out how modernity, through technology and culture brought about new infrastructures, a 'hidden city' of sewages and hydraulic systems running under streets and built masses, which allowed sanitary conditions to be dramatically improved. Other forms of infrastructure – roads, highways, reservoirs, garners, waste management stations, etc. – also remain fundamental for the functioning of contemporary cities. The food system is one example where both visible and hidden infrastructures concur. A study of urban (spatial) food systems would benefit greatly from including the infrastructural conditions of cities and their surrounding areas.

With respect to architecture and urban planning, Vijoen et al. (2005) point out the potential of urban agriculture for the creation of a 'productive multifunctional landscape' with spatial, social and environmental implications.

Urban form, understood as the configuration of fixed metropolitan elements, comprises several important features of cities, including density, compactness and land-use, the importance of which is very considerable within the food system.

Yet, design solutions for such spatial dimension of the food system require further attention (as recalled by the *Urban Design* Journal issue number 140 from 2016) as well transdisciplinary research in long-term projects that effectively assess the sustainability of urban changes (Baccini et al. 2008).

Architecture emerges therefore as an important tool, or an opportunity, to explore such design issues and enlarge our understanding of the urban forms that integrate food system functioning, including infrastructures. A methodological approach to such exercise could draw from visual characterization of existing built structures, making use of photographic records and systematizing identified elements according to its

different types and territorial situations. This approach has been explored in studies of urban metabolism, while articulating cartographical sources and photography with methodologies used by engineers, such as Materials Flow Analysis (Marat-Mendes et al. 2016). Reconsidering the role of architecture in basic human activities may also provide a way for architects to escape their alienation from urban planning debates (Figueira 2016).

### 1.3 *Structure, methodology and aim*

To ascertain relations between the food system and urban design, this article is divided into four parts. Following this introduction, two sections retrieve food-related structures from two of 20th century architectural surveys, the 'Inquérito sobre a Arquitectura Regional Portuguesa' (IARP), started in 1955 and published in 1961 as 'Arquitectura Popular em Portugal' (AAVV 2004); and the 'Inquérito à Arquitectura do Século XX em Portugal' (IAPXX), started in 2003 and published three years later (AAVV 2006). The first studied vernacular, popular and traditional architecture in Portugal. The second focused on representative examples of 20th century architecture. For each one, we provide an overview of food-related examples. A comparative reading will be presented in the Discussion, while the Conclusion will briefly discuss how visual characterization may help integrate the food system into urban design and architecture practices.

As will be exposed, both analysed surveys sought to present extended overviews of specific realities of the Portuguese territory, and thus constitute key contributions for assessing the History of Architecture in Portugal. But given the materials they include, they may also suggest ways to make future architecture and urban design more sustainable.

## 2 THE SURVEY ON PORTUGUESE REGIONAL ARCHITECTURE (IARP)

### 2.1 *Context, goals and methodology*

After the International Union of Architects Congress in Lisbon 1948, the influence of the Modern Movement was incorporated in Portuguese architecture, despite resistance from the dictatorial regime. However, the perception of the Portuguese on modernism started to change soon, and concerns shifted towards a 'humane' architecture, which included an interest in local traditions and relations between built and natural environment (Tostões 1997). This shift is signalled by architect Francisco Keil do Amaral (1947) in his 1947 article 'Uma iniciativa necessária' (*A necessary initiative*), which defended the need for a survey on regional architecture. The article follows a suggestion by Brazilian architect Lúcio Costa (1938), who wrote in 1938 an article, 'Documentação necessária' (*Necessary documentation*), claiming that autochthonous architecture in Portugal was a high-quality universe which the Portuguese had yet failed to acknowledge.

Surveys on vernacular, popular and traditional architecture were conducted in several European countries in the mid-20th century, including Germany, France, Italy, England, Spain and Greece (Dimitsantou-Kremesi & Marat-Mendes 2012). In Portugal, geographer Orlando Ribeiro had coordinated surveys on rural settlements, aiming to establish regional habitat typologies, according to natural and historical evolution, property regimes and communities' life (Cabrita & Marat-Mendes 2013). Moreover, architect Fernando Távora has written on the problem of the 'Portuguese house' since 1945, which he believed could provide lessons for 'new intentions' in architecture (Cabrita & Marat-Mendes 2013).

It took nearly a decade for Keil do Amaral to obtain permission and financing to conduct this survey. In 1955, Eduardo de Arantes e Oliveira, then the Minister of Public Works, accepted the proposition.

The country's territory was divided into six zones – Minho, Trás-os-Montes, Beiras, Estremadura, (including the Lisbon Region), Alentejo and Algarve – to which six team of architects was assigned. Their aim was to collect, through drawings and maps, but mostly photography, a characterization of traditional, vernacular and popular architecture in Portugal, with a particular focus on the countryside. Over 10 000 photographs were collected. Results were presented to Oliveira Salazar, in April 1958 (AAVV 2004). The idea that a typical 'Portuguese house' would result from this survey was disproved, as regional realities were astonishingly specific (Tostões 1997).

The 'IARP' is a key moment for the development of a Modern Architecture in Portugal, whose influence extends to the present. Although the 'IARP' seemed to serve the interests of the regime, namely an appreciation of an architecture with national identity and a focus on rural territories (Cabrita & Marat-Mendes 2013), for architects, its use was more pragmatic. It allowed a critique of the rationalist excesses of the Modern Movement, showing that vernacular buildings contained their own rational organization of space, as well as articulations between territories, buildings and communities (Tostões 1997). This may explain why, despite the general guidelines, no coherent methodology was followed, and no systematization of surveyed materials was attempted, as it had been, for example, in the geographical surveys of Ribeiro (Cabrita & Marat-Mendes 2013).

The 'IARP' allowed Portuguese architects to envision new articulations between international modernism and local realities, as seen in the Portuguese presentation at CIAM 10 (Congrés Internacionaux d'Architecture Moderne) in Dubrovnik 1956. A collective housing estate for a rural community was presented, drawn from examples in Zone 1 (Minho) of the 'IARP' (Marat-Mendes & Borges 2017), thus providing new readings of urban form and human activities, as is the case of food production and the spatiality of the food system. More recently, a 'IARP' website was created to provide more photographs (http://www.oapix.org.pt/300000/1/index.htm).

## 2.2 A sample of a photographic portray on food & urban form in IARP

In the 'IARP', it is possible to identify several building types and settlements connected with the food system and water provision. In the Lisbon Region, these include farms, rural housing (mostly individual, but also collective), as well as windmills and watermills, haystacks, public wells and fountains, saline and commercial facilities. Although the Zone 4 (Estremadura) of the 'IARP' included the Lisbon Region, most surveyed examples are not located in urban centres. In the particular case of food system structures, nearly all of them are located in rural areas, showing that by the mid-20th century, a considerable part of the Lisbon region territory was dominated by food-production.

The images show a region where agrarian activities are often untouched by industrial transformation. Scale of buildings is usually contained, and landscape is highly valued for its productive capacities. It is interesting to observe the photographs as such. Framing is fundamental, and most photographers made a clear effort to portray the situation of buildings in their surroundings. Land is a fundamental extension for many buildings (Images 2, 3, 6, 11, 14 and 15 in Figure 1), a direct consequence of their agrarian context.

## 3 THE SURVEY ON THE 20TH CENTURY ARCHITECTURE IN PORTUGAL (IAPXX)

### 3.1 Context, goals and methodology

Four decades passed from the research of architect Nuno Portas who, funded by the Calouste Gulbenkian Foundation (c. 1960), identified architectural examples considered significant by him, accompanied by brief comments and one or two photographs. Later, this work informed the final chapter of the Portuguese edition of Bruno Zevi's 'Storia dell' Architecttura Moderna' (Portas 2006). Portas selected examples of Portuguese modernist and modern architecture (Toussaint 2009). For many years, Portas' article, local architectural guides (Ferreira et al. 1987; Berger et al. 1994; Fernandes & Cannatà 2002) and monographs on specific architects established an idea of twentieth-century urban architecture in Portugal, while vernacular and popular architecture remained fundamentally covered by 'IARP'.

A survey on the 20th century architecture in Portugal, 'IAPXX' was promoted in September 2003 by Ordem dos Arquitectos (Portuguese Institute of Architects), in partnership with the Mies van der Rohe Foundation and the Instituto das Artes (Arts Institute), with financing from Interreg III – SUDOE. With scientific coordination by Ana Tostões, the survey intended to represent 20th century architecture, helping to draw up strategies for safeguarding Portuguese built heritage.

The work, conducted until April 2006, had the methodology applied in 'IARP' as reference. Consequently, the territory was divided in six regions – North, Centre, Lisbon and Tagus Valley, South, Azores,

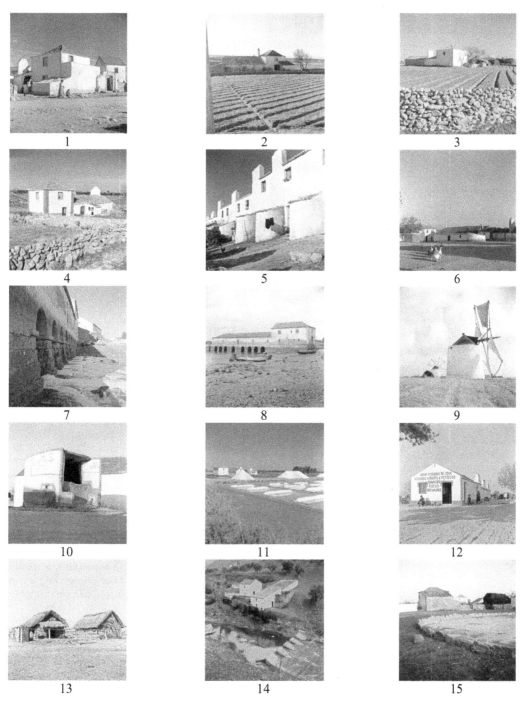

Figure 1. *Inquérito sobre a Arquitectura Regional Portuguesa (1955–1960)*, food-related structures in Lisbon Region: **1** – Rural house in Cascais [PT-OA-IARP-LSB-CSC00-012]; **2** – Rural house in Assafora, Sintra [PT-OA-IARP-LSB-SNT00-070]; **3** – Rural house in Assafora, Sintra [PT-OA-IARP-LSB-SNT00-014]; **4** – Settlement in Sintra [PT-OA-IARP-LSB-SNT00-049]; **5** – Ilheus housing in Picanceira, Mafra [PT-OA-IARP-LSB-MFR13-002]; **6** – Public square in Fontanelas, Sintra [PT-OA-IARP-LSB-SNT00-025]; **7** – WatermiU in Rouxinol, Seixal [PT-OA-IARP-STB-SXL00-001]; **8** – WatermiU in Seixal [PT-OA-IARP-STB-SXLOO-005]; **9** – Windmills in Ericeira, Mafra [PT-OA-IARP-LSB-MFR06-003]; **10** – Public covered well in Fontanelas, Sintra [PT-OA-IARP-LSB-SNT00-008]; **11** – Saline in Alcochete [PT-OA-IARP-STB-ACHO1-002]; **12** – Tavern in Pegoes, Montijo [PT-OA-IARP-STB-STB00-002]; **13** – Haystack and servants' house in Vila Franca de Xira [PT-OA-IARP-LSB-VFX00-003]; **14** – WatermiU in Venda do Pinheiro, Loures [PT-OA-IARP-LSB-LRSOO-001]; **15** – Threshing floor in Arneiro dos Marinheiros, Sintra [PT-OA-IARP-LSB-SNT00-056]. © Ordem dos Arquitectos.

Madeira – and each was assigned a team of architects. Each team had available for the fieldwork (circa 10 months) cars, computers, digital cameras, a pre-designed database and a software for GPS identification. Examples included both vernacular and popular or author architecture in all Portuguese territory, meaning cities, towns and villages anywhere, including the countryside. 180 000 km were covered. In a total of 308 municipalities, 290 were covered by IAPXX. The idea was not to build a History of Portuguese Architecture of the 20th century, but rather to bring architecture closer to civil society, emphasizing its quality.

Researchers recognized architectural work as belonging to different typologies, including bandstands, houses, buildings, factories, water reservoirs, train stations, urban plans, among many others related to functioning of the food system. In the end, more than 5000 architectural works were identified and 100 000 photographs were collected in the database, later posted online (http://www.iap20.pt/Site/Front Office/default.aspx). A summary was published in book form (AAVV 2006). Some examples were signed by renowned Portuguese and foreign architects, nevertheless, this survey acknowledged unknown works and designers, as well as representative buildings in a high state of degradation. One of the strengths of 'IAPXX' is its recognition of the plurality of architecture in Portugal, beyond the boundaries of dominant critical discourse. Just like 'IARP' showed great variety within autochthonous construction, so 'IAPXX' accounts for a century of architecture far more eclectic than historiography would usually concede. Furthermore, it is only possible to promote the safeguarding of paradigmatic architectural works when the totality of the built patrimony is known. Thus, 'IAPXX' must be understood as a tool for the Direção-Geral do Património Cultural (Directorate General of Patrimony), the Portuguese institution for recognition and classification of real estate.

### 3.2 A sample of a photographic portray on food & urban form in IAPXX

Although that was not the intent of 'IAPXX', it is possible to identify urban forms associated to food system and water provision. The Lisbon Region is covered in the inventory from the Lisbon and Tagus Valley team, coordinated by João Vieira Caldas and José Silva Carvalho, and the South team, coordinated by Michel Toussaint and Ricardo Carvalho. Here, we highlight markets, factories, cooperatives (wine/oil), water springs, water tanks, canteens, houses/farms with a sustenance agriculture area, etc., located in urban centres, others in the countryside.

The images show several scales of buildings. Some equipment justified a collection of photographs and drawings; nevertheless, some images do not do justice to the quality of architectural works. It also happens that many food-related urban forms may have escaped this inventory. For instance, sustenance gardens in family urban houses or farms, in some cases, may have not been even photographed, but we know that they existed (Images 7 and 8 in Figure 2). In the case of the manufacturing structures linked to the food system, many were located in peripheral areas of the cities, near the riverbed or railway stations (Images 4, 11 and 12 in Figure 2), however, many examples are today abandoned and some explored for tourism. The water infrastructures serve the population clusters or these manufacturing structures (Images 12 and 15 in Figure 2). Now, the land is no longer an extension of buildings, especially since it is much more valuable as urban property.

Another important aspect is the variety of architectural aesthetics encountered, ranging from traditional designs (Images 3, 6, 7 and 8 in Figure 2) to modern ones (Images 2 and 5 in Figure 2), to the characteristic style of the New State, called 'Português Suave' (Soft Portuguese), a mesh of neoclassic and Art Deco aesthetics (Vieira de Almeida & Fernandes 1986) visible in Image 9 in Figure 2.

## 4 DISCUSSION

For urban design to integrate the food system, one main challenge is to recognize its inherent spatiality. Figures 1 and 2 show examples of built structures, mostly buildings, and, to a lesser extent, settlements and equipment, which help clarify this spatiality. Particularly in the 'IARP', some photographs show land-uses and their relations with buildings. In 'IAPXX', examples are predominantly architectural.

Comparing the two surveys, one encounters a profound change in the territory of the Lisbon Region. Whereas in the 'IARP', most food-related structures are characteristic of a technologically simple agrarian production system (Figure 1), the examples from 'IAPXX' shows the appearance of industrial facilities and a new relevance for food-consumption spaces (Images 9, 10, 11, 12 and 15 in Figure 2).

This exposes how the socio-metabolism of the Lisbon Region has changed between these two surveys. On the first, solar energy and animal labour were the dominant energy source for agricultural activities. On the second, industrial production allowed new flows of energy and materials within the Region, including electricity and fossil fuels. The comparison of surveys reveals how the socio-metabolic aspect of the territory is intrinsically marked by human activities in the natural and built landscape.

Large-scale facilities for the food system are inexistent in the 'IARP', but there are plenty in 'IAPXX'. The specific territorial arrangements linked to agriculture were once a structuring force in the Lisbon Region, but land-use and urban planning have change considerably since then and a greater segregation between urban and rural is now evident with repercussions in spatial planning and the territory itself (Marat-Mendes et al. 2018).

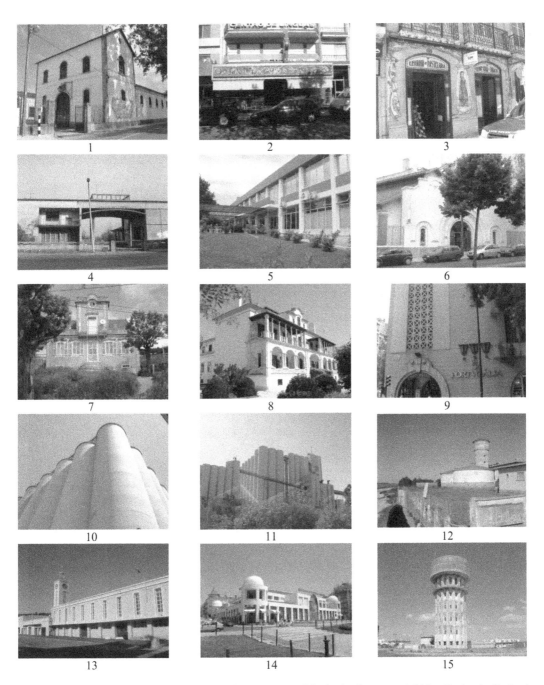

Figure 2. *IAPXX – Inquérito à Arquitectura do Seculo XX em Portugal*, food-related structures in Lisbon Region: **1** – Regional Winehouse in Colares, Sintra [L100501]; **2** – Galeto Snack Bar, Lisbon [LI00781]; **3** – Milk house 'A Camponesa', Lisbon [L200394]; **4** – Municipal slaughterhouse, Vila Franca de Xira [L100355]; **5** – University Canteen, Lisbon [L200246]; **6** – Public economic kitchen, Lisbon [L200312]; **7** – Vila Amelia sustenance garden, Odivelas [L300214]; **8** – Rio Frio Manor, Palmela [S200293]; **9** – Portugalia Beer Factory, Lisbon [L200322]; **10** – CUF Mill, Almada [S100658]; **11** – Grain silos, Almada [S100670]; **12** – Oyster depuration centre, Moita [S200482]; **13** – Fish selling lot, Setiibal [S200168]; **14** – Campo de Ourique Marketplace, Lisbon [L100671]; **15** – Water reservoir, Barreiro [S200918]. © Ordem dos Arquitectos.

Agricultural labour in most of the photographs from the 'IARP' (See images 4, 5, 6, 10, 11, 12 and 15 of Figure 1) seemed to provide its own form of conviviality around food-related activities. No food-related public equipment is present in the 'IARP', showing that concerns expressed by Parham (2016) on the convivial aspect of food are particular to present times, marked by urbanization and consumption. This contemporary notion of food-based conviviality is illustrated by 'IAPXX' examples of marketplaces, restaurants and cafes (See images 2, 3, 5, 6, 13 and 14 of Figure 2).

If Viljoen et al (2005) have suggested a 'Continuous Productive Urban Landscape' of allotments and urban farms to ensure environmental quality and food-provision in cities, these Portuguese surveys expose that the conditions for achieving this may have decreased with the reduction of agrarian areas and urbanization. Such move was necessary, as in 1960s, Portugal was under-industrialized and needing modernization in many social aspects, including the territory and the production system. However, this bygone rural reality, reflected in 'IARP', might contain possible lessons for establishing a necessary urban agenda for sustainability. In 'IAPXX', the diversity of built structures reveals opportunities for solidifying links between urban and rural activities.

## 5 CONCLUSIONS

Although these two surveys were guided by different aims, they allowed retrieving some representative examples of the food system spatial dimension. These show how ubiquitous the food system is in human activities and in the territory. Technology made surveys possible, specifically by photography, analogic in the 'IARP' and digital in the 'IAPXX'. These photographs have great aesthetic importance – the 'IARP' allowed Portuguese architects the development of a specific interpretation of modernism, and 'IAPXX' presents a far-reaching overview of 20th century taste and sensibility, both popular and erudite. However, these materials are no less important as the other documents. Susan Sontag (2008) claims that scientists use photography to produce an inventory of the world, which was certainly the methodological approach of both analysed surveys. They were expected to give a comprehensive account of specific forms or timeframes in Portuguese architecture.

However, as Sontag (2008) also claimed, photography is a fragmentary moment cut off from time, a quotation, turning a photography book into a book of quotations. Thus, many other quotations would be possible within the same territory. The diversity of food-related structures identified here shows that a survey specifically aimed at the food system of the Lisbon Region would be possible.

Considering the important role of the food system in the socio-metabolism of territories (Marat-Mendes et al. 2018), such surveys are increasingly important. For architecture and urban design they are an opportunity to rediscover elements of urban form that may accommodate sustainable changes in cities. Thus, it is necessary to counteract the deficit of urban form design solutions for the overall food system, allowing further improvements on the ground and on urban design practice itself.

The examples discussed here occur in the territory in several scales, associated with different uses and with specific relations to the land. As such, they are highly diversified. More effort is therefore needed from architects and urban designers to fully acknowledge such diversity and bring to the debate new creative design solutions to enhance the role of food in urban systems.

'IARP' and 'IAPXX' show that food-related structures have a considerable mark in the landscape and in the collective memory that forms around such landscape. When observing these images, it is important to understand their meaning in our perception: as Sontag (2008) reminds us, photographs change our notions of what is worth looking at and what we can observe, and thus constitute an ethics of seeing. Observing certain aspects of the world through photography promotes further understandings of it and allows imagination to creatively transform it, towards better built and natural environments. The examples extracted from these two surveys are inspiring starting-points for imagining how food can help us design our way into sustainability.

## FUNDING AND ACKNOWLEDGMENTS

The authors were financed by Grants (SFRH/BPD/117167/2016) financed by the National Funds through the Foundation for Science and Technology Portugal (FCT) and the Community budget through the European Social Fund (ESF) and (POCI-01-0145-FEDER-016431) financed by the European Structural and Investment Funds (ESIF) through the Operational Thematic Program for Competitiveness and Internationalization (COMPETE 2020) in its European Regional Development Fund and by National Funds through the Foundation for Science and Technology Portugal (FCT).

The authors also thank the Portuguese 'Ordem dos Arquitectos' for the permission to use the images included in this text.

## REFERENCES

AAVV. 2004. *Arquitectura Popular em Portugal*. Lisboa: Ordem dos Arquitectos.
AAVV. 2006. *IAP XX Inquérito à Arquitectura do Século XX em Portugal*. Lisboa: Ordem dos Arquitectos –CDN.
Amaral, F.K. 1947. Uma iniciativa necessária. *Arquitectura: Revista de Arte e Construção*, 2(14): 12–13.
Baccini, P & Oswald, F. 2008. Designing the Urban: Linking Physiology and Morphology in Hadorn, G. et al. (eds.) *Handbook of Transdisciplinary Research*: 79–88. Switzerland: Springer.

Berger, F. G. & Toussaint, M. & Bissau, L. 1994. *Guia de Arquitectura Lisboa 94*. Lisboa: Associação dos Arquitectos Portugueses.

Brinkley, C. 2013. Avenues into food planning. *International Planning Studies*, 18(2): 243–266.

Cabrita, M. A. & Marat-Mendes, T. 2013. Inquéritos à arquitectura popular em Portugal – uma aproximação metodológica. *Colóquio Internacional Arquitectura Popular – conference proceedings, Arcos de Valdevez, 3–6 April 2013*. Arcos de Valdevez: Casa das Artes.

Costa, L. 1938 [1997]. Documentação necessária. *Registro de uma vivência*. Rio de Janeiro: Empresa das Artes: 457–462.

Dias, A. M. 2018. *The shape of food – an analysis of urban agricultural shapes in Lisbon's Greater Area*. Unpublished MSc Thesis, Instituto Universitário de Lisboa – ISCTE, Portugal.

Dimitsantou-Kremesi, C. & Marat-Mendes, T. 2012. Issues on Architectural Surveys – The Inquérito à Arquitectura Regional Portuguesa. *Surveys on vernacular architecture – their significance in 20th century architectural culture* – conference proceedings, Porto, 17–19 May. Porto: ESAP.

Fernandes, F. & Cannatà, M. 2002. *Guia da Arquitectura Moderna – Porto*. Porto: Asa.

Ferreira, F. C. & Carvalho, J. S. & Ponte, T. N. & Silva, F. J. 1987. *Guia Urbanístico e Arquitectónico de Lisboa*. Lisboa: Associação dos Arquitectos Portugueses Secção Regional Sul.

Figueira, J. 2016. *Arquitectanic – Os dias da Troika*. Lisboa: Note.

Fischer-Kowalski, M.; Haas, W. 2014. Exploring the transformation of human labour in relation to socio-ecological transitions. Beblavý, M; Maselli, I.; Veselková, M (eds) *Let's get to work! The future of labour in Europe* – vol. 1: 56–84. Brussels: Centre for European Policy Studies.

Gandy, M. 2004. Rethinking urban metabolism: water, space and the modern city. *City*, 8(3): 363–379.

Kennedy, C & Pinceti, S. & Buhe, P. 2010. The study of urban metabolism and its applications to urban planning and design. *Environmental Pollution*: 1–9. Doi: 10.1016/j.envpol.2010.10.022

Kostof, S. 1991. *The city shaped. Urban patterns and meanings through History*. London: Thames Hudson.

Marat-Mendes, T. & Cunha Borges, J. 2017. Sustainability in Portuguese Architectural Higher Education: its contribution to the social role of the Architect. Presentation in *Designing the city with the community: notes on participative projects, FAUL, Lisboa, June 8th*.

Marat-Mendes, T. (coord), Mourão, J., Bento d'Almeida, P. & Niza, S. 2015. *Water and Agriculture Atlas: Lisbon Region in 1900–1940*. Lisboa: Instituto Universitário de Lisboa – ISCTE/ DINAMIA'CET-IUL.

Marat-Mendes, T., Mourão, J. & Bento d'Almeida, P. 2016. Access to water in the Lisbon region in 1900. *Water History*, 8 (2): 159–189.

Marat-Mendes, T., Cunha Borges, J., Dias, A.M. & Lopes, R. 2018. Food system and Spatial Municipal Planning – analysis of its integration in the 18 municipalities of the Lisbon Metropolitan Area. Presentation in *Dinâmicas socioeconómicas e territoriais contemporâneas IV – ISCTE, Lisboa, December 17th*.

Ordem dos Arquitectos. IAP 20 Inquérito à Arquitectura do Século XX em Portugal, acessed 26 April 2019, http://www.iap20.pt/Site/FrontOffice/default.aspx

Ordem dos Arquitectos. OAPIX – Inquérito à Arquitectura Popular Portuguesa, acessed 26 April 2019, http://www.oapix.org.pt/

Parham, S. 2016. *Food and Urbanism. The convivial City and a sustainable future*. London: Bloomsbury.

Portas, N. 2006. A oportunidade do IAPXX e uma interpretação dos Anos 40, in AAVV. *IAP XX Inquérito à Arquitectura do Século XX em Portugal*. Lisboa: Ordem dos Arquitectos – CDN.

Pothukuchi, K. & Kaufman, J. L. 2000. The food system – a stranger in the planning field. *Journal of the American Planning association*, 66(82): 113–124.

Sontag, S. 2008. *On Photography*. London: Penguin.

Steel, C. 2013. *Hungry City: How Food Shapes our Lives*. London: Vintage Books.

Tostões, A. 1997. *Os verdes anos na Arquitectura Portuguesa dos Anos 50*. Porto: FAUP.

Toussaint, M. 2009. *Da arquitectura à teoria e o universo da teoria da arquitectura em Portugal na primeira metade do século XX*. PhD presented to Universidade Técnica de Lisboa Faculdade de Arquitectura. Accessed in 30 April 2009, https://www.repository.utl.pt/bitstream/10400.5/1411/1/DISSERTA%c3%87%c3%83O_Michel%20Toussaint.pdf.

Vieira de Almeida, P. & Fernandes, J.M. 1986. O arrabalde do céu. *História da Arte em Portugal*. Lisboa: Alfa.

Vijoen, A., Bohn, K. & Howe, J. 2005. *Continuous Productive Urban Landscapes: Designing Urban Agriculture for Sustainable Cities*. Amsterdam: Architectural Press.

29

*Experiencing Food: Designing Sustainable and Social Practices – Bonacho, Pires & Lamy (Eds)*
*© 2021 Taylor & Francis Group, London, ISBN 978-0-367-49414-8*

# Gastronomic potential and pairings of new emulsions of vegetable origin

A.T. Silva, C. Morgado, N. Félix, C. Brandão & M. Guerra
*ESHTE, Escola Superior de Hotelaria e Turismo do Estoril, Estoril, Portugal*

G. Lima & C. Laranjeiro
*ESAS, Escola Superior Agrária de Santarém, Santarém, Portugal*
*Instituto Politécnico de Santarém, Santarém, Portugal*

ABSTRACT: Five innovative emulsions prototypes (preserving expensive or seasonal raw materials and value surplus or regional by-products) were analyzed: 1 strawberry, 2 bell pepper (red and yellow) processed differently, with aqueous vegetable phase and 2 mustards with red fruits or beet. An initial sensory evaluation was carried out (hedonic scale 1–9) with a panel of specialist tasters and the online Foodpairing® tool was also used. The panel positively evaluated all emulsions (global appreciation mean values between 5.6 and 7) but none was pointed out as having potential gastronomic use by itself, but always as an ingredient of some composition. There were 33 combinations of ingredients with the Foodpairing® tool. The opinion of the food professionals was quite important and useful, but not always coincident with the ingredients proposed by the application Foodpairing®. Global food innovation includes characterization of new products, including their potential in terms of gastronomic use, and sensorial acceptability, basing further developments.

## 1 INTRODUCTION

### 1.1 Food industry and innovation

The agri-food and beverage industry is the main activity sector in Europe (FoodDrinkEurope, 2018), characterized by the numerous changes that have led to an increasing innovation in the production and supply of food. The new needs of consumers – both final or intermediate (professional cooks) translate into the design and availability of the food produced and idealized to suit them. This is done from the nutritional point of view, health and well-being, from the point of view of convenience and practicality, reliability and quality, through the sustainable management and ethics of the resources used in its production (PlantFoods, 2018). Pushed by the industry needs and also by the demand of consumers, the use of surplus production (primary and food processing sectors) and by-products are a trend. This, objectively, play an important role in terms of local producers income; local products valorization and constitutes one of the chains of the circular economy aiming an optimum use of natural resources, raw materials and products and re-using them (Rood et al., 2017; EMF, 2018).

These challenges provide an opportunity for the development of new products and the creation of new market niches.

### 1.2 Spreads and mustards

The spreadable creams are essentially water-in-oil emulsions. The lipid phase is usually a mixture of vegetable oils and, or oils and fats of animal origin containing natural dyes (β-carotene), stabilizers, emulsifiers, flavorings, antioxidants, lecithins and fat-soluble vitamins. The aqueous phase contains proteins, skim milk, where small amounts of other ingredients, such as salt, preservatives, thickeners and water-soluble vitamins (Nylender et al., 2008).

Spreads have, like traditional butter, several applications: breaded, toasted, crackers and other bases, and can be used as an appetizer or accompaniment and, or confection of other foods including cold meat, roast beef and grilled meat or fish (Lima, 2014).

Mustards are emulsified, oil-in-water (o/w) type vinegar products, in which the continuous phase is water and the phase disperses oil. The lipid phase is an oil of vegetable origin. The milled mustard seeds release surfactant phospholipids which help to stabilize the emulsion formed. Mustard creams are used as a seasoning and, or accompaniment of salads, fried and grilled meats, sandwiches or in the confection of sauces. Mustards are used to add flavor to several dishes and to enhance the piquancy and texture of several types of sauces (Hriddek, 2014).

### 1.3 Consumer trends and sensory evaluation

Today, new lifestyles, higher incomes and consumer awareness are creating consumer demand for a year-round supply of high-quality, diverse and innovative food products (Traynor, 2013). But, higher demand for new products is not a guarantee for their success. In fact, many factors contribute to the acceptability of new launched products both in the market and in the food service industry. Among factors like trends, price or brand, arises the organoleptic attractiveness of the product and also its convenience in use, which also includes technological suitability of culinary preparations for domestic consumers and also for professional in the catering (food service) industry. Sensory evaluation is therefore an important step in the food development process as it is the potential gastronomic use. Sensory characteristics comprising appearance, odor, flavor and texture are included within the important attributes that contribute for the perceived quality of food products (IFT, 1981). The sensory acceptance assessment by food specialists may contribute to the understanding of the potential of the food being developed and, in a context of consumers test, to the prediction of the overall success of the product.

## 1.4  *Food pairing and the online tool*

Food Pairing is a scientific method for identifying which foods and beverages work well together. The taste sensation is easily connected to our taste experience. When we taste food, we detect the 5 basic flavors in our mouth and in our tongue: sweet, salty, bitter, sour and umami. Flavors are the main drivers of our taste experience and therefore are crucial for the synergy of food and drinks. Up to 80% of what we call taste is aroma. The aroma profile of the culinary ingredients is the starting point of the Foodpairing® computer application and this scientific research. Ingredient that does not have aromatic combination are not possible matches. Ingredients that can give rise to contrasting flavors and textures must be added in order to be able to obtain a well-balanced recipe (Ahn, 2016; FoodPairing, s/d).

The main objective of this study was to assess the gastronomic potential and possible uses of water-in-oil (60% to 65% lipid phase) innovative inverse emulsion prototypes previously developed (Lima et al., 2017; Laranjeira et al., 2018), using both sensory evaluation and the Foodpairing® tool.

## 2  MATERIALS AND METHODS

### 2.1  *Samples*

Five samples were analyzed – 3 emulsions of strawberry and bell pepper (one red and one yellow) processed differently, with aqueous vegetable phase and 2 mustards with red fruits or beet. These products were recently prototyped and are characterised for the additions of vegetables and, or fruit syrups, with no tradition of manufacture or consumption in Portugal, preserving expensive and, or seasonal raw materials and value surplus and, or regional by-products and for having nutritional quality. These emulsions have a vegan or lactovegetarian profile, which can be used as substitutes for butter (fat phases using cocoa butter or coconut oil). Traditional mustards (in vinegar) are distinguished by ingredients, flavors and unusual colors (Lima et al., 2017; Laranjeira et al., 2018).

## 2.2  *Gastronomic potential evaluation*

### 2.2.1  *Sensory evaluation*

In order to a first sensorial characterization of each of the samples and to determine the perception of the respective potential of gastronomic use, a hedonic test was performed using a panel of tasters (specialist – 6 Chefs and 3 food professionals), previously established.

The general attributes were considered from the descriptors previously generated by the researchers. The individual parameters selected were as follows:

– visual appearance and color (on appearance); smell and, or odor, flavor and aroma, taste persistence (gustatory smell): used a 9-point scale with defined terms situated between "poor" and "excellent";
– texture, ointment and acidity (for mustard fruity creams): used 9-point scale with defined terms situated between "extremely unpleasant" and "extremely pleasant".

An overall assessment item (using a 9-point scale with terms defined between "poor" and "excellent") was also presented.

In the scope of the test were also measured:

– consumption potential and purchase intention: a 5-point scale was used with definite terms between "definitely no" and "certainly yes";
– the culinary potential of the samples per se and as a basis for other preparations: a 5-point scale with definite terms placed between "definitely without application" and "certainly with application";

It was also asked to identify the emulsion fat in the case of the first 3 samples and comments on the potential culinary applications of all creams.

The samples were coded using a three-digit code and analyzed in the laboratory at a temperature of about 20°C, similar to the one that is customary to use with natural fluorescent lighting.

### 2.2.2  *Foodpairing assessement*

The online Foodpairing® tool was used. Through the data obtained in the sensorial analysis performed on the samples, the main aroma of each sample was identified. This identified ingredient was selected in the online application. Then the other ingredient (s) that composed the emulsions were selected. In view of future developments, it was previously established the context of use of a possible delicacy: for Food Service or for domestic consumption, since the level of difficulty of producing the recipe, and the type of ingredients used would have to be different. Then it was considered the order to appear in a possible menu – sauce, canapé, cold starter, hot starter, main course of fish, meat main course, garnish and dessert.

In the continuation one or more ingredients were selected from the presented results, calculated by the application algorithm, as being "best aromatic combination".

## 2.3 Statistical analysis

Data were treated using the Statistical Package for Social Sciences (SPSS), IMB software version 24.0 and Excel spreadsheet software, Microsoft Office 365, version 16.0.

The results were presented in mean ± standard deviation (SD) and frequency. Emulsions were accepted when they obtained an average ≥ 5.0 (equivalent to the hedonic term "neither good nor bad").

## 3 RESULTS AND DISCUSSIONS

### 3.1 Gastronomic potential revealed

The results of the hedonic sensorial evaluation showed that the panel of experts appreciated positively all the creams, except for the strawberry emulsion. These tasters preferred the yellow bell pepper spread on all aspects except for the smell and odor; in this parameter the preferred one was the red bell pepper cream (Figure 1).

The least appealing in terms of the visual appearance, color and greasiness was the strawberry cream. Tasters noticed a lack of the characteristic color of this fruit and high viscosity at room temperature.

The second less appreciated was the beetroot and raspberry mustard cream, again by the visual aspect and the color little appealing and also because it is not homogeneous, being the presence of the seeds a depreciative factor, not only in this sample, but like in the others which also had this aspect (strawberry emulsion and raspberry and blueberry mustard).

There was less dispersion in the views of the overall appreciation for the bell pepper and raspberry mustard cream (MFM code) samples and a greater dispersion

for the strawberry emulsion and the beetroot mustard cream (MBF code) (Figure 2).

Fats used in the emulsions were always identified (data not shown) (cocoa butter or coconut oil) and apparently led to satisfactory aroma and flavor acceptance levels (>6). Studies related to cocoa butter have shown that it can be used to alter the introduction of fats into margarines and chocolates, making them healthier, with a view to reducing the epidemic problem of global obesity by manipulating the percentages in their emulsions (Norton & Fryer, 2012).

The sensory results obtained in this study may be seen as an important contribution to the future commercialization of the products, since they gives us a perspective of the potential consumer acceptance (Mohamed & Shalaby, 2016), specially the food service prespective. A number of studies have been carried out during the development of the products in order to achieve an optimum formulation from the consumer's point of view. Several findings on similar products, confirm the importance of conducting acceptance tests during the development process, even leading to recommendations of reformulations or improvements of the sensorial characteristics of products to be better accepted by the consumer (Nwosu, 2014). Other studies reveal that appearance and color are aspects that influence the appreciation of products, which is in accordance to our findings.

In our opinion, the study also benefit from using individuals experienced in tasting food, as they more easily were able to identify and name the flavours in the new products.

In relation to the possible gastronomic use of the emulsions (data not shown), none was pointed out as having great potential on its own, to be used alone, but always as an ingredient of some composition. Strawberry sour cream has been suggested only for desserts or sweet compositions; the yellow bell pepper spread was singled out as a flavoring potential for a white rice or a cooked dough, to finish off risotto or curry such

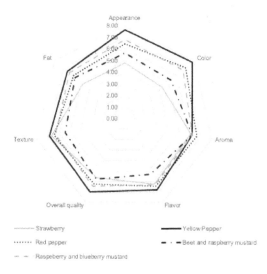

Figure 1. Hedonic sensory evaluation parameters and average scores, analyzed by the panel of experts, using a 9-point scale with defined terms situated between "poor" and "excellent".

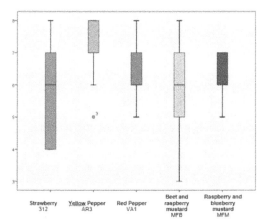

Figure 2. Box-plot of the values of the hedonic sensorial parameters of the samples analyzed by panel of experts.

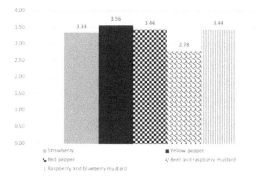

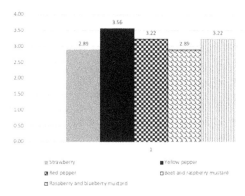

Figure 3. Consumption potential of the samples analyzed by panel of specialists using a 5-point scale with definite terms placed between "definitely without application" and "certainly with application".

Figure 4. Purchase intention of the samples analyzed by panel of experts using a 5-point scale with definite terms between "definitely no" and "certainly yes".

Table 1. Example of the combinations given by the Foodpairing® tool regarding the yellow bell pepper spread.

| Meal course | Ingredientes point out in the Food Parking tool |
| --- | --- |
| Sauce | egg yolk; olive oil, virgin; red wine vinegar; mustard |
| Couvert | cream cheese; cheddar sharp shiso; crab meat; pepper caiena; ciabatta; french fries |
| Vegetarian main course | Pasta; walnut; basil |
| Fish main course | Turbot; sake; soy miso; egg yolk; eggplant; cauliflower; onion; olive oil virgin; blueberry vinegar; cilantro; raisin; garlic |
| Meat main course | Beef; olive oil, virgin; cognac |
| Garnish | Rice; pasta |

as roasted meat seasoning or sauces ingredient; the red bell pepper cream was the least appreciated in terms of culinary potential because it was compared to the mass of bell pepper and its consequent use; beetroot and raspberry and raspberry and blueberry mustard creams were used as ingredients for vinaigrettes or for spreading on roasted meats, the latter being the second most appreciated in this sensory evaluation.

Having the possibility of using a panel experienced in culinary arts and food production permitted a broader view on gastronomic possible uses of the tested products, as this professionals can easily anticipated technical proprieties (both in a catering and household environment) and also anticipates the final consumer reactions and acceptance.

Addressing the consumption potential (Figure 3), on average the yellow bell pepper (AR3 code) was the sample that showed the best results. The red bell pepper emulsion (VA1 code) and the MFM showed intermediate results, followed by the strawberry emulsion (132 code) and with the worst result, the beetroot mustard cream MBF, however, all the samples revealed, on average, a consumption potential.

In what regards to the relation to the intention to buy, on average (Figure 4) the yellow bell pepper AR3 was the sample that showed the best results. The red bell pepper emulsion VA1 and beetroot and raspberry mustard cream MFM showed intermediate results, the strawberry emulsion 132 and the beetroot mustard cream MBF having the worst results, however, all the samples revealed, on average, a positive purchase intention.

### 3.2 Foodpairing possibilities

There were 33 combinations of ingredients with the Foodpairing® tool for the 5 prototypes considering possible meal courses. Given the extension of the results, a single example is provided in Table 1 for the combination of ingredients suggested for the yellow bell pepper spread.

The opinion of the chefs was not always coincident with the ingredients proposed by the application of Foodpairing®. We are aware that the suitability of the ingredients for inclusion in recipes or food pairings depends on a myriad of ingredient characteristics in addition to their flavor profile. Flavor is not necessarily the main role of ingredients, recipes also rely on ingredients to provide the final textures and the overall structure of a given dish (Ahn et al., 2011). Actually, according to the above mentioned authors, shared flavor compounds represent one of several contributions to fitness value, while shared compounds clearly play a significant role in some cuisines, other contributions may play a more dominant role in other cuisines. Western cuisines, for example, show a tendency to use pairs of ingredients that share many flavor compounds, supporting the so-called food pairing hypothesis.

### 4 CONCLUSIONS

The new prototypes have potential multiple food applications. The opinion of the chefs was quite important and useful, but not always coincident with the ingredients proposed by the application of Foodpairing®.

This tool together with the sensory results and with the available knowledge can be associated with the work of a chef (or other food producer) who demonstrates his experience and ability to generate recipes, techniques and confections, knowing in advance which ingredients will have higher potential of combination. Given the increasing availability of information on food preparation, this data-driven research has opened new avenues for a systematic understanding of culinary practice, that can be oriented towards a specific food product, like the emulsions and spreads tested.

Further studies will be carried on for the production of several recipes allied to consumer studies.

## ACKNOWLEDGEMENTS

Project financed within Agrio et Emulsio – Desenvolvimento de Novos Produtos LISBOA-01-0145-FEDER-023583.

## REFERENCES

Ahn Y. et al. 2011. Flavour pairing and network principles of food pairing. *Scientific Reports*, 1, 1–7.

EMF. 2018. Cities and the circular economy for food. UK: Ellen Macarthur Foundation. https://www.ellenmacarthur foundation.org/assets/downloads/Cities-and-the-circular-economy-for-food-1.pdf.

Dickinson E. & McClements, J. 1996. Advances in food coloids. UK: Blackie Academic & Professional. pp. 333.

FoodDrinkEurope. 2018. Data and Trends 2018. Belgica: FoodDrinkEurope. https://www.fooddrinkeurope.eu/uploads/publications_documents/FoodDrinkEurope_Data_and_Trends_2018_FINAL.pdf [04/05/2019].

FoodPairing (s/d) "Food Pairing Blog. http://blog.foodpairing.com/ [14/09/2017].

Hrideek, T. K. 2004. Mustard. Herbs and Spices, Edition: first, Chapter: 12. UK: Woodhead Publishing Limited. pp. 332.

IUPAC. 2002. International Union of Pure and Applied Chemistry. Guia IUPAC para a Nomenclatura de Compostos Orgânicos. LIDEL, September.

Guiné, R. P. F. et al. 2016. New Foods, New Consumers: Innovation in Food Product Development *Current Nutrition and Food* Science, 12(3), 175–189.

Laranjeira, C. et al., 2018. Agrio et Emulsio – development of fruity mustard creams. (POCI-01-0145-FEDER-023583). In: FOODBALT 2018 – 12th Baltic Conference on Food Science and Technology. Abstracts. Kaunas, Lithuania, May 17–18. p. 72. https://epubl.ktu.edu/object/elaba:28855510/28855510.pdf

Lima, M. 2014. Caracterização reológica e microstrutural de emulsões água em óleo para uso alimentar, Évora: Instituto De Investigação e Formação Avançada da Universidade de Évora Tese de Doutoramento https://dspace.uevora.pt/rdpc/bitstream/.../Tese%2025%20de%20Novembro%202014.pdf

Lima, M. et al. 2017. Agrio et Emulsio – New Products Development. (POCI-01-0145-FEDER-023583). XXIII Encontro Galego-Português de Química, Ferrol de 15–17 Novembro. p. 143. http://newfoodnewtech.ipsantarem.pt/wp-content/uploads/2019/01/222-Abstract-p149-2017-11-LIBRO-XXIII-ENCONTRO-FINAL-Galego-portugues-p-149.pdf.

Mohamed, A. G. & Shalaby, S. 2016. Texture, Chemical Properties and Sensory Evaluation of a Spreadable Processed Cheese Analogue Made with Apricot Pulp. *International Journal of Dairy Science*. 11(2):61–68.

Norton, J. E. & Fryer, P. J. 2012. Investigation of changes in formulation and processing parameters on the physical properties of cocoa butter emulsions. *Journal of Food Engineering*. 113, 329–336.

Nwosu, J. N. et al. 2014. Evaluation of the Proximate and Sensory Properties of Spread Produced from Cashew Nut and Groundnut Blend. *Austin Journal of Nutrition and Food Sciences*. 2(6): id1031.

Nylander T. et al., 2008. Protein/emulsifier interactions. In Hasenhuettl, G. & Hartel, R. (Eds.) in: Food emulsifiers and their application. Chap 5. New York: Chapman & Hall, 89–171.

PlantFoods. 2018. Desenvolvimento de alimentos e bebidas não-lácteas de origem vegetal (Projeto para a cimeira nacional de inovação na agricultura, floresta e desenvolvimento rural 2018) Rede rural nacional. https://agroinovacao.iniav.pt/images/Posters/cereais/PLANTFOODS.pdf

Rood T., et al. 2017. Food for the Circular Economy. PBL Netherlands Environmental Assessment Agency, The Hague.

Traynor, M. 2013. Innovative Food Product Development using Molecular Gastronomy: a Focus on Flavour and Sensory Evaluation, Dublin: Dublin Institute of Technology (PhD thesis), https://arrow.dit.ie/cgi/viewcontent.cgi?article=1025&context=tourdoc.

*Experiencing Food: Designing Sustainable and Social Practices – Bonacho, Pires & Lamy (Eds)*
*© 2021 Taylor & Francis Group, London, ISBN 978-0-367-49414-8*

# #Foodporn vintage, food depiction – from symbolic to desire

A. Jorge Caseirão
*Lisbon School of Architecture, Universidade de Lisboa, Lisbon, Portugal*

ABSTRACT: The aim of this paper is to analyze a set of images, especially paintings from various periods of food and meal scenes depiction, antagonistic or with some parallelism between them, and thus demonstrate that the phenomenon of graphic recording of meals and foodporn is not as contemporary as it seems. It's not a painting of a genre, like still life, but it anchors in some paintings of that genre. Meals and food images arise in a natural way as a scene. Images are presented in parallel discourses, without chronological concerns and assume a symbolic content while others are presented merely as objects of desire.

## 1 WHAT IS #FOODPORN?

### 1.1 *Religious and symbolic approach*

It's a very popular hashtag used in social media that accompanies the posting of showy and supposedly delicious food images which present a visual glamor. From exotic dishes that arouse the desire of experiencing to high-fat foods, from beautiful dishes to ranch pans, every food as a place in food pornography in the form of a provocative photo, somewhere between fashion, glamor or naked photography.

When the expression appeared in the late 1970s it was used to describe foods that weren't healthy, paralleling it with pornography itself. Yet, the expression gained a new meaning being used to describe foods presented in an attractive fashion. With the internet, the expression evolved into a way of documenting the meals recognized by its looks and glamor. Examples of this can be found on Instagram, Flickr, Snapchat, Facebook, Reddit, and Twitter.

The use of the hashtag connects users with information about culture, calories, presentation, preparation, taste, etc.

The expression transferred from social media to other platforms as TV shows, with a myriad of culinary shows and contests, magazines, blogs, etc.

Communication through social media became viral, a means to convey desire. There are numbers, percentages and studies of who posts the images, what they eat, and to what age group they belong. The collection of this information results in studies that help the industry to develop food trends.

In 2016, Cornell University's Food and Brand Lab published a study entitled Food Art does not Reflect Reality in which they analyze paintings and photographs depicting 500 years of meals, notably from 1500 to 2000. Considering that they didn't had access to all the paintings, the study compared the frequency in which a food was depicted and the frequency of its consumption. Amongst several findings, they concluded that 39% of the paintings from the Discovery Period depicted sea food, having also appeared in a fifth of German paintings despite the country's scarce costal area. They also concluded that the depiction of rare foods like lobsters and artichokes was very popular as well as the depiction of the vulgar like hazelnuts and lemons. They concluded that 28% of the paintings from the Enlightenment Period depicted lemons and that grapes were depicted in 26% of the paintings from the same period. They concluded that this type of depiction in art was used essentially to convey wealth or even the talent of the painter than to display what was actually ingested.

However, this study by Cornell's University does not take under consideration that the Baroque Period is a time of allegory and metaphors, where the depicted gains meaning.

Thus, in the light of Do Tratado do Significado das Plantas, Flores e Frutos que se referem nas Sagradas Escrituras, published in Lisbon on 1622 by Friar Isidoro Barreira, the lemons represent will and, mainly, willpower, while the white grapes represent the essence of Christ or the "water that springs from the wounds of Christ" and the red grapes represent the Eucharistic blood. But other values could still be considered given that within this theme duel the forces of Reform and Counter-Reform which may carry some weight in the meanings of the depicted items. It's believed to be the case of Lucas Cranach's painting which depicts the head of St. John the Baptist with the same composition, as in the painting on Lisbon's Museu Nacional de Arte Antiga, where the painter depicts the offering of the essence of Christ with a bunch of white grapes.

Once concluded the religious and symbolic approach of the theme, we'll begin this study with Leonardo da Vinci's Last Supper. The paint certainly needs no introduction. It's a fresco from 1495–96, a depiction of a scene described in John 13:21 where Christ announces that someone amongst the dinners will betray him, customary in monastic dining halls. The key focus is a meal with thirteen figures, one at the center with six on each side, share bread and wine…the water having already been turned into wine by Christ at the marriage at Cana in Galilee.

Food sharing and ingestion became secondary to the attitudes and poses of the figures, being relevant the distribution of the diners across the table. In a social meal it would be logical that everyone sit around the table, whether squared or round, around a central focus. In the Last Supper, and in all its versions, all figures stand facing the beholder. The focus is not the sharing of the meal, instead it's the central figure, Christ, usually with arms wide open.

"I am the true vine", Christ states (Jo 15:1). At the last supper, Christ took the cup, gave thanks and gave it to his disciples saying: "Drink from it, all of you. This is my blood of the covenant, which is poured out for many for the forgiveness of sins.

The Last Supper is a meal covered with symbolism, and of great importance within the sacred depiction. Marriage is also always accompanied by a huge feast and images to prove it. The Wedding Banquet by Brueghel the Elder (1567–68) is an example. It portrays a peasant scene in a barn where tables mimicking easels are surrounded by rough benches. As for the festivities, a woman offers a beer or wine mug to a man in red while another man, with his back turned, drinks another beer or wine mug. There are several empty jugs. The meal is abundant with plenty of food and drinks, pancakes, bread, soup or porridge. Next to the table there's a character with a bagpipe. In the foreground a child licks an empty goblet.

Another meal is Eduard Manet's Déjeuner sur l'herb from 1862. The painting that caused scandal at the time depicts a picnic scene with two fully clothed men and a naked woman. A fourth female figure appears in the background. Manet's original painting was later reproduced by other artists, and perhaps it even inspired William Burroughs in the title of his autobiographic novel Naked Lunch, first published in 1959, and of which David Cronenberg directed a movie with the same name. Neither the book nor the film are about any naked lunch.

In Manet's paintinh the naked figure contrasts with the elegance of the two dresses men. The model, Vitorine Meurent, was the artist's favorite, and appeared in several of his works including Olympia, another canvas that caused scandal.

The naked figure is sited on the grass with one man in front of her and another by her left side. In front of them, the woman's clothes, a basket of fruit, and a round loaf of bread are displayed. Her skin tone is extremely bright which grants light to the whole canvas, arising as a shot in the dark in Parisian society, so prude at the time.

A still-life composed by the basket, the dress, the hat, and other elements close to the naked figure's right side names the masterpiece. Focusing on the basket it appears it contains peaches, figs and cherries or sour cherries. On the side, a bred, not a Parisian baguette. Close by, a metal box or a glass, suggesting a kettle and more food. Interestingly, there are no beverages nor cups nor mugs.

The still-life is more than an allegory and each depicted object has a meaning. A still-life acts as a manifestation of reality for the eyes delight and as an ornament of dining halls and rooms in convents and palaces or, furthermore, to conceal or reveal other meanings and intentions.

As a sequel to Manet's picnic we present the photograph of a surreal or Dada picnic, or simply a celebration of life in a war-torn Europe, known as Hedonistic Picnic at Mougins from 1937, where we can find some parallelism with Manet's painting through the dressed men and semi-naked figures. In the photo by Lee Miller (who was to bathe in Hitler's bathtub at Berlin's liberation) we recognize Nusch Eluard, Paul Eluard, Roland Penrose, Man Ray, and Ady Fidelin.

In this brief approach to the universe of photography I would like to refer to Jimmy Hendricks drinking Mateus Rosé, Marilyn Monroe in bed, eating breakfast in a diet that the world sought to discover its secrets, with a tray where we can see a litter of milk and several raw mixed eggs, and, at last, David Bowie, king of glamor, having lunch in a wagon restaurant, eating slices of steak, small stewed potatoes and a huge portion of sautéed peas.

Still, as stated before, the victuals' depictions don't exactly match what is regularly eaten. So, we'd like to present two lobster paintings from different painters and different periods. Better said, we'd like to present three different paintings, the first two from the same artist, Clara Peeters, a Flemish painter (1594–c.1657), with a similar composition. The first is a still-life with seafood and eggs from 1608. The second was painted approximately 30 years later and it's also a still-life with a crab, prawns and lobster, and can be seen at the Houston Fine Arts Museum. The first painting still presents the meal as something sacred in a long table with white lace, the lobster is inside a plate. At the center, inside another plate, small prawns from the coast, a crab or stuffed crab, several white eggs, half a cheese, probably Gouda, a white bread, a dark bread, a corn bread, a trough, a bowl with a brown paste, biscuits, and, judging by the color, butter or fried eggs, a glass, a pitcher, and some kind of chandelier with what we believe is salt. Thirty years later, the artist repaints the same composition with some differences. Without any kind of artistic appreciation or comparison, it's inevitable to realize that the painting is darker or, we shall say, more Flemish, according to the taste of the period, more Mannerist. The composition is more triangular and richer with more elements: the number of cheeses in the center and in pile triples, an element that would become one of the greatest Flemish productions, the eggs appear to be white but there also quail or partridge eggs. There's also another kind of biscuits, a metal jug, and a slim glass. It's important to mention that the bread is now at the center of the composition e covered with a napkin which may either suggest some hygiene habits at the table or a symbolic link to the reformation and counter-reformation period of the Catholic Church.

The third painting mentioned above is Eduardo Viana's A Lagosta from 1953 that's in permanent display at the Museu Soares dos Reis, Oporto. The depicted animal has generous proportions and is displayed in a platter accompanied by a simple lemon and a series of lemon tree leaves. We know that Eduardo Viana used plastic models such as flowers and fruits as well as ceramic objects. In Bordallo Pinheiro's pottery there's a lobster that could very well have been the model to this painting.

In contrast to foodporn's richness, glamor and luxury and of all the images of desire, we present Van Gogh's The Potato Eaters, from 1885, which is in permanent display in the Van Gogh Museum in Amsterdam.

The painting in dark shades aims to be a depiction of the most unprotected and rural classes. The picture shows five people sitting around a rough wooden table. The oldest man in the scene is the father, Joseph Roulin, who was a postman. The younger woman holds a platter with smoking hot potatoes and is serving the portions with an interrogative look on her face. The older woman in front of her pours coffee in the mugs, surely barley coffee. The old peasant drinks. A peasant family gathers for this frugal meal. An oil lamp radiates a faint light, displaying the great poverty of the scene.

This family represents the social class of the place where the artist was living, as the Roulin family was friends with the painter who used them as models without individualizing them. There are five identical canvases within the same theme and featuring the same characters as central figures, which demonstrates Van Gogh's interest on the social aspects of life.

In a letter to his brother Théo, when referring to this work, he says: "(…) I really have wanted to make it so that people get the idea that these folk, who are eating their potatoes by the light of their little lamp, have tilled the earth themselves with these hands they are putting in the dish, and so it speaks of manual labor and — that they have thus honestly earned their food."

In Portugal we cannot dismiss Júlio Pomar's O Almoço do Trolha, a unique masterpiece of national neo-realism. Due to a mistake was on sale for a thousand escudos, the Portuguese currency at the time. However, the price lacked a zero and should have for sale by ten thousand. The first time it sold for five thousand escudos, something like 25€ at current values. On its latter transaction it was sold for three hundred and fifty thousand euros. It's considered a national treasure and cannot leave the country. The artist said that he remembered the workers sitting on the street floor near their construction site with their lunches that were often delivered by their wives. In this painting, the worker has the wife and the son next to him in a sacred family symbolism. By analyzing the lunch we realize that it's a packed lunch, something to eat with a spoon, characterized by the upper circle, thus certainly a soup or some light or watery stew.

Pop-art has trivialized victuals' images, some of them as the spirit of the time and the beginning of a consumption society and the search for comfort and speed. Consider the example of Andy Warhol's canned soups, packages with the same color but different soups or packages only with tomato soup with different colors. Also by Andy Warhol the ketchup box, another product from a consumption society and pop culture. With the same idea of a quick meal Roy Lichenstein presents a sandwich and a soda. From the same period the representations of hot dogs and hamburgers will thrive.

It's with Wayne Thiebaud that the image begins to convey desire, perhaps even the pornographic spirit of the image offered. Thiebaud does not consider himself (he's still alive, born in 1920) a pop-art artist. He became famous for is paintings of sweets, cakes and desserts as well as smoothies and pies, tarts and sweets from Californian cafes in the most gluttonous and pornographic spirit with its creams and butter castles. As a young man in Long Beach he worked in a cafe called Mile High and Red Hot, where "Mile High" was an ice-cream and "Red Hot" a hot-dog. In 1949, he earned a master's degree in art and started to teach at California University at Davis. His paintings depict colored sugar, creams and butter, glitter and glamor, objects of desire and pure gluttony. We can find a parallel with the paintings from the Portuguese artist Josefa de Óbidos. Her paintings from 1676 depict sweets and cheeses, queijadas, sponge cakes, tijeladas and other desserts. There's also something identifiable with the Eastern folar, almond candy and a box with sweets.

There's certainly a great difference between victuals' paintings and the pornfood selfie photos shared on social media. While the former work essentially towards the future, selfies clearly record and share the present.

## REFERENCES

AAVV, *Diálogo de Vanguardas*, Fundação Calouste Gulbenkian, 2006.

Bronowsky, J., *Arte e Conhecimento – Ver, Imaginar, Criar,* Edições 70, Lisboa, 1983.

Calabrese, O., *Como se lê uma obra de arte*, Edições 70, 1997.

Changeaux, J.-P., *Razão e Prazer*, Lisboa, Instituto Piaget, 1994.

Genette, G., *Work of Art: immanence and transcendence*, London, Conuell Up, 1997.

Merleau-Ponty, M., *Phénoménologie de la Perception*, ed. Éditions Gallimard, France, 1945.

Wollheim, R., *A Arte e os seus Objectos*, tradução de Marcelo Brandão Cipol.

*Experiencing Food: Designing Sustainable and Social Practices – Bonacho, Pires & Lamy (Eds)*
© 2021 Taylor & Francis Group, London, ISBN 978-0-367-49414-8

# Where interaction design meets gastronomy: Crafting increasingly playful and interactive eating experiences

Ferran Altarriba Bertran, Rosa Lutz & Katherine Isbister
*Social Emotional Technology Lab, University of California Santa Cruz, Santa Cruz, CA, USA*

ABSTRACT: In this paper, we respond to recent calls for more playfulness in gastronomy by discussing Interaction Design inspired strategies to craft food experiences that are more social, emergent, and fun. First, we discuss the state of play in gastronomy, highlighting opportunities for an increasingly interactive approach to food design. Then, we present six well-established Interaction Design principles that can help reconfigure gastronomy in increasingly playful ways. Finally, we illustrate how those concepts can be implemented through a case study of our own work: *The Mad Hatter's Dinner Party*. Our contribution will empower chefs to enrich the experiential palette of their designs by embracing social interaction and play as core elements of a meal.

## 1 INTRODUCTION

Over the last years, gastronomy has been discussed as yet another form of design. Designers are increasingly interested in food as a design material, and in food practices as a space for intervention. Restaurants and culinary artists in commercial settings use design thinking to craft their food. The intersection of gastronomy and design is also receiving attention from academia, with an emergence of specialized conferences and journals connecting food and design, e.g. EFOOD (Bonacho et al., 2018a) or the International Journal of Food Design (Zampollo, 2016).

Within that context, we see diverse connections between design and gastronomy, e.g.: Using graphic design principles to inspire the visual aesthetics of food and dishes, e.g. (Bonacho et al., 2018b); Exploring the material properties of food through the lens of material design, e.g. (Genomic Gastronomy, 2010); Learning from multi-sensory research to design more holistic food experiences, e.g. (Spence, 2017); Or using design thinking to critically reflect on current gastronomy and speculate about future directions, e.g. (Stummerer & Hablesreiter, 2014). Whether the focus is on the aesthetics of food and surrounding objects, the multi-sensory perception of a meal, or the creative concept motivating all of these, design can help chefs craft experiences that are more compelling to diners.

In this paper, we focus on a form of design practice that—we argue—has not yet received much attention in gastronomy: Interaction Design (IxD). IxD studies and crafts interactions between people, objects, and spaces. Rather than focusing on aesthetics *per se*, or on the concept behind a design, IxD pays most attention to the way the design enables, promotes, and supports activity. Here we argue that there are numerous IxD principles that can inspire chefs to enrich their work in ways that are currently underexplored.

Our work builds on, and responds to, previous calls for more interactive and playful avenues in gastronomy—an interest shared by diverse stakeholders but generally unaddressed by restaurants. To advance gastronomy in new and playful directions, we provide actionable strategies to design for active and playful engagement with food: we present a series of IxD principles we believe can empower chefs and other gastronomy designers to craft food experiences that are not only tasty, beautiful, and conceptually sound, but also compelling from a social engagement perspective. We illustrate those principles through a case study of our own work, *The Mad Hatter's Dinner Party,* giving concrete examples of how they can be applied to design meals that are more social and fun.

Overall, in this paper we reflect on how carefully crafting interactions with and around food can add value to, and enrich the social dimension of, gastronomic experiences. We hope that our work will provide chefs and other food designers with actionable tools to design food experiences that are not only beautiful, tasty, and inspiring but also interactive, social, and fun, and thereby enhance the diversity of gastronomy in playful ways.

## 2 DESIGN AND GASTRONOMY

### 2.1 *Gastronomy: experiences that transcend food*

Over the last years, gastronomy has increasingly been framed as a holistic experience that transcends the scope of taste. Zampollo and Peacock's (2016) research on the composition of food design as a field illustrates the diversity of factors to be considered when crafting food experiences. While food and drinks are key to gastronomy, a myriad of other factors shape a meal, e.g.: the shape of utensils, the sound ambiance in the dining space, or the interactions between diners, among others. Over the last years, scholars have studied some of those factors, mostly from the perspective of cross-modal psychology.

Cross-modal psychology is concerned with how humans perceive multi-sensory stimuli, and how those stimuli have an impact on each other, e.g. how sound stimuli impacts taste perception (Knoeferle et al., 2015). A prominent figure in this space is Charles Spence, who coined the term *Gastrophysics* (2017) to define the area of research that explores the impact of multi-sensory stimuli on food experiences. Illustrative works in this space are: a study of how the form factors of food containers impacts taste perception (Harrar et al., 2011); or a study of how the ambient sounds of a restaurant impact taste perception and eating behavior (Zampini & Spence 2010).

Gastrophysics is very relevant to food design, as it unpacks the effects of multi-sensory stimuli on the diner's perception of a meal. That knowledge is invaluable for chefs: it can help them carefully craft dishes (and their surrounding elements, e.g. utensils or space) in ways that they afford the experience targeted by the chef. However, Gastrophysics does not necessarily account for the interactive qualities of food experiences. It is more focused on the effects of concrete, measurable stimuli than on the complex interactions that might happen during a meal. Therefore, it is less informative when it comes to designing playful food interactions. Here, we argue, is where Interaction Design principles come to play.

## 2.2 *The state of play in gastronomy*

We see a parallel between Gastrophysics' focus on multi-sensory stimuli and the types of gastronomic experiences proposed by most gastronomic restaurants that are considered to lead the culinary *avantgarde*. Multi-sensory approaches to gastronomy are often focused on how food and its surrounding objects and spaces are perceived by the diners. They are less concerned with the actions people do with, or around, that food. In other words, they are more dish- than eating-centric—the object of design is the dish, its surrounding elements, and how they are perceived; and less attention is paid to *how* the dish is eaten.

An example of a well-known gastronomic proposal that leveraged multi-sensory design is *El Somni,* a single-time event created by Franc Aleu and the world-renowned restaurant El Celler de Can Roca (2013). Framed as an attempt to achieve the ultimate essence of gastronomy, the dinner consists of a number of beautifully prepared dishes that are surrounded by multi-sensory cues (e.g. projections or sound). Each dish is a scene of a story, and all the multi-sensory stimuli are directed towards focusing the diner's attention towards their food. The multi-sensory universes around the dishes are carefully crafted to the smallest details, but it is interesting to see how the interactions around them are left aside. In each course, diners use all of their senses to contemplate the piece of art that

is presented to them; but they are not given a chance to interact with it, beyond just eating the food that is being served. This creates a clear tension, to the point that two diners eventually begin discussing the dish, which thereby creates an unexpected disruption that compromises the immersive nature of the experience. In other words, the chefs of El Somni paid a lot of attention to crafting dishes that are extremely compelling from a multi-sensory point of view, but failed to acknowledge (and design for) the natural interactions that commonly emerge during a meal. We argue, and in this paper illustrate, that in doing so they missed various opportunities to enrich the dining experience and promote an even stronger feeling of immersion.

The multi-sensory ethos of El Somni has inspired a number of chefs around the world. More and more, restaurants are starting to use emerging technologies to afford immersive multi-sensory experiences. A good example is *Sublimotion* (Roncero, n.d.), a restaurant that projects visuals across the dining room to captivate and delight the diners. Both El Somni and Sublimotion succeed in leveraging the multi-sensory potential of food and its surrounding elements to wonderfully stimulate diners' senses. However, they pay little attention to providing diners with opportunities to actively engage in interesting ways, both with their food and with other diners.

There are also examples of gastronomic proposals that are explicitly framed as playful, e.g. what Regol describes as *play-food* (2009): dishes that look one way but taste another; feasting as a theatrical event; or elaborations imbued with a narrative. Those proposals often gravitate towards contemplative rather than interactive play. Active diner engagement is rarely harnessed as an asset to enrich the experience. As Regol explains (2009): the role of diners is to "sit and contemplate," while the restaurant provides them with an experience that must not be disrupted. Recent research on play and gastronomy (Altarriba Bertran & Wilde, 2018) demonstrates that there is much more to play than what restaurants currently offer.

## 2.3 *The chef- and dish- centric model*

The dominant chef- and dish-centric approach to gastronomy responds to chefs' tendency to use food as a medium for creative expression. According to recent research (Altarriba Bertran & Wilde, 2018), mainstream gastronomic proposals, e.g. El Somni or Sublimotion, are often very unidirectional—chefs present diners with dishes that consist of short, highly predefined experiences where diners play a rather passive role. Such an approach to gastronomy design limits the diversity of experiences afforded by restaurants. Most importantly, it does not always resonate with the desires of diners and other stakeholders in gastronomy, who see social interaction as a key aspect of a gastronomic experience. Arguably, overly chef- and dish- (rather than diner- and eating-) centric approaches to gastronomy might be undermining the diversity of the current gastronomy scene.

Building on Altarriba Bertran and Wilde's work, we argue that interactions are a fundamental aspect of a meal—both those with food, and those emerging between diners. We thus suggest that chefs might benefit from paying careful attention to the activity their dishes afford, promoting and supporting interactions that add value to the overall experiential texture of a meal. As much as they design their dishes to be tasty, beautiful and surprising, chefs might want to consider how to make them engaging, social, and fun. Otherwise, they might miss opportunities to expand the palette of eating experiences offered in their restaurants.

While there are interesting cases of innovative restaurants that propose novel and disruptive ways of interacting around food (e.g. the increasingly popular dinners in the dark), the set of food and gastronomic designs that put interaction at the forefront of the eating experience remains limited. In their research on food and play, Wilde and Altarriba Bertran (2019) highlight 3 examples of exceptionally playful *New Cookery* (Adrià et al. 2006) dishes: elBulli's *Las especias* challenges diners to guess the names of different spices positioned around their plate (Adrià et al., 2005); Alinea's (2012) *Balloon* is a floating, helium-filled sugar bubble that you eat by sucking its surface; and El Celler de Can Roca's *Tocaplats* transforms the color of food on the plate into musical tones, to 'play' with changes in food composition as the meal is eaten (Carulla et al., 2016), extending previous works that augment food experiences with sound such as Blumenthal's (2015) *The Sound of the Sea*. In food design, Guixé and Knolke's (2010) *Mealing* shows how a playful food disruption can add value to a social setting: a cup with snacks attached on its surface rewards people with small treats as they perform specific social interactions in public events. In game design, Jenn Sandercock's (2018) *Edible Games* show how game rules can be embedded into dishes to craft highly playful and interactive eating experiences.

Inspired by those and other examples of interactive and playful designs, we propose that, to continue enriching the palette of gastronomic experiences available in restaurants, it might be interesting to promote a move from dish- to eating-centric approaches to gastronomy design, where not only the dish but also its surrounding activity is at focus. To that end, in the following section we present 6 concepts that have guided the work of interaction designers in other areas than gastronomy. We argue, and in this paper show, that these principles can help food designers craft gastronomic experiences that are not only tasty and artful, but also engaging, social, and fun.

## 3 TOWARDS AN INTERACTION DESIGN INSPIRED APPROACH TO GASTRONOMY

Interaction Design (IxD) is a form of design practice concerned with crafting compelling interactions between people, objects, and spaces. Rather than focusing on a design's aesthetics *per se*, or its underlying concept, IxD pays most attention to how the design enables and supports activity. As such, interaction designers have long-standing expertise on how to promote social and playful engagement. We believe that chefs could learn from how interaction designers conceptualize their work—it might help them enrich their designs with more interesting forms of interaction, both between diners and their food, and among diners themselves. Here we present 6 design principles proposed by interaction designers that we have found useful for designing gastronomic experiences. In Section 4 we illustrate and exemplify how those theoretical principles can be useful to gastronomy designers through a case study of our own work.

### 3.1 *Activity as the ultimate particular of interaction design*

Design practice is often generative (Gaver, 2012) and local (Bertelsen et al., 2018)—that is, it is best suited to create "specific solutions to particular problems—*the ultimate particulars*" (Waern & Back, 2017). What differentiates Interaction Design from other disciplines is that its *ultimate particulars* are not artifacts but activities (Waern & Back, 2017). Even though IxD often resorts to the design of artifacts as a way to mediate interactions (Buchanan, 2001), its end goal is not the artifacts themselves but the interactions they enable. Gastronomy design could benefit from that activity-focused ethos: by opening the focus beyond the object (a dish) and highlighting the activity (eating), chefs might be more likely to explore alternative forms of interaction around food.

### 3.2 *Crafting immersion through real activity*

Within Interaction Design, there are communities that are particularly focused on designing highly immersive and multi-sensory experiences. For example, the designers of pervasive games. Those games, designed through the lens of activity rather than artifact discussed above, resort to a variety of elements to afford highly immersive and believable experiences. In other words, they create what Waern et al. (2009) describe as a "360 illusion" of realism that keep players engaged and immersed through intrigue and fun. We believe that such immersion can be a desirable thing in gastronomic meals, especially those that are surrounded by some kind of overarching narrative. A key strategy to achieving such immersive illusions is giving players the chance to "act for real" (Waern et al., 2009). That is, offering possibilities for interacting with diegetic objects—objects that are meaningful within the narrative universe of the experience—in ways that feel real and authentic. According to Waern et al. (2009), designing for real activity implies offering players a real, authentic environment, where there is some degree of role-play, physical contact, and movement that makes them feel more absorbed in the environment created in the experience.

### 3.3 *Ambiguity as a design resource*

From a perspective of usability and ease of use, ambiguity is often thought of as an undesirable quality in design. However, (Gaver et al. 2003) argue it might be an interesting quality in situations where free-form exploration could add value. Dealing with an ambiguous object forces us to think about how we might personally use it, or interact around it. It encourages us to try things out, to explore, and to see what happens as a result (Gaver et al. 2003). In other words, ambiguity is a design quality that gives us opportunities to be creative with how we interact with the world that surrounds us. As such, in IxD, ambiguity is considered as a resource for design that can be useful to encourage close and personal interaction within an experience (Gaver et al. 2003). We believe that in gastronomy, where exploration and learning are desirable, designing dishes that afford ambiguous interaction could enhance the experience.

### 3.4 *Transformative play*

Another interesting concept for interaction design is allowing space for user appropriation. That is especially true for cases in which the object of design is a somewhat playful experience. The reason, Back et al. argue, is that while complying with established rules and structures allows players to enjoy a predefined experience, creatively disrupting those norms and structures allows them to appropriate the experience and to transform it in ways that it feels like it is their own (Back et al., 2017). Allowing players to break past the designed confines of an experience by "transforming" its structure leads to more interactivity and higher enjoyment. Back et al. (2017) highlight ways in which that can be promoted by design: allowing space for exploration, promoting creative attitudes towards the limits of the experience, and making it possible for users to transgress those limits, thereby fostering the "transformative power of play" (Back et al., 2017). We argue that those qualities might help "loosen up" the sometimes overly-serious nature of high cuisine, where diners sometimes feel that the structure of a meal is too tight and does not allow them to engage in the ways they want—as Altarriba Bertran and Wilde (2018) note.

### 3.5 *The pleasures of disputation*

Another interesting concept from the perspective of fostering compelling interactions is Wilson's (2012) idea that certain kinds of intentionally provocative interactions can help nurture "distinctly self-motivated and collaborative" forms of playful engagement. By designing experiences that are surprising, disruptive or even, to some extent, uncomfortable, the designer can provoke situations where people self-organize and team up to work around the system. According to Wilson (2012), it is interesting to carve opportunities for players to be subversive within an experience, as the very act of bending the rules is likely to make them feel empowered and be more engaged. More to the point, creating those moments of "rebel action" can be a way of promoting laughter and carefree fun, something that we argue is often desirable in gastronomy.

### 3.6 *Game-inspired affordances*

When it comes to designing experiences that are playful and fun, interaction designers often resort to looking at how games function—what Isbister et al. (2018) call "game design affordances". A defining trait of games is that they often invite players to inhabit what Huizinga (1971) calls a *magic circle*—that is, an ephemeral universe within which all game actions make sense and that might not have much to do with what happens outside of the game. We suggest that thinking of a gastronomic meal as a magic circle, where everything—not only the food, but also the accompanying activity—adds up to a common theme might help chefs craft interactions that are not only fun and interesting but also strongly coherent with the food that is being served. Further, it might support immersion within the experience, something we argue is desirable in gastronomic experiences. In this context, it is important to think about how the rules and social interactions that will structure the experience are unique and can lead to the emergence of meaning and relations that might help diners live the experience of being momentarily away from the real world.

## 4 CASE STUDY: THE MAD HATTER'S DINNER PARTY

*The Mad Hatter's Dinner Party* (Altarriba Bertran et al., 2016) is a pop-up playful dining experience designed by a group of researchers at the University of Southern Denmark. Themed after the diegetic universe of Alice in Wonderland, it presents a combination of storytelling, multi-sensory stimulation, and playful interaction as the core structure of a 7-course dining experience. Here we describe key parts of the experience to illustrate the interaction design concepts presented in the previous section. Our reflections are based on the analysis of four diners' interactions throughout the meal[1], as well as on their reflections during a post-meal focus group.

### 4.1 *The Magic Potion*

Looking at the dinner in a chronological order, "the adventure begins" when a waiter appears in the hall where the diners are waiting, bearing a platter with 4 hats (Figure 1). Each diner is invited to choose one of the hats. With each hat comes a poker card and a small beverage in the form of a "magic potion". The poker cards give diners a personal identifier they will carry

---

[1] See *http://bit.ly/2GLIDQ2* for a short video description; and *http://bit.ly/2GCj1nv* for a video of the full dinner.

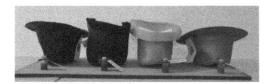

Figure 1. The Magic Potion: each diner received a potion, a had and a poker card.

throughout the meal and will help them find which dishes and utensils belong to them.

Upon their arrival, diners are told that one of them will play the role of the evil Queen: "You are about to enter the universe of Alice in Wonderland. You are going to be part of the Mad Hatter's Dinner Party. One of you will be the Queen. Now, the Queen needs to hide, she needs to make sure that she is not discovered, while the others have to find out who she is. Because the Moment of the Truth will come and at that point you will have to guess who the Queen is; otherwise, the Queen will win."

The role of the Queen is kept secret from the onset. The *Magic Potion*, apart from being the first appetizer, is the mechanism through which one of the diners will be assigned the role of the Queen. That happens without the other diners noticing: all the potions are sour besides the Queen's, which is sweet. This situation sets the right conditions for the emergence of the first hilarious moment of the meal: the Queen is forced to disguise her role by pretending her drink is sour, blending in with all the other diners to whom the sour drink will likely put a face of disgust.

The Magic Potion and all its surrounding paraphernalia (Alfred, the hats and the cards) exemplify how a *magic circle* of play can be built through *real activity*: the distribution of roles is done in a way that allows diners to enter the diegetic world of The Mad Hatter's Dinner Party through an activity that is meaningful both gastronomically and narratively (drinking a magic potion). Building on the notion of activity as ultimate particular of Interaction Design (Waern & Back, 2017), the Magic Potion also shows the benefits of framing food as an activity rather than just a static dish: diners are put in a specific narrative context thanks to a game-inspired (Isbister et al., 2018) action that prepares them for an interactive experience that is separate from their everyday lives.

## 4.2 The Cards

Shortly after drinking their potions, diners are brought to the dining room. When Alfred opens the door, diners walk into a dark dining room with a table at the center, illuminated with bright projections, and covered with of strange-looking objects and foods (Figure 2). A musical soundtrack is playing in the background. As diners approach the table, they meet the waiter, who embodies the character and personality of the Mad Hatter, and who greets them speaking cheerfully

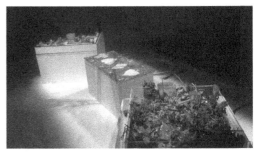

Figure 2. Initial table setup, including dishes and projections.

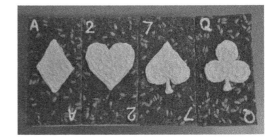

Figure 3. The Cards: poker card-looking crackers.

and eagerly. The waiter will be in charge of facilitating the rest of the meal, in a similar way to how both a maître d' (in restaurants) and a game master (in board games) often do: sometimes participating and sometimes stepping aside, always focused on making sure that the experience flows nicely. The combination of projections, soundtrack, elements on the table, and the strange-acting waiter help solidify the *magic circle* of the experience. It is a magic *mise en scene* that absorbs the diners and creates an immersive environment, similar to that of pervasive games.

At that point in the dinner, the Mad Hatter serves the second appetizer: the *Cards* (Figure 3). Each diner receives a cracker, shaped as their card identifier. In addition, each diner receives a mysterious object that will give them a special 'power' which they can use in specific moments of the meal. The four objects are as follows: a knife, a magnifying lens, a labyrinth map, and a cup with a broken bottom. Importantly, the utility of the objects, or the ways in which they can be used, is not clear from the onset: the waiter presents them in a rather mysterious manner, leveraging the potential of *ambiguity* to promote exploration and curiosity. The broken cup is the only object that is useful from the very beginning and until the very ending of the meal. A proximity sensor allows the broken cup holder to pour tea when a cup is placed close to the teapot. The person bearing the cup, then, is given the role of taking care of all the other diners' drinks. Importantly, the Mad Hatter does not impose clear rules on how to deal with that situation: that is a deliberate design choice aimed at affording space for *transformative play* that allows diners to appropriate the experience and figure

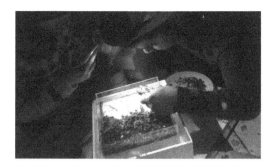

Figure 4. Diners using a lens to read a clue in the Magic Forest.

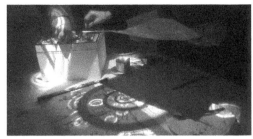

Figure 5. Diners trying to find their way through The Labyrinth.

out their means of participation, e.g. the broken cup bearer can play their role in radically different ways, for example being nice and nurturing other diners or being mischievous and pouring drinks only when it yields benefits to her.

### 4.3 *The Magic Forest*

Another important aspect of the meal is that there are various clues throughout its duration that point towards the identity of the Queen. Such design choice hints at the problem-solving aspect of the experience, which contributes to approaching it as a holistic activity rather than as fragmented engagement with different dishes. In other words, the whole meal is *activity-centered*, rather than just a compilation of beautiful and tasty dishes. In each of the courses, a clue is introduced, either by the waiter through a riddle, or through a hidden message in the dish. For example, the Mad Hatter presents the third course of the meal, the *Magic Forest* (Figure 4), using the following words: "In search of a good clue, in the forest you'll be immersed. If you are looking for the truth, it will be under the last taste." From the riddle, the diners deduce that they must look for the clue.

The Magic Forest is a forest-looking salad, with a base made of crumbled bread, parmesan cheese, and black colorant to simulate soil. Under the soil, there is a tiny piece of text with a clue pointing at who the Queen is. At the beginning of the course, diners hesitate to transfer the salad to their plates and to start eating the salad, as they seem uncertain about how to begin finding the next clue. Slowly, however, they begin discussing ways they might discover the clue, and start eating the salad more confidently. As the diners explore, they creatively co-create their own strategies for finding the clue; here, *ambiguity* is key again, in this case induced through the mysterious riddle-clue. One of the effects of that ambiguous situation is that it is initially perceived as confusing (or, as Wilson (2012) would put it, "broken") which over time leads to collaboration that creatively transgresses the lack of clarity on how to progress through the experience—an important design quality in Wilson's notion of *pleasures of disputation*. This is an important aspect of this dish: the ambiguity ends up generating a sense of teamwork,

which brings players closer to one another. Here, there is also an element of role-play: the diner bearing the lens is in charge of using their special ability to read a clue that is too small to be read with the naked eye.

The Magic Forest's ambiguity is intimately connected with a call for, and guide to, action. As described by Gaver et al. (2003) ambiguity "[pushes] us to imagine how we might personally use" an artefact, in this case the dish—it allows us to be creative with how we handle or interact within an experience. This, in addition to the fact that eating the dish is true *real activity*—it feeds diners and leads them towards the clue—supports immersion and keeps the *magic circle* at the forefront. Another factor that contributes to shaping immersion is the combination of projections and soundtrack, curated specifically for each dish—in the case of the Magic Forest, to provide feelings of captivation and relaxation.

### 4.4 *The Labyrinth*

The Magic Forest is followed by the *Labyrinth* (Figure 5). The transition is supported by an abrupt change in the projection and soundtrack: all of a sudden, an animation evoking time-travel is projected onto the table, enhanced through the sound of a ticking clock. While remaining in full character, the waiter introduces that dish with another clue: "throughout the precious labyrinth, precious rewards you will get. But get fast to the center, otherwise you'll eat dry bread." In other words, players must navigate a small maze under a time constraint in order to get the full meal, collecting small pieces of bread throughout. If they manage to arrive at the center of the maze, they will be served two bread dippings; otherwise, just one. To do that, they can be guided by the person bearing the labyrinth map. This is a very intense moment of the dinner, because not only are players overwhelmed by fast-paced sound cues and distracting light projections, but the food they eat depends on their ability to finish a task within a certain amount of time. All those conditions, the combination of rules and ambient stimuli, contribute to creating a hectic situation. Though stressful, this environment appears to keep the diners very engaged in the activity, something that is consistent with Wilson's (2012) suggestion that the *pleasures of disputation* can be leveraged to support immersion.

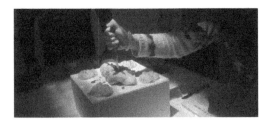

Figure 6. A diner killing The Dragon.

Upon completion of this task, diners are rewarded with all intended components of the meal, as well as with a transition to calm music and clearer lighting, returning the mood of the dinner to a positive and satisfying one. That, in itself, creates a feeling of reward, an aspect of games Isbister et al. (2018) suggest can inspire designers to craft experiences with a compelling *magic circle*.

### 4.5 *The Dragon*

After diners have taken their time to enjoy their well-deserved food earned in the Labyrinth, the next course is served: *The Dragon* (Figure 6). The clue reads: "A fierce dragon you'll encounter in the middle of your path. Don't fear it for a second, you'll defeat it with the knife". The waiter brings out a piece of meat on a flat surface, and the light projections turn a danger-resembling red color, and flapping dragon wings are projected on top of the meat. In addition, the Mad Hatter is yelling for somebody to "do something!". Here, the diner bearing the knife is compelled to heroically kill the dragon—it is nothing but an example of an action that feels *real*. At the same time, it is somewhat *ambiguous*: no one tells diners how to kill the dragon—in fact, the Mad Hatter appears to be scared and out of control, which pushes diners to figure out how to kill the dragon themselves. Once the Dragon is dead, diners can enjoy its meat.

### 4.6 *The Dragon's Blood*

As a show of gratitude for killing the Dragon, diners are served the *Dragon's Blood* (Figure 7). Here the clue states: "As a gift to thank your courage, you'll be given dragon blood. Be aware of your reactions as they might be the last clue". In this course, the diners must pick a spoon bearing a blood-looking edible sphere, placed next to their corresponding poker card identifier. That reminds the players about the game objective of finding who the queen is, bringing the *activity-centered* nature of the meal to the forefront again: the *Moment of the Truth* is approaching, and therefore they are running out of time to discover the Queen. One by one, the players consume the Dragon's Blood; the Queen's is the only one that is spicy. Here, there is a sense of competition: all diners look at each other in search of a reaction that uncovers the hidden Queen. Here, again, Wilson's (2012) notion of the *pleasures of disputation* is used to foster social connectedness.

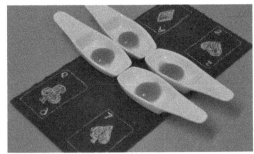

Figure 7. The Dragon's Blood, assigned to each diner through their card identifiers.

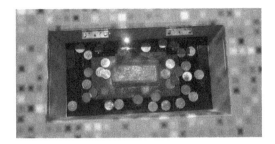

Figure 8. The Moment of the Truth, a gold ingot-looking cake.

### 4.7 *The Moment of the Truth*

Finally, the last course of the meal is the *Moment of the Truth* (Figure 8), the dessert. Rather than being served, that dish is uncovered: the Mad Hatter removes all objects from the table and then, theatrically, he removes the tablecloth. Under the tablecloth there is a transparent door, inside of which lies a golden ingot looking cake surrounded by chocolate coins. At that point, it is time to guess who the Queen is, otherwise the treasure will be gone. A key is needed to open the compartment, and the key will be given to the winners of the game—that is, to the Queen or to the rest of the dinner party. Once again, the diners' food consumption is directly tied to, and determined by, their actions and decisions. Most importantly, here, the activity is purposefully *ambiguous* and *transformative*: the winners can choose whether to keep the treasure for themselves or share it with the party who lost, thereby appropriating the experience and making their own rules.

## 5 CONCLUSION

Using an Interaction Design approach was key to designing The Mad Hatter's Dinner Party, a dining experience that was described by the participating diners as highly immersive, enjoyable, and fun. In a post-meal focus group, one of the participants noted that she had not felt "such immersion into a fantastic world since childhood". Similarly, another diner mentioned that while he came with a clear agenda of sating his hunger—he was starving, he recognized—he soon forgot about it and got immersed in the story. Overall, diners agreed on the fact that they perceived the dinner as a coherent experience where eating and playing blended in smoothly, to the point that they became one same thing. Among the experiential qualities diners highlighted were: fantasy, challenge, subversion, humor, discovery, exploration, relaxation, captivation, thrill, fellowship, and suffering.

Arguably, a key success factor to The Mad Hatter's Dinner Party was that it was designed beyond the flavors and aesthetics of the dishes, looking at the meal as an activity and crafting it to afford a diverse palette of social and playful emotions. This sets the Mad Hatter's Dinner Party apart from contemporary practices in gastronomy, e.g. El Somni (see section 2.2), where meals revolve around multi-sensory stimulation, and social or unexpected interactions are often seen as disruptions to the experience intended by the chef. We argue that exploring increasingly playful types of gastronomic experiences, such as The Mad Hatter's Dinner Party, might have a positive impact on the current state of gastronomy: it would diversify the palette of experiences available to diners, thereby responding to a latent desire for more playful and interactive forms of engagement with and through food.

In this paper, we described concrete examples of Interaction Design concepts that can facilitate the design of such kinds of highly playful, interactive, and social gastronomic experiences:

First, inspired by Waern and Back (2017), we proposed looking at food experiences as activities rather than as compilations of dishes, thereby focusing design not only on the qualities of the dishes but also on eating, and on how diners interact with one another around food.

Second, we suggested that immersion can be built by affording eating interactions that diners perceive as *real activity* (Waern et al., 2009), where playing and eating intertwine in ways that one cannot be dissociated from the other, e.g. when clues in the Magic Forest could only be found by eating the forest.

Third, building on Gaver et al.'s (2003) ludic design work, we argued that *ambiguity* might be a useful design quality in experiences where curiosity, exploration or surprise are desirable, e.g. when diners received objects they did not know when to use, and had to discover how to use them throughout the dinner.

Fourth, we discussed the importance of embracing a *transformative* approach to designing for play (Back et al., 2017), offering diners chances to appropriate the experience and adapt its unfolding to their own will, e.g. when the diner holding the broken cup could decide whether to be nice and serve drinks to others, or to be mischievous and use that power to his advantage.

Fifth, we saw how affording space for *disputation* (Wilson, 2012) can help promote active participation during a meal: carving opportunities for diners to be subversive and encouraging them to play around the rules empowers and engages them, e.g. when diners are told there is a clue hidden in the Magic Forest, and have to figure out their own strategy to find it because the Mad Hatter offered none.

Finally, we have seen how using *game-inspired social affordances* (Isbister et al., 2018) (e.g. the time-pressure in the Labyrinth, or the social role-play competition of guessing who the Queen is) can contribute to building and maintaining a *magic circle* (Huizinga, 1971) of immersion around the meal.

Those are just 6 of the many Play and Interaction Design concepts that could inspire chefs to make their food designs more interactive. We suggest that future work should explore more of those concepts to expand the set of strategies available to chefs to design gastronomic experiences that are more emergent, social and fun. We hope that the concepts we presented here, made tangible through a case study, are useful to chefs and other food designers. Ultimately, we hope that they empower them to take actionable steps towards further enriching their work, so that the future landscape of gastronomy becomes increasingly interactive, social, exciting, and fun.

## ACKNOWLEDGEMENTS

We would like to thank Mirzel Avdić, Asbjørn Grangaard Erlendsson, Lennart Schlüter, Thomas Neville Valkær and Andrés Lucero for their participation in the design of *The Mad Hatter Dinner Party*.

## REFERENCES

Adrià, F., Soler, J., and Adrià, A. 2005. 'El Bulli: 1998–2002', RBA Libros.

Adrià, F., Blumenthal, H., Keller, T., and McGee, H. 2006. 'Statement on the "new cookery"', The Guardian, https://www.theguardian.com/uk/2006/dec/10/foodand drink.obsfoodmonthly, Accessed May 2018.

Aleu, F. and El Celler de Can Roca. 2013. El Somni.

Alinea n.d., 'Edible Balloon', https://alinearestaurant.com/ site/portfolio/edible-balloon/, Accessed May 2018.

Altarriba Bertran, F., Avdić, M., Erlendsson, A. G., Schlüter, L., and Valkær, T. N. 2016. "The Mad Hatter's Dinner Party": Enhancing the Dining Experience Through the Use of Game Thinking. In 12th Student Interaction Design Research Conference (pp. 126–129). IDM, Malmö University.

Altarriba Bertran, F. and Wilde, D. 2018. Playing with food: reconfiguring the gastronomic experience through play. In Experiencing Food, Designing Dialogues: Proceedings of the 1st International Conference on Food Design and Food Studies (EFOOD 2017), Lisbon, Portugal, October 19–21, 2017 (p. 3). CRC Press.

Back, J., Márquez Segura, E., and Waern, A. 2017. Designing for Transformative Play. ACM Transactions on Computer-Human Interaction, 24, 1–18.

Bertelsen, O. W., Bødker, S., Eriksson, E., Hoggan, E., and Vermeulen, J. 2018. Beyond generalization: research for the very particular. Interactions 26, 1 (December 2018), 34–38. DOI: https://doi.org/10.1145/3289425

Blumenthal, H. 2015. Sound and food. In Olive Magazine.

Bonacho, R., Pinheiro de Sousa, A., Viegas, C., Martins, J. P., Pires, M. J., and Estêvão, S. V. (Eds.). 2018a. Experiencing Food, Designing Dialogues. Proceedings of the 1st International Conference on Food Design and Food Studies (EFOOD 2017), Lisbon, Portugal, October 19–21, 2017.

Bonacho, R., Pires, M. J., and Viegas, C. 2018b. "A Saudade Portuguesa". Designing a dialogical food narrative. In Experiencing Food, Designing Dialogues. Proceedings of the 1st International Conference on Food Design and Food Studies (EFOOD 2017), Lisbon, Portugal, October 19–21, 2017 (p. 41). CRC Press.

Buchanan, R. 2001. Design research and the new learning. Design Issues 17, 4:3–23.

Carulla, A., El Celler de Can Roca, and Harbisson, N. 2016. 'Music to the tastebuds', http://www.acidstudio.com/works/tocaplats, Accessed May 2018.

Gaver, W. 2012. What should we expect from research through design? In Proceedings of the SIGCHI conference on human factors in computing systems, 937–946.

Gaver, W., Beaver, J., & Benford, S. 2003. Ambiguity as a Resource for Design. CHI 2003, 5, 233–240.

Genomic Gastronomy. 2010. Glowing Sushi. Accessed on April 3, 2019 at http://www.glowingsushi.com/

Guixé, M. and Knolke, I. 2010. Food designing. Corraini Edizioni.

Harrar, V., Piqueras-Fiszman, B., and Spence, C. 2011. There's more to taste in a coloured bowl. Perception, 40(7), 880–882.

Huizinga, J. 1971. Homo Ludens: A Study of the Play-Element in Culture. Beacon Press.

Isbister, K, Márquez Segura, E., and Melcer, E. F. 2018. Social Affordances at Play: Game Design Toward Socio-Technical Innovation. CHI 2018, 1–9.

Knoeferle, K. M., Woods, A., Käppler, F., and Spence, C. 2015. That sounds sweet: Using cross-modal correspondences to communicate gustatory attributes. Psychology & Marketing, 32(1), 107–120.

Regol, P. 2009. 'Los maestros de la cocina sacan de la chistera sus abracadabras comestibles.! Playfood', Vino y gastronomía, (229), pp. 6–18., transl. by author.

Roncero, P. n.d.. Sublimotion. Accessed on April 15, 2019 at https://www.sublimotionibiza.com/

Sandercock, J. 2018. Edible Games. Accessed on April 17, 2019 at https://ediblegames.com/

Spence, C. 2017. Gastrophysics: The new science of eating. Penguin UK.

Stummerer, S., and Hablesreiter, M. 2014. Honey and Bunny. Accessed on April 12, 2019 at https://www.honeyandbunny.com/

Waern, A. and Back, J. 2017. Activity as the Ultimate Particular of Interaction Design. CHI 2017, 3390–3402.

Waern, A., Montola, M. and Stenros, J. 2009. The Three-Sixty Illusion: Designing For Immersion in Pervasive Games. CHI 2009, 1549–1558.

Wilde, D. and Altarriba Bertran, F. 2019. From playing with food to participatory research through design: a designerly move towards more playful gastronomy. In International Journal of Food Design, Volume 4.

Wilson, D. 2012. Designing for the Pleasures of Disputation -or- How to make friends by trying to kick them! Chapter 4: In Celebration of Low Process Intensity. Dissertation,109–119.

Zampini, M. and Spence, C. 2010. Assessing the role of sound in the perception of food and drink. Chemosensory Perception, 3(1), 57–67.

Zampollo, F. 2016. Welcome to Food Design (Editorial). International Journal of Food Design, 1(1), 3–9.

Zampollo, F. and Peacock, M. 2016. Food design thinking: a branch of Design Thinking specific to Food Design. The Journal of creative behavior, 50(3), 203–210.

Experiencing Food: Designing Sustainable and Social Practices – Bonacho, Pires & Lamy (Eds)
© 2021 Taylor & Francis Group, London, ISBN 978-0-367-49414-8

# Sustainability on the menu: The chef's creative process as a starting point for change in haute cuisine (and beyond)

S. Parreira
*CIEBA, Faculdade de Belas-Artes, Universidade de Lisboa, Lisbon, Portugal*

ABSTRACT: The sustainability of the food system should be an urgent global objective in a planet facing challenges on how to feed a growing population without destroying its natural resources. In haute cuisine, intricate dishes are hardly the first example of sustainable practices in the food industry. Mapping the creative process of five chefs, from Michelin-starred restaurants, uncovers the dynamics of the creative mind and unveils the chef's role in changing food habits and purchasing behaviors. Taking the mackerel campaign for sustainable fish consumption in Portugal as an example, the chef's creative process as a tool for sustainability is discussed in haute cuisine but also to a broader audience at home who identify with the chef as a food 'celebrity' to follow.

## 1 INTRODUCTION

Sustainable futures in food offer environmental, economic, and social challenges considering how our food is grown, processed, and distributed, both locally and globally. An important part is concerned with food choices, diet trends, and the narratives created around ingredients, products or consumer habits. What we eat nowadays can be defined by the way "technological advances, business and economic changes, and government policies are transforming entire food chains, from farm to fork" (Ranganathan et al., 2016: 1). Being able to communicate ideas rather than brands has become an essential asset to make information available to large groups of people, thus producing a change in how food is consumed and what most eaters choose to have on their tables.

In haute cuisine, the chef's role in the way cooking (and a dish or an ingredient in particular) is perceived has become more and more important as food and chefs assumed front row in the media (e.g. cookbooks, television cookery shows, social media posts) (Scarpatto, 2002). Using that special status to start a conversation about sustainability or sustainable choices is already done at their restaurants by chefs like Eneko Atxa of Azurmendi (recipient of the most sustainable restaurant award by The World's 50 Best Restaurants in 2018) or Dan Barber, Blue Hill. Food sustainability has been seen as a path for major discussion about relevant matters like climate change or hunger as much as a signature for haute cuisine's chefs with a personal interest in social welfare, environmental activism or new sustainable food trends.

Given that chefs actually validate certain choices when creating dishes, our present food culture has granted chefs a potencial of influence, including the opportunity to innovate whilst communicating possible alternatives. The chef's responsibility reached a new high with the current media presence and growing popularity earned by the profession. With a voice to create awareness for the need to adopt different food habits, "restaurateurs and chefs have the power to change opinions and have highly influential roles to play in shaping the gastronomic desires of society to a more sustainable future (Sloan et al., 2015: xvi). Changing eating habits to offer more efficiency to food chains and the environment was acknowledged in 2018 by the United Nations as one of the Sustainable Development Goals.

"What if chefs create dishes that not only taste good but also generate good for the planet and for the people?" That question has been posed to chefs by considering a different way of cooking, writing a menu or sourcing an ingredient. The creative process is an important part on how sustainable a dish is and its general impact on the food scene. A chef's creative process usually begins with the chef deciding what to cook, then gathering the necessary materials or ingredients, and finally, creating something that has not yet been created and which translates into value for the client and for society. How can the creative process accommodate a more sustainable perspective of the dish? How can sustainability enter the creative process in haute cuisine?

## 2 CREATIVITY IN HAUTE CUISINE

### 2.1 Understanding creativity in food and design

Creativity is the ability to come up with new ideas, an opportunity to transform a possibility into something concrete, and to establish connections between seemingly disconnected realities. The concept is intangible and difficult to define, it can be applied diversely and found in different disciplines and activities (Sternberg, 2006). Professionals in various areas use creative processes: creativity translates into generating ideas and developing alternative proposals for solving problems. As in design, creativity in food considers the complex relationship between the individual, the general structure (where the creative process takes place) and a broad context (or field of action). Often associated with artistic areas, creativity is essential for the designer and the chef, sharing a common territory.

The analogy between creative processes in design and food, particularly in haute cuisine, can be acknowledged when design principles are used similarly in both fields (Parreira, 2014). Considering design and haute cuisine are activities user or client-oriented, what results from the creative process must follow a function or meet the expectations created. The generation of ideas, development and execution of a dish presents analogies with the design process — the two fields have the notion of project in common. This parallel becomes more evident in haute cuisine, where each dish has to meet a wider set of expectations (e.g. experience as a gastronomic dimension). In this type of cuisine the chef's role is preponderant (assuming most creative and leadership decisions) and the outcome of the process (i.e. the dish) is an experience with symbolic, cultural and economic value.

## 2.2 Mapping the chef's creative process

The process of creating a dish (from the initial idea to the final result in a menu, to the idea's evolution and to all the technical and technological steps) represents recognizable guidelines in the work of all the chefs in this study. In general, each chef explains the work from their own personal values and perspectives, focusing on the process from the outset (when the first idea comes) to the end (when the dish comes to the table and is, or not, well accepted by the customer).

The initial idea triggers the entire process and underlies all the procedures required to create the dish, after that tests are made and the final result is a dish with a concept and all the technical definitions duly consolidated. The chef follows a set of steps in sequence — from the abstract to the concrete — starting the process with an idea and ending with the final dish. It is a process with multiple components in the conception, development and implementation, to which cultural, technical, and emotional dimensions converge.

Through every creative process in haute cuisine, four important moments can be identified: (1) the initial idea; (2) the concept's definition (the chef's individual thinking is very present at this stage); (3) the development procedures (extended to the team); (4) the final dish is tested in real context. Only at the end of the process, all dimensions (conception, technique, technology and public acceptance) work

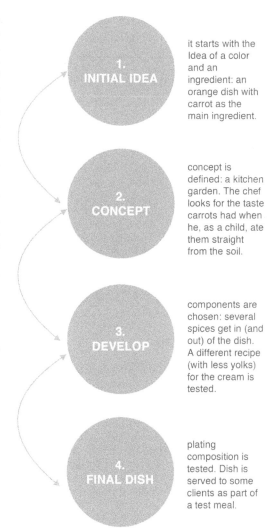

Figure 1. The chef's creative process (with an example of a dish by chef Leonel Pereira).

together to form a credible whole, validated by the chef and the client.

The sequential appearance of those four steps is misleading since the process isn't always linear or straightforward: advances and setbacks throughout the process may occur. For example, different experiences may bring a new technique, discard one ingredient, or at the end of the process, after full development and tests, the chef may decide not to put the dish in the menu (this can happen for several reasons, including technical issues, customer acceptance or the chef's lack of satisfaction with the dish)

Back at the beginning of the process, where do ideas come from? For ideas to emerge, the chef's experiences, imagination, and natural, technical and intellectual abilities are determinant; the creative process integrates food memories and the chef's personal and professional experiences. Although it is not always possible to define with precision the essential conditions required, the ideas generated are often related to: (a) the chef's personal characteristics and abilities (e.g. imagination, perseverance); (b) the experience and knowledge developed over time; (c) the surrounding (i.e., the near and extended context); (d) the emotional dimension of the process (i.e. the chef's motivation).

The definition of a concept from the idea chosen usually represents the next step of the creative process. A concept synthesizes the initial idea into a word or theme; may arise in the form of a question or refer to a distant or imaginary story. It may result from something unimaginable or difficult to accept and that becomes possible only at the moment when this idea is formalized. Nevertheless, conceptualization may simply correspond to the identification of a situation that already occurs and to which a new name is attributed, which, when accepted, constitutes a new reality. Or it may be a deconstruction or reconstruction of something that already exists, where the shape and not the basic nature of the dish is changed. In this latter approach the concept involves altering the appearance of the ingredients used in a dish, enhancing the intensity of the flavors and transforming presentation, textures and shapes (e.g. the use of temperatures different from those used in the "original" dish).

When the idea is outlined and the concept determined, the process of developing a dish goes through the definition of all the specific needs, techniques and actions for its realization. Specifications made available to the team for each dish should explain in detail the execution, composition and presentation. These procedures are essential in daily management in the restaurant, so even when the chef is not present, the dish is served according to the same parameters of rigor and quality.

The process' conclusion is marked with a test period in a real context (or as similar as possible), where the details are fine-tuned and possible technical or logistical issues are verified, as well as the public's reactions. The different variables are managed together to ensure the dish's reproduction over time and at the flexibility to consider changes needed.

## 2.3 Methodology

The study focused on the creative work of five chefs whose work is classified as high cuisine: all are Michelin stars' holders working in Portugal. Phenomenology was used to map the creative process; the profile of each chef was built using their statements, directly to the researcher, in interviews and in-depth conversations, and participation in public presentations and in publications and documents available.

As research method, phenomenology focus on a theme (i.e. identifies a topic to be discussed), seeks to understand the phenomenon by putting it in suspension (i.e. discards all existing preconceptions before starting the discussion). Thus, it is possible to advance

to the essence (or structure) of the theme, which is present in the chefs' discourses. In their descriptions, chefs describe the phenomenon as they perceive it and communicate their perceptions of it (Finlay, 2008).

In order to map the chef's creative process, 39 themes emerged from the applied research method: how the variables interact with each other, and in what phase of the creative process in which they intervene is only suggested by the chefs' statements and previous literature review. The researcher only offers an interpretation after observing and following the description of the experience, identifying the most recurrent patterns, and reflecting on possible meanings within the context.

## 3 SUSTAINABILITY ON THE MENU

### 3.1 Sustainable haute cuisine?

Haute cuisine is not the best example when sustainability is on the table: food cost is usually high, dishes come with a huge carbon footprint and leave behind plenty of waste. Plus, being an intensive hands-on cuisine (with many hours of work in each dish) makes kitchens hard for staff, visible in the French haute cuisine culture. But recent years brought new visions to Michelin-starred restaurants: an eco-conscious approach often includes the use of local products, ethical business practices, the fair treatment of staff and respect for consumer's rights.

Historically, the new Nordic cuisine, showcasing the day's freshest ingredients from the restaurants' premisses, made way for a product-centered approach. That alternative vision has been cooked from the start in the chef's creative process, with sustainability in the center of the dish. By doing so chefs like René Redzepi (from Noma) started a new conversation around local grown ingredients and more efficient (energy wise) technics of cooking and serving dishes at the restaurant. The creative process accommodates sustainability in every step, from the idea to the concept, during development and whilst validating the final dish. One can even consider a sustainable model where the chef's creative process backbone relies on those principles and values, from start to finish. Even though recent food trends that originate from Nordic chefs' cuisine show a better path concerning the sustainability of the dish, food is far from having an environmentally friendly position, and the chef's role couldn't be more relevant. Moreover, sustainable futures call for out-of-the-box ideas that can change the current status quo, and that's what haute cuisine chefs do.

### 3.2 How chefs can contribute to change: the 'mackerel campaign' in Portugal

In the present, chefs can create value outside their kitchens as their visibility in the media gives them a voice. Indirectly, when a chef uses innovative products

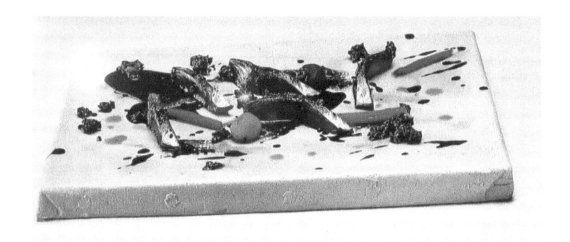

Figure 2.    Smoked mackerel belly, pickled vegetable puree and confetti (2013) — José Avillez (photography by Raul Lufinha).

and techniques those tend to find their way to other contexts, such as home cooking (e.g. rocket/arugula is now consumed in every Portuguese household but, just a few years ago, before being popularized by chefs it was almost unknown in Portugal).

In the beginning of the decade (2012), Docapesca (a public organization under the Portuguese Ministry of the Sea) started a program to promote sustainable fish. Horse mackerel and mackerel are cheap and abundant in Portuguese waters but consumers don't usually consider it a first choice. Traditionally, this fish was mostly bought by the tinned fish industry to be transformed into low value products. With the promotion program (and the increased importance of tourism in Portugal), mackerel consumption has been a growing market.

The campaign was developed in partnership with municipalities, tourism and hospitality schools, producers, traders, food distribution and canning industry. Several chefs were asked to use mackerel as a core ingredient in order to increase consumption and fleet profitability, fair remuneration of the fisherman and responsible economic consumption. Many haute cuisine dishes were created featuring mackerel as a core ingredient, José Avillez's (Figure 2) being one of them. When ready to choose his best dishes from Belcanto (two Michelin stars) in the last 10 years, the chef included a "Smoked mackerel belly, pickled vegetable puree and confetti" first served in 2013.

More recently, chef Henrique Sá Pessoa (Alma, two Michelin stars) used mackerel in a tasting menu's dish. "Mackerel, vegetable escabeche, mussel broth and barnacles, sea lettuce" was the initial dish in "Coast to Coast menu – exclusively inspired by the sea". Not exactly an approach centered on sustainability but certainly a sustainable choice concerning the fish in the dish. To this day, chef Henrique Sá Pessoa has been using mackerel frequently.

When these chefs accepted the challenge to cook with mackerel and use it in haute cuisine dishes they were also accepting the responsibility to communicate a sustainable fish to a broader audience. Getting a chef's sign of approval on a specific product holds the ability to influence more than ever before; celebrity chefs stimulate our interest in food (Hopksinson & Cronin, 2015). A dish is no longer just something to be consumed but simultaneously an expression of self, a form of communication.

## 4    CONCLUSION

Combining sustainability and haute cuisine has been a task difficult to carry out. Usually, not only dishes have a high food cost but their sustainable record often falls short. With imaginative dishes and careful planning, chefs are hoping to renew industry practices – and to put sustainability on the menu. The chef's creative process assumes special relevance as it considers all possible options and chooses the path to follow. If sustainability is part of that process, different sustainable futures become possible from the beginning: (1) the idea emerging initially originates from the sustainability spectrum (e.g. ancient techniques such as fire, local products) and marks the remaining process; (2) the concept itself, on step two, may be determined as sustainable following an initial idea (e.g. "zero waste", "nose-to-tail"); (3) through development, sustainable practices can be integrated independently from the idea and the concept previously determined; (4) the final step may consider optimizing the whole process with sustainability as as goal. From the first moment of the creative process, during its multiple steps or any time throughout the entire process, putting sustainability on top of concerns and objectives offers a chance to change the chef's perspective, the restaurant profile or the food chain itself.

To be able to change consumer habits has as much to do with price, convenience (e.g. being easily available)

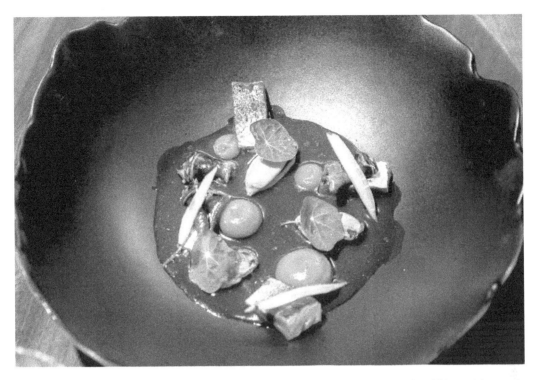

Figure 3. Mackerel, vegetable escabeche, mussel broth and barnacles, sea lettuce (2016) — Henrique Sá Pessoa (photography by Pedro Cruz Gomes).

and identity (i.e. culturally accepted and validated) as with trends. The movement toward chefs as celebrity figures has changed the culture of the food industry, influencing consumer patterns (e.g. cooking habits, purchasing behaviors). When a personal connection between the audience and a chef is achieved, a phase of influence takes place. What the 'mackerel effect' in Portugal shows is how important the chef's creative process is, by developing a personal signature and a new way of cooking in haute cuisine, but more than that how the chef's voice can be heard outside haute cuisine, starting change in other food industry's levels (like the tinned fish factories), not to mention home cooking and everyday fish that gets to the table.

## REFERENCES

Finlay, L. (2008). "Debating phenomenological research methods". *Phenomenology & Practice*. Vol 3, pp. 6–25.

Hopkinson, G.C. & Cronin, J. (2015). "When people take action ....' Mainstreaming malcontent and the role of the celebrity institutional entrepreneur", *Journal of Marketing Management*, 31:13–14, 1383–1402, DOI: 10.1080/0267257X.2015.1068214

Margolin, V. (2012). "Design Studies and Food Studies: Parallels and Intersections", *Agroindustrial Design: 2nd International Product and Service Design Congress and Exhibition on Agricultural Industries – Mediterranean/Food/Design. Proceedings*, Izmir University of Economics, pp. 19–32.

Parreira, S. (2014). *Design-en-place: Processo de design e processo criativo na alta cozinha*. (PhD thesis), Universidade de Lisboa: Lisboa.

Ranganathan, J., Vennard, D., Waite, R., Dumas, P., Lipinski, B. & Searchinger. T. (2016). "Shifting Diets for a Sustainable Food Future." *Working Paper, Installment 11 of Creating a Sustainable Food Future*. Washington, DC: World Resources Institute.

Scarpatto, R. (2002). "Sustainable gastronomy as a tourist product", in Anne-Mette Hjalager & Greg Richards. *Tourism and Gastronomy*. London: Routledge, pp. 132–52.

Sloan, P., Legrand, W. & Hindley, C. (eds) (2015). *The Routledge handbook of sustainable food and gastronomy*. New York: Routledge.

Sternberg, R. (2006). "The Nature of Creativity". *Creativity Research Journal*. 18(1), pp. 87–98.

*Experiencing Food: Designing Sustainable and Social Practices – Bonacho, Pires & Lamy (Eds)*
© *2021 Taylor & Francis Group, London, ISBN 978-0-367-49414-8*

# 'Squid Inc': Designing transformative food experiences

S.J. Marsden

*Independent Researcher, Edinburgh, Scotland*

ABSTRACT: Artists working with food, use innovative and interdisciplinary methods to engage people, an approach which could help contribute to greater food literacy amongst the public. This paper explores how artist-led projects can engage the public with the complexities of food, using a case study. The 'Squid Inc' events, organised by the Slow Food Youth Network are described as an 'artistic and gastronomic experience' based on three elements: 'the squid, the ink and the paper'. Interviews and a focus group were used to gain insights into the aims of stakeholders and the experiences of participants, which in turn could be used for future educational Food Design methodologies.

## 1 INTRODUCTION

Our relationship with food is intrinsically complex and relevant to socio-economic, environmental and political issues at both a global and local level. The study of food, including its "physical, emotional and symbolic resonance" allows us to understand and tackle these complexities, and in turn, can create innovative solutions which could impact our roles as citizens within the food system within daily life (Parasecoli, 2017, p. 15).

As the new disciplines of gastronomy and food studies emerge, it has become acknowledged that there is a need for interdisciplinary study to create interdisciplinary solutions to these complexities of food, as well as to investigate opportunities to re-examine how we most effectively educate and engage with people about food (Reissig, 2017).

Much of the existing research on the idea of engaging the public with food focuses predominantly on health goals, although our relationship with food is inherently more complex and nuanced. Despite the visibility of artist-led Food Design projects, there is limited specific academic research that addresses how the educational ambitions of these projects are experienced by participants. Therefore, the rationale for the study was to bridge gaps in the literature, posing the research question: *"How do artist-led projects engage members of the public with the complexities of food?"*

To explore these broad interdisciplinary themes, the researcher utilised an artist-led project entitled 'Squid Inc', that they had coordinated in Scotland as a case study, to create achievable, measurable outcomes. The 'Squid Inc' events, organised by artist Eduard Pagès Rabal, and the Slow Food Youth Network, are described as an 'artistic and gastronomic experience based on three elements: 'the squid; the ink

and the paper', and combine a presentation about the historic tradition of gyotaku printing with an artistic printmaking class, followed by instruction in preparing and cooking calamari.

A holistic approach was taken to select key literature appropriate to this study, to effectively examine both the educational and aesthetic ambitions of the 'Squid Inc' events.

## 2 FOOD EDUCATION

### 2.1 *The need for a holistic and transformative food education.*

Roberts (2016) and Reissig (2017) both acknowledge the peculiarity of a lack of a provision of a meaningful and holistic food education within our current educational landscape. Roberts (2016) advocates for experimental teaching methods that allow for engagement with food in a fun and imaginative way, that engages all the senses. He purports that the methods of doing this are equally important;" teaching ourselves *how* to learn about food is the perfect match to teaching ourselves *what* to learn about food" (Roberts, 2016).

Reasons for a lack of holistic food education are given as an 'invisibility of food' as well as the 'invisibility of food connections', both within the classroom but also within public and governmental discussions (Roberts, 2016), as well as a convention of reducing food education to elements concerning public health and nutrition (Contento, 2001, cited in Goldstein, 2016, p. 94).

### 2.2 *Discourses on food literacy*

Food literacy can be described as the idea of "proficiency in food-related skills and knowledge"

(Truman et al., 2017), although varying definitions have resulted in different applications and some confusion as the definition of the term (Vidgen & Gallegos, 2011; Truman et al., 2017). Food literacy is an important concept to both define and understand as food is both relatable and a tangible, powerful way of understanding and communicating other aspects of modern life. Truman et al. (2017) investigated the varying use of definitions within existing literature by carrying out a scoping review in which it was found that the "majority of definitions of food literacy emphasize the acquisition of critical knowledge (55%) over functional knowledge (8%), although some incorporate both (37%)" (p. 365).

Goldstein's (2016), research, summarises discourses in literature as falling into two different paradigm; that of a 'neoliberal consciousness model' as opposed to a 'critical consciousness model'. The 'critical consciousness' paradigm definition correlates with work by researchers (e.g. Janhoven et al., 2016; Kimura, 2011; Sumner, 2013), who claim that accomplishing true food literacy goes beyond that of just increased knowledge – requiring active engagement in democratic practice within the food system to nurture ecological health, and disrupt current food practices whilst considering cultural, social, ecological and environmental factors – a definition more in line with theories of "ecoliteracy" (Stinson, 2010 cited in Goldstein, 2016, p. 185).

## 2.3 Food literacy through transformative learning and creativity

Although Goldstein claims there is little evidence that food literacy leads to food system change, she agrees with Roberts (2016), Kimura (2011) and Sumner (2013) that the method of learning is paramount and that 'transformative learning' could be a useful tool in helping to procure food literacy and facilitate food citizenship. Transformative learning, originally coined by Jack Mezirow (2011) occurs in a process of adult education as a process of adult learning through "critical reflection, engaging in discourse, and taking action" (cited in Goldstein, 2016, p. 196).

Additionally, Massari (2017) acknowledges a gap in literature concerning food system education, citing a "lack of studies or curricula that highlight the importance and role of *creativity* as a learning object." (p. 121). Massari's findings exemplify how creativity is understood and utilised by different subsets working within the food system to study how design may be utilised into "formal and informal and unconventional formats of food system education" (Massari, 2017, p. 121).

Research by both Goldstein (2016) and Massari (2017) acknowledges there is limited research in this area and suggest there is potential to further investigate the role of creativity and transformative learning in relation to alternative food education.

## 3 THE COMPLEXITY OF FOOD

The word complexity is one that is commonly utilised to both describe and explain the inherent characteristics of food; be it the food system; the cultural and social significance of food; or the difficulties in providing education or achieving food literacy which accurately reflects the convoluted 'nature' of food (Biderman, 2017; Reissig, 2017; Parasecoli, 2018).

Complexity is generally described as a non-linear model or system which can be emergent, path and context-dependent and is subject to irreversible 'tipping' into new eras (Boulton et al., 2015; Kavalski, 2015). Reissig (2017) states that the complexities of the current foodscape and changes to family structures and dynamics have further inhibited our food knowledge and practice, which traditionally was handed down through generations by family or social praxis. Evitts et al. (2010, cited in Boulton et al., p. 5) call for a "radical shift in perceptions, thinking and values", arguing that thinking in systems and interconnectedness can facilitate and accelerate a transition to a broader, more holistic worldview.

Despite the emergence of complexity theory as a discipline, there is limited literature which addresses complexity theory specifically in relation to Food Design, although Spence (2018) reviews the way in which complexity can be used as a design tool and signaled for within a tasting experience.

Biderman (2017) argues for the importance of embracing complexity within the discipline of Food Design stating it is the responsibility of a designer to consider the complexities of food – be it systemic or cultural – within their practice. He also argues for food education that is mindful of this complexity, but acknowledges the challenges of combining interdisciplinary epistemologies and pedagogies when working in this manner.

## 4 DESIGNING MEANINGFUL FOOD EXPERIENCES

### 4.1 *Food design as a methodology for food education*

The concept of Food Design is also often misunderstood, but within the literature is summarised thus; industrial design and design-led innovation; a more 'eater-focused' role centered mostly on conceptual, artistic or sensorial experiences (such as the 'Squid Inc' project); or a strategic and research-based approach including systems thinking (Parasecoli, 2018) as well as social innovation and process design (Reissig, 2017). Biderman (2017) argues that design may not necessarily require a tangible outcome in the form of a product, and sometimes 'intent to influence behaviour' is one such intangible design.

Perrone & Fuster (2017) stress the potential of food to be used as an "educational force" due to the following factors; "the accessibility of the real product;

direct access to certain level of knowledge; it's being the node of a complex system of relationships; ability to 'rapid prototype' (this medium) with a high degree of reliability and immediate testing of results on individuals and environment" (p. 71). Furthermore et al. (2015) and Zampollo (Zampollo & Peacock, 2016), have created a set of food design methodologies to specifically address the issues of designing for and with food. However, the transformative potential of Food Design is debated by art critic Lucas Verweij (2017), who postures that all aspects could be considered as just branding or advertising, and that an 'eating design' cannot do any more than "raising awareness" of an issue, although he does concede that raising awareness may be an important first step in making changes to a complex food system.

## 4.2 *Multisensory experience design*

In Western society, it can be argued that consumers now exist within an 'experience economy' (Pine & Gilmore, 1999) – a progression to selling a 'total product' rather than just a 'tangible (or edible) product' (Spence, 2017, p. 376). The integration of experience design within 'Food Design' may be one such way to enhance outcomes, out with that of purely 'the consumer'. Research into cross-modal and multi-sensory science has demonstrated the potential to use experience design which incorporates innovative use of sight, sound, touch and smell which may inform our hedonic expectations of our eating experiences including, but not limited to, dining and taste (Spence, 2017) and could be potentially utilised to transmit values of a culture or society (Perrone & Fuster, 2017).

Utilising Pine and Gilmore's (1999) notion of an 'experience economy'; Moore & Bruce (2015) summarise that experiences can be classified into four domains, within two dimensions; those of participation and connection. The domain of participation ranges from passive participation at one end of the spectrum to active participation at the other, whereas connection can be sorted into the categories of absorption and immersion. For example, a PowerPoint presentation on the history of papermaking would usually be categorised as absorption, whereas a gyotaku printmaking workshop would be usually classified as immersion. Furthermore, Moore & Bruce (2015) utilise Pine & Gilmor's (1999) key principles of experience design to identify ways in which innovative and engaging educational experiences could be created. These key principles are; (a) theme the experience; (b) harmonise the experience with positive cues; (c) eliminate negative cues; (d) mix in memorabilia and (e) engage all the five senses.

From a phenomenological perspective, Klein (2018), envisions a framework which can be to nurture transformative learning experiences, utilising the senses. She defines this as a three-stage process; beholding, immersion and reflection. The emphasis of the senses is of paramount important to both authors

in relation to both effective and transformative experiences, be it for entertainment or for educational purposes.

## 5 METHOD

The research design was centered on a case-study which would incorporate two artist-led educational food workshop events in May 2018 in Glasgow, CCA, and Edinburgh, Quay Commons entitled 'Squid Inc'. The objective was to collect and analyse data on the stakeholder's intentions for the 'Squid Inc' project and how these are experienced and interpreted by the participants of the event, using qualitative, semi-structured interviews. Full ethical approval was given by Queen Margaret University, Edinburgh, and steps were taken to ensure that both the interviews and focus groups were compliant with ethical considerations (Morgan, 1997), and all participants gave their informed consent.

The researcher was aware of the existence of the threat of reflexivity (Yin, 2014). during the data collection and analysis stages, and used a questioning route to cultivate consistency throughout the interviews and focus groups.

A framework approach was used to organise and effectively analyse the data for thematic content analysis (Seale, 2018). This was done in spreadsheet form to allow for cross-disciplinary thematic management of emergent categories and codes (Saldaña, 2015). The respondents were anonymised and can be identified in the following text by location 'E' for Edinburgh workshop attendees and 'G' for Glasgow attendees), and by number (1–4).

Individual interviews were carried out with the stakeholders of the events; the project artist, Eduard Pagès Rabal, and the chef, Caroline Rye, who led the event, and a volunteer in attendance at both events. The focus groups were designed as two one-hour focus groups, each with between 4–6 participants. The criteria for inclusion in 'Squid Inc' focus groups was participation in the events in either Glasgow or Edinburgh locations, this predetermined the possible sample pool with 7 attendees at the Glasgow CCA event, and 16 in attendance at the Edinburgh event.

The small sample sizes within the Glasgow and Edinburgh group resulted in some limitations in data collection. Firstly, it wasn't possible to coordinate a convenient focus group with the minimum desired number of four Glasgow workshop participants. Therefore, three Glasgow workshop respondents were interviewed individually utilising the same question framework as the Edinburgh focus group. With regards to the demographic of the sample, there were limitations in which it could be imperative to exercise caution when making generalisations based on results of the data (Silverman, 2013). Firstly, only females responded to a request for focus group participation resulting in a potentially biased set of data. Additionally, it was observed that most participants appeared to, or reported, having been educated at higher or postgraduate level.

# 6 RESULTS AND DISCUSSION

## 6.1 Skills and knowledge

The Squid Incc event had unique educational aims, combining sessions on the history and culture of both hand-made paper making, gyotaku and cyanotype print-making, as well as practical instruction in gyotaku printmaking, how to fillet and prepare a Squid Inck calamari recipe.

### 6.1.1 Functional knowledge: Deskilling and everyday barriers

An overarching theme during the interviews was of the skills and knowledge gained by the participants at the events. When questioned on her aims, the chef at the two events had expectations of what she hoped the participants would learn; *"I hoped that they would take away...a bit more...confidence and knowledge of how to prepare both the squid from scratch or even you could buy cleaned and chop yourself.... also, I hope that now they've seen the squid being dissected and prepared that they might get them to think that other species are...potentially not that difficult to tackle"*

When questioned about their experience of preparing and cooking squid, five of the seven participants hadn't filleted a squid before, and four of seven participants hadn't made calamari before. Most participants enjoyed this process, finding it easier than expected, with one stating; *"I really enjoyed gutting the squid and I was thinking...I can really do this..."* and was keen to retain her new skills; *"I guess it was a really good educational process because I'm wanting to do it again and so I should do it sooner rather than later so I don't forget anything!"* (E2). Another participant explained how the experiential, practical instruction appealed to her, *"if you are shown rather than reading in a book – it's so much quicker – quite a tactile thing...perfect for a workshop"* (E4).

In discussion with participants and stakeholders about their skills and knowledge in cooking and consuming squid, key points which emerged were how cultural differences affected confidence and ability in cooking with seafood as well as barriers which may affect participant's likelihood to cook squid. This phenomenon is referred to as 'consumer deskilling' by Jaffe & Gertler (2006). The chef identified the barriers to knowledge and confidence in cooking with squid and seafood in general as being three-fold; sourcing, preparing and cooking the squid stating: *"it's not just the cooking, it's the buying...the fishmonger is definitely a barrier whether it's a shop, a van or a counter in the supermarket"*. The chef cited issues with pricing, weighing and embarrassment at lack of knowledge, as all being potential hurdles for the consumer. These sentiments were echoed by the participants, who reported they rarely cooked squid at home or lacked confidence

and knowledge in sourcing squid. As cited by Goldstein within the literature, Jaffe & Gertler (2006) stress the re-introduction of some of these missing skills as being of imperative value within food system transformation, stressing those that who empower themselves *"represent a challenge to dominant development trajectories and to conservative doctrines of necessity and inevitability"* (p. 158).

There are two ways of interpreting the acquisition of these skills and knowledge at these events in relation to food literacy. Firstly, applying Goldstein's model of 'neoliberal consciousness', it is likely that the participant's application of this 'functional knowledge' gained at a one-off event such as 'Squid Inc' would be considered as 'reskilling' (Jaffe & Gertler, 2006), and would not meet the criteria of Goldman's critical consciousness model.

If the skills and knowledge passed on at the Squid Incc event, is only likely to create 'functional, technical knowledge' (Goldstein, 2016). Nevertheless, as Goldstein herself acknowledges "it is simpler and easier to teach concrete food skills and individual behavior modification for health and well-being than to shape active citizens who can critically engage with contemporary food systems issues" (p. 159).

### 6.1.2 Food literacy: taking action

Alternatively, the responses from participants could also be interpreted within the secondary paradigm, as some participants discussed a desire to share knowledge – reporting that they had shared their experiences with others, and a few expressing that they would be confident in passing some of these skills on; *"I felt I learnt a lot of different skills...different knowledge...and also learnt a lot that you can actually use again...I think I could actually show someone else how to cut up a squid and how to print with the squid"* (G3).

This desire to *take action* in sharing knowledge and empowering others (Jaffe & Gertler, 2006) could be seen to display critical consciousness in relation to food literacy. Furthermore, this notion of 'taking action' corresponds with Mezirow's theory of transformative learning (Mezirow & Taylor, 2011).

## 6.2 Transformative experiences

### 6.2.1 Space and atmosphere

The Squid Incc workshops took place at two different venues and with a variety in the number of participants; with 7 participants at the CCA, Glasgow and 16 at the Quay Commons, Edinburgh. The CCA space was a blank canvas allowing flexibility for the room set up whereas the Quay Commons event was within a cafe space with working bakery, requiring some rearrangement of furniture and decor to display the artist's gyotaku prints. Having performed the 'Squid Inc' workshop and gyotaku events at several different locations in over three countries, the artist stressed the importance of the suitability and design of the spaces for the gyotaku in relation to the space atmosphere; *"the first thing that gives me piece of mind is like having a kitchen close to where we're doing that, and of course the architecture of the place, the atmosphere, the lighting if it's beautifully arranged...the better you're going to feel...the better you're going to print."* For him, the importance of designing a successful experience goes beyond that of just visual aesthetics, instead, being integral to the underpinning of Japanese aesthetic and philosophy of the gyotaku printmaking technique itself; *"it's really a meditative process...when a relaxed mind will give you better results..."* This statement suggests that the overall atmosphere at the event was of utmost importance to the artist, to nurture a meditative state for the participants during their gyotaku printmaking experience. Certainly, the stakeholders who were present at both events noticed a distinctive difference between the two events, with the Glasgow event seeming calmer and more focused than the Edinburgh counterpart. However, participants did not report any noticeable differences in how they evaluated their response to the atmosphere in the different locations, a limitation when dealing with subjective experiences.

Additionally, it transpired that the artist intended the display of his gyotaku and cyanotype prints to not only provide visual stimulus to the space, but was often utilised to prompt participants to discuss the seafood depicted. This stimulus allows an exchange of ideas both as a tool, and as an important discussion of the work itself. Therefore, it could be pertinent to consider how the educational ambition to create conviviality within the space also aligns with the morality of the Japanese 'Zen' philosophy (Saito, 2007). This highlights the complexities and philosophical implications of aesthetics and the ethical implications when designing cross-cultural arts projects and educational experiences.

### 6.2.2 *Intimacy with the medium*

The next concept that arose when discussing the hands-on nature of the event, was that of intimacy and connection to the squid as a medium.

The choice of the medium seemed integral to the experience of the event, with participants and stakeholders describing squid as being novel in form, using words such as *"mildly-terrifying on the inside"*, *"alien"* and *"other-worldly"*. The event chef believed this *"added to the drama and intrigue of the event"*, and enhanced engagement with the filleting process as (with fish) *"they know it's a fish...but with a squid they're like...where do you start...?!"* It could be suggested that these reactions are due to neophobia – a common fear of unknown foods (Rozin, 1979; Wilson, 2017), with one Vietnamese-American participant commenting on a differing approach to fish within her culture, in which it is common to eat fish in its entire form; *"I think it's easy to get squeamish the more removed you are from preparing your own food."* (G1).

The technique of gyotaku required a lot of time immersed in close contact with the both the medium of the washi paper and the squid. All participants agreed that this was quite a smelly and messy process, but it appeared all participants enjoyed both these elements. One participant explained her experience thus; *"I like touching things and I love the fact that it... looked very messy and kind of shapeless maybe when in the bowl but actually it's a beautiful shape to it...that kind of made me look at Squid Inc a completely different way"* (G2).

This exposure to squid during the printmaking process appeared to make participants more connected to the medium with one participant reporting a feeling of intimacy, another stating they were *"really fond of my squid"* (E1), a third agreeing; *"you take ownership of it"* (E2) This sense of connection also heightened respect for the creature with one participant reflecting; *"...it almost makes you pay attention to the animal a bit more...respect it a bit more...you end up remembering the parts..."* (E2).

These expressions of 'intimacy' correlate with research on the sense of touch by Gallace & Spence (2014), in which it is discussed that the active kinesthetic, rather than passive aesthetic experience of touch may be a much more emotional or intimate aesthetic experience than that of a visual aesthetic experience. Driscoll (nd) describes tactile art as being "intimate, drawing us into relationship with what we are touching" (Driscoll in Gallace & Spence, 2014, p. 5). Participants also described how the experiential process of handling the squid during the printmaking process helped them within the process of filleting the squid; *"I think once you'd spent the whole evening handling the creature then actually preparing it, it didn't seem so daunting"* (G3).

The other factor integral to the experience was the smell of the medium; both the fresh squid and the cooked squid. When questioned, the artist explained he thinks this *"helps them to be more present"* during the process, and indeed the two smells were described differently with the smell of the squid during the printmaking as being *"kind of fresh"* (G2), whereas the smell during the cooking process encouraging hunger.

Interestingly, one participant (G2), reported how these multi-sensory experiences had affected her hedonic expectations of taste; stating the calamari she ate on the evening was *"delicious"*, despite having previously not enjoyed the taste, smell or texture she had experienced when previously consuming calamari within restaurants; *"Knowing food inside out, where it comes from, slows you down and makes you appreciate it"* (G2).

This participant, who was attracted to the event due to the printmaking element, did not participate in the squid filleting due to her dislike of seafood, reflectively expressed regret in not filleting the squid during the event. In this example, it is possible to see how Klein's (2018) framework for transformative learning through sensory appreciation could (possibly) be interpreted;

firstly her 'beholdment' of the squid a 'mindful awareness driven by wonder'. Secondly, immersion in the experience; which acts to enhance the participant's appreciation of touch and smell enabling her to capture ' "nuanced and complex" details (Klein, 2018, p. 22). Thirdly on reflection, she has stepped back to achieve perspective and distance on her decision which makes connections beyond that of the experience (Bresler, 2013, p. 22, in Klein, 2018).

Such responses from participants would suggest that Klein's (2018) transformative learning theory is, overall, more aligned with the participant's experiences than Mezirow's (2011) three step theory of 'transformative learning' (critical reflection; engaging in discourse; and taking action). This could have interesting implications as they are more sensory-based than the critical pedagogical model of Mezirow (2011). Therefore, there is potential for further research on creative multi-sensory food education for adults.

### 6.3 From 'medium' to larger food system complexit

These examples suggest that this close and intimate contact with the squid as a medium, prior to consumption could help attendees of the event understand the medium as a complex entity. Certainly, when questioned, the artist indicated that his gyotaku praxis had widened his knowledge and understanding of the biodiversity of species available for sale in fish markets in different parts of Europe. He also believes this is a way to help encourage participant's knowledge; *"...with every gyotaku every species I printed I wanted to know the Latin name, I wanted to know where these fishes came from, I wanted to know what was the best way of cooking them...I wanted to know different recipes and the culture of them."*

When discussing whether participants thought that the event may help them understand the concept of food as being a complex entity, most participants reported a holistic understanding of a range of factors that would influence and impact the food they consumed. Although none of the participants referenced the concept of biodiversity in direct relation to the squid, a few did mention increased understanding of anatomy. The majority however, did confirm that the cross-disciplinary nature of the event was useful in increasing understanding of a range of factors that impacted the two mediums; the paper and the squid; *"It gave the squid like a few more layers...it was squid functioning at all these kind of levels...history where you got the squid from, the usage and how it is as a being...gave it a whole other real...not just bit of fried calamari y' know!"* (E1.)

Additionally, participants reported that a key element they gained new knowledge on, was the history of papermaking; the causal connection between global plant diversity and the development of different styles of traditional handmade paper around the world, which was used for different purposes; *"I didn't realise that the sort of like...plants landscape of an area actually affects the types of materials that are produced from it"* (G2).

One participant described how the event may inform her understanding of complexity, by intellectually dissecting and articulating individual components that make up the overall event; *"when you...kind of start breaking things down...it helps you start noticing things that maybe you wouldn't know. It was an eye opener!"* (G2.)

It could be suggested that this statement echoes Roberts (2016) statement on the need for deepening and widening of the visibility of food and the food system. It is difficult to conclude whether transformative learning experiences can, in *themselves*, lead to a greater understanding of complexity per se. However, the researcher posits that this could also be interpreted as an *embracement of complexity*. Furthermore, it is the researcher's suggestion that appreciation of the food medium as a complex entity could indeed have potential to help to engage the public with a broader understanding of food and food system complexities by providing greater insight into complex systemic interactions of individual components that form a wider food system.

## 7 CONCLUSION

In this investigation, the aim was to use the 'Squid Inc' events as a case study to critically evaluate how artist-led projects engaged the public with the complexities of food. This study has established that artist-led projects such as 'Squid Inc' can be a valuable way of providing food education to the public. However, utilising discourses on food literacy found within the literature, it has become apparent that it is essential to exercise caution to ensure that these do not reinforce or contribute to paradigms of neoliberal consciousness within gastronomy. The second finding was that the role of the artist is integral in designing meaningful food experiences that both *sensitively* and *effectively* combine aesthetic and educational goals. However, it is pertinent to add that seeking to 'enhance' experiences using a Western business approach may hinder the aesthetics of the project.

Overall, this study has established that artist-led projects such as 'Squid Inc' show the potential to engage the public with the complex, interwoven, powerful and nuanced themes of Gastronomy using Klein's (2018) transformative learning experiences theories as a framework. Due to the small-scale and exploratory nature of this research, further studies in the following areas would be recommended:

– A better holistic, academic understanding of complexity in relation to food should be developed, to embrace both the complex nature of food, and the implications of food education.
– There is potential for further research on the utilisation of multi-sensory experience design for adult food education.

- Further studies on artist-led projects that deal with food would be recommended, to gain additional insights that could help create enhanced transformative learning experiences.

## REFERENCES

Adria, F. & Pinto, J.M., 2015. SAPIENS: A Methodology for Understanding Gastronomy. First explanation (work in progress). *Temes de disseny*, (31), pp. 10–21.

Biderman, J.L. 2017. Embracing complexity in food, design and Food Design. *International Journal of Food Design*, 2(1), pp. 27–44.

Boulton, J., et al. 2015. Embracing complexity: strategic perspectives in an age of turbulence. OUP. Oxford.

Gallace, A. & Spence, C. 2014. *In touch with the future: The sense of touch from cognitive neuroscience to virtual reality*. OUP Oxford.

Goldstein, S. 2016. Youth and Food Literacy: A Case Study of Food Education at The Stop Community Food Centre. In Sumner, J. ed., 2016. *Learning, food, and sustainability: Sites for resistance and change*. Springer.

Guthman, J. 2008. Neoliberalism and the making of food politics in California. *Geoforum*, 39(3), pp. 1171–1183.

Jaffe, J. & Gertler, M. 2006. Victual vicissitudes: Consumer deskilling and the (gendered) transformation of food systems. *Agriculture and human values*, 27(2), pp. 143–162.

Janhoven, K. Mäekelä, J. and Palojoki, P. 2016. Food education: from normative models to promoting agency. In *Learning, Food, and Sustainability* (pp. 93–110). Palgrave Macmillan, New York.

Kavalski, E. ed., 2015. World politics at the edge of chaos: *Reflections on complexity and global life*. SUNY Press.

Kimura, A.H. 2011. Food education as food literacy: privatized and gendered food knowledge in contemporary Japan. *Agriculture and Human Values*, 28(4), pp. 465–482.

Klein, S.R. 2018. Coming to Our Senses: Everyday Landscapes, Aesthetics, and Transformative Learning. *Journal of Transformative Education*, 16(1), pp. 3–16.

Massari, S. 2017. Food design and food studies: Discussing creative and critical thinking in food system education and research. *International Journal of Food Design*, 2(1), pp. 117–133.

Mezirow, E. J. & Taylor, E.W. 2011. Transformative learning in practice: insights from community.

Moore, L.L. & Bruce, J.A., 2015. Teaching Leadership in the Experience Economy Paradigm. *Journal of Leadership Education DOI, 1012806*(V14/I4), p. I3.

Morgan, D.L, 1997. Focus group kit: vol. 1. The focus group guidebook. 1997. London: SAGE.

Parasecoli, F. 2017. Food, Research, Design: What can food studies bring to food design education? *International Journal of Food Design*, Volume 2, Number 1, pp. 15–25(11).

Parasecoli, F. 2018. Food, Design, and Innovation: From Professional Specialization to Citizen Involvement. *The Bloomsbury Handbook of Food and Popular Culture*, p. 155.

Perrone, R., & Fuster. A. 2017. Food as a system and a material for the creative process in design education. *International Journal of Food Design*, Volume 2, Number 1, pp. 65–81(17).

Pine, B.J. & Gilmore, J.H. 1999. *The experience economy: work is theatre & every business a stage*. Harvard Business Press.

Reissig, P. 2017. Food Design Education. *International Journal of Food Design*, Volume 2, Number 1, pp. 3–13(11).

Roberts, W. 2016. Afterword: Food 360: Seeing our way around learning about food. In Sumner, J. ed., 2016. *Learning, food, and sustainability: Sites for resistance and change*. Springer.

Rozin, P. 1979. Preference and affect in food selection. In J. H. A. Kroeze (Ed.), *Preference Behavior and Chemoreception* (pp. 289–302). London: Information Retrieval.

Saito, Y. 2007. The moral dimension of Japanese aesthetics. *The Journal of aesthetics and art criticism*, 65(1), pp. 85–97.

Saldaña, J. 2015. The coding manual for qualitative researchers. Sage.

Seale, C. ed., 2018. Researching society and culture. Sage.

Silverman, D. 2013. A very short, interesting and reasonably cheap book about qualitative research. Sage.

Spence, C. 2017. Gastrophysics: The New Science of Eating. Penguin UK.

Spence, C., 2018. Complexity on the Menu and in the Meal. *Foods*, 7(10), p. 158.

Sumner, J. 2013. Food Literacy and Adult Education: Learning to Read the World by Eating. *The Canadian Journal for the Study of Adult Education (Online)*, 25(2), p. 79.

Truman, E. Lane, D. and Elliot, C. 2017. Defining food literacy: A scoping review. *Appetite*, 116, pp. 365–371.

Verweij, L. 2017. *Food Design is nothing but advertising*. [online] [viewed 15 June 2018] Available from: http://lucas-berlin.blogspot.com

Vidgen, H.A. & Gallegos, D. 2014. Defining food literacy and its components. *Appetite*, 76, pp. 50–59.

Wilson, B. 2015. *First bite: how we learn to eat*. Basic Books.

Yin, R.K. 2014. *Case study research: design and methods*. 5th edn. Los Angeles: SAGE.

Zampollo, F. & Peacock, M. 2016. Food Design Thinking: A Branch of Design Thinking Specific to Food Design. *The Journal of creative behavior*, 50(3), pp. 203–210.

# Beyond product-market fit: Human centered design for social sustainability

N. Bender
*Falk School of Sustainability, Chatham University, Pittsburgh, Pennsylvania, USA*

E. Rovira
*Square 41 Studios, Barcelona, Spain*

ABSTRACT:   While claims about design thinking have been shown to benefit the process of new product development, little research has studied how leveraging design thinking in the new product development process can lead to sustainable behavior change. When product developers are considering three pilar models of sustainability, economic concerns are often dealt with first. Increasingly, environmental concerns are being addressed. But social concerns are often afterthoughts (if even considered at all). Here, the authors propose that incorporating human centered design thinking methodologies will not only encourage social sustainability, but cause long-lasting shifts in culture that benefit both communities and the planet.

## 1   A NOTE ON BEGINNINGS

It is worth noting that this research is built on, and make suggestions about for-profit businesses that are interested in leveraging a product to make a long-term change for good. It is also worth noting that some of the words in this work – namely "economic sustainability", "environmental sustainability", and "social sustainability" – have varied meanings depending on their use. Because this can easily obscure the meaning of these words and undermine the work of this research, we begin by outlining the terms as they are used here.

### 1.1   *The sustainability of 3 pillars thinking*

Whether starting with Malthus' panic about food scarcity (1798), Hotelling's "peculiar problems of mineral wealth" (1931), or any number of earlier anthropogenic theories on how humans extract resources – sustainability deals with the long-term viability of action.

Modern discourse around sustainability often starts with the Brundtland Report. This document, published by the UN in 1987 was a way to elucidate elements of sustainability and frames it as a multifaceted concept that deals with a variety of aspects including food security, ecosystems, energy, and economics.

Throughout the document, sustainability is presented as a framework to better tackle development and deals specifically with understanding how we might measure the continuation potential of a given human activity. It also divides sustainability into three major themes – environmental, economic, and social – which are later referred to as the "three pillars" of sustainability.

While the Brundtland Report lays groundwork for the modern discourse around sustainability, it is a document meant to guide UN decisions on policy. It is not meant to serve as a definitive text. What's more, even the report itself specifies that "no single blueprint of sustainability can be issued because particular needs are different in every country" (Brundtland, 1987).

With that said, the concept of the three pillars of sustainability is a commonly used framework when talking about sustainability because it deals with a high level understanding that there are several key factors in measuring the long term impact of resource extraction to deliver goods and services.

In a 2011 publication showing how each of the pillars relate to development, Moldan et al. give readers a clearer idea of how these three terms might be better defined.

**Economic** – sustaining various kinds of capital, optimizing resource management, and potentially conceiving a new economy free of the pressures of growth.

**Social** – values/identities/relationships/institutions that can continue well into the future due to healthy environments and vibrant economies.

**Environmental** – encompasses economic and social development while protecting finite ecological resources and decoupling environmental pressures from economic growth.

Though these concepts have been presented in equal terms and are suited for development, Kuhlman and Farrington (2010) argue that sustainability should only be thought of in a simpler – and more direct – way as the "well-being of future generations".

They contend that thinking about the three pillars separately "risks diminishing the importance of the environmental dimension". In fact, when we focus on aspects of sustainability, it's easy to stray from systems thinking.

The authors of this research agree with the critique of the three pillars model that it when the individual aspects of sustainability are examined in isolation, it's easy to forget about one or another. The metaphor, itself, suggests that if the right pillar is removed, that the other two standing may still be able to support the structure. Further, it is also worth noting that for-profit companies are most invested in addressing the concerns of Economic sustainability. Though the degree to which they address it is up for scrutiny, the nature of a for-profit business is to maintain financial capital and manage resources.

As it stands, for-profit companies tend not to consider environmental needs. If they do, they are often doing so in a tangential peripheral way.

The authors of this paper argue that the blind push towards environmental sustainability is a push away from social and economic sustainability. All three have to be considered holistically in order to enact any kind of long-term change.

However, they take a shape and precedence because it is social sustainability that drives at the heart of users. It is social sustainability that resonates in the everyday lives of people.

It is our hope that we can tap into long-term and impactful environmental change by focusing product design on social sustainability.

### 1.2 *Human centered design*

A product or trend is observably more successful when it is catered toward human needs or wants. Keeping that in mind, designers ought to create products and experiences that respond to social sustainability, by minding the particular circumstances of their intended audience, while also bear the responsibility of ensuring its environmental sustainability.

It has been shown that human centered design has a positive impact on new product development because it aligns business and market needs while also bringing together disparate disciplines for collaboration (Veryzer, 2005).

Indeed, in a progressively more globalized market environment, it becomes of increased value to cater to the sociological context of a region and, by proxy, understanding its environmental impact. Traditions have been in place for long spans of time because of their sustained durability and melding with the existing resources.

### 1.3 *New product development*

There are several approaches and understandings about what new product development is and how it should take place in a company. Of course, the goal of any NPD process is to mitigate risks of launching a new product into a new market.

Here, we will talk about two popular approaches: IDEO's innovation process and the Stage-Gate system.

While there are other methods for developing new products, we found these to be the most predisposed to engage with the needs of the user.

Coming from a product market focus, the Stage-Gate system develops the product in tandem with the user. That is, there are several phases, or *gates*, along the system that are meant to confirm the usability of the product with the end-user before launching the product into the market. But, in principle, the initial design is likely based on an assumption about the user's needs (Cooper, 1990).

Coming from a design focus, the IDEO process spends a lot of time gathering information about user before breaking down their particular needs and formulating an idea based on these needs. Then, once they formulate the idea, they test and re-iterate along with the user (Moen, 2001).

While both methodologies serve the same purpose – to mitigate risk – and spend a lot of time validating information with the user during and after development of the product, there is one key difference between the two methodologies. IDEO formulates the solution to be tested around their initial observations, whereas the Stage-Gate system builds a solution based on an assumption (or observation) about the user's needs.

IDEO's initial investigation vehemently pushes against focus groups and depends a great deal on resources of time to do initial interviews, information gathering, and observation.

The Stage-Gate system is more aligned with businesses that are short on time and need to validate assumptions about their users as soon as possible.

Both processes depend on rapid prototyping and allow the product developer to focus on the needs of the user to create socially sustainable design, but Stage-Gate aligns more easily with economic sustainability.

### 1.4 *Product-market fit*

After a product has been launched, people often talk about Product-Market Fit. The clearest definition of this concept comes from Dan Olsen in his book *The Lean Product Playbook* (2015). In the book, he outlines a pyramid of considerations that build on top of each other.

The bottom two layers of the pyramid are the market layers. These layers consist of "Target Customer" and "Underserved Needs". These layers are the foundation of the entire pyramid; and so, Olsen posits, if you change either of these layers, you will need to change the entire pyramid.

The top three layers of the pyramid are the product layers. These layers consist of the "Value Proposition", the "Feature Set", and the "UX" of the product.

Product-Market fit is a way to validate that the product that was developed was the product needed by the target market. The idea is that once you have identified core users and their needs (the market layers) you can confirm that the specifics of the product (the product layer) are delivering on those established needs.

As there are phases of product-market fit, each product should be evaluated and re-evaluated against the criteria that was set out during development. If something isn't working, then it needs to be iterated until product-market fit is achieved.

## 2 THE FILET-O-FISH PARABLE

### 2.1 *JFK: America's first Catholic president*

In the 1960 US presidential campaign, there were two main candidates running for office: incumbent Vice President Richard Nixon and then-senator for Massachusetts John F. Kennedy. While there was coverage and conversation around policy, voting records, and platform positions, there was also heavy coverage and lots of conversation surrounding Kennedy's religion.

Kennedy was a practicing Catholic. And, to date, there had never been a Catholic president in office. The conversation around Kennedy's religion suggested that a Catholic president would potentially put the concerns of the Vatican before the concerns of the United States. He addressed these concerns heavily on the campaign trail.

In one particularly famous speech – given to the Houston Ministerial Association in Texas – Kennedy assures voters that "contrary to common newspaper usage, I am not the Catholic candidate for president. I am the Democratic Party's candidate for president, who happens also to be a Catholic. I do not speak for my church on public matters, and the church does not speak for me."

He goes on in that same speech to reaffirm the separation of church and state under the US Constitution. "I believe in an America where the separation of church and state is absolute, where no Catholic prelate would tell the president (should he be Catholic) how to act, and no Protestant minister would tell his parishioners for whom to vote; where no church or church school is granted any public funds or political preference; and where no man is denied public office merely because his religion differs from the president who might appoint him or the people who might elect him." (NPR, 2007).

The speeches were enough to convince American voters that his religion was a secondary issue in the matters of the presidency, and on January 20, 1960, he became the first Catholic elected president of the US. But the national conversation around religion and the ways that Americans practice their religion endured.

### 2.2 *(No) fish on Fridays*

In 1962, Lou Groen, was a McDonald's franchise owner in a largely Catholic area of Cincinnati, Ohio. While reviewing his monthly sales, he noticed that his numbers always dropped on Fridays during Lent. Lent is a religious celebration for Christians that falls before Easter – usually in March.

As a practicing Catholic, he knew that Catholics (and other Christians) tend to abstain from eating meat from land animals on Fridays during Lent. This meant that McDonald's mainstay of hamburgers was not an option for most practicing Catholics in the greater Cincinnati area.

Since fish was an acceptable meat to consume on Fridays during this religious celebration, Groen decided to innovate a product that would appeal to his observant audience. The Filet-O-Fish was born (Kroc, 1992).

The sandwich was tested at his location as a prototype in 1961 before being pitched to the McDonald's headquarters. After a round of development about the thickness of the filet, type of batter, and other considerations, the sandwich was finally accepted. In 1965 it had a nationwide roll out. It is now a mainstay of the menu; the only seafood item available year-round in all markets. To this day, McDonald's sells 25% of their yearly Filet-O-Fish numbers during Lent (Berger, 2019).

### 2.3 *Prices and participation may vary*

It's worth mentioning that Groen wanted to use Alaskan Halibut, but it was too expensive for the margins that McDonald's allowed. So they had to change to cod (Kroc, 1992).

This is an example of economic sustainability being the forefront of consideration for a for-profit company. The question in response to the type of fish used for the sandwich was "Which has the least environmental impact?", it was "How much will it cost?"

### 2.4 *See store for details*

While Groen's particular business was geared or more open towards its community, the broader enterprise was and still is very much driven by its economic sustainability, which comes to light when one digs deeper into the particularities of how the Filet-O-Fish came to be. Human needs were met, but the product was put through a design process, however straightforward or primitive it may be seen in today's landscape.

## 3 PUTTING IT ALL TOGETHER

Though we can think about the three pillars separately, we need to examine the ways in which they interact with each other. It is common to think about economic and environmental sustainability working together. We see this frequently with conscious capitalism.

Groen's Filet-O-Fish story is an example of economic sustainability working together with social sustainability. The sandwich was evaluated prior to its release and understood to be an economically sustainable choice. Due to the need that it was fulfilling for consumers, it was also a socially sustainable choice.

Diners were now able to enjoy the convenience and affordability of McDonald's while also practicing their religion. There is no conflict. And the behavior maintains social dynamics for the foreseeable future.

What we would ideally want would be a focus on both the environmental and social aspects of sustainability. That is to say, when we evaluate product market fit we look to understand adoption of the product that has been developed. In this way, we can build on product market fit by examining the social sustainability of the product.

This is a capitalist system; the economic sustainability of products is one of the first things evaluated when developing a product: does it make money? Is it priced appropriately for this particular market? Are the margins correct for the sale of this product?

But if we can design for environmentally sustainable products that maintain the social dynamics of a market, designers will be able to make long lasting behavioral change.

It has been shown that consumers are not motivated by sustainability alone when making purchase decisions (Verbeke, 2007). It has also been shown that consumers are confused about sustainability-related terms on products (Grunert, 2014). So while we must design for environmental sustainability, and the economic sustainability should be taken into account – the real challenge of the designer lies in developing products that engage with the social aspects of sustainability.

With human centered design to focus on the needs of the user, Stage-Gate innovation process to validate development, and product market fit as a baseline to understand how well the product is doing in the market, designers have a structure to make positive, long-lasting changes.

## 4 CONCLUSION (BRING IT ON HOME)

Thankfully, people are now looking to solve more problems of environmental sustainability. It is on the forefront of people's minds, on their social media timelines, and a growing part of public discourse.

In 2019, we are globally entrenched in a capitalistic system that values economic sustainability. We are not looking to upend this system in a single paper. But with the development of goods/services in an economically/environmentally sustainable model, we need to use human centered design to innovate products that are socially sustainable as well.

With this approach, any designer can make the next Filet-O-Fish, and it will save the planet.

## REFERENCES

Berger, Arielle 2019. Here's why McDonald's Filet-O-Fish sales skyrocket in March. *Business Insider*

Brundtland, G. 1987. Report of the World Commission on Environment and Development: Our Common Future. United Nations General Assembly Document A/42/427

Cooper, Robert G. 1990. Stage-Gate Systems: A New Tool for Managing New Products. *Business Horizons*

Grunert, Klaus G et al. 2014. Food products: Consumer motivation, understanding and use. *Food Policy* (44), 177–189

Hotelling, Harold 1931. The Economics of Exhaustible Resources. *The Journal of Political Economy* (39) 137–138

Kroc, Ray 1992. *Grinding it Out: The Making of McDonald's.* Chicago, IL. Contemporary Books

Kuhlman, Tom and Farrington, John 2010. What is sustainability? *sustainability* (2), 3436–3448

Moen, Ron 2001. Review of the IDEO Process. *Research and Negotiations in Design*

Moldan, Bedrich et al. 2012. How to understand and measure environmental sustainability: Indicators and targets. *Ecological Indicators* (17), 4–13

NPR (National Public Radio) 2007. Transcript: JFK's speech on religion

Olsen, Dan 2015. *The Lean Product Playbook.* Hoboken, NJ. John Wiley & Sons

Verbeke, Wim et al. 2007. Perceived Importance of Sustainabilty and Ethics Related to Fish: A Consumer Behavior Perspective. *Ambio* (36), 580–585

Veryzer, Robert W. and Borja de Mozota, Brigitte 2005. The Impact of User-Oriented Design on New Product Development: An Examination of Fundamental Relationships. *The Journal of Product Innovation Management* (22), 128–143

*Experiencing Food: Designing Sustainable and Social Practices – Bonacho, Pires & Lamy (Eds)*
*© 2021 Taylor & Francis Group, London, ISBN 978-0-367-49414-8*

# Designing menus to shape consumers' perception of traditional gastronomy: Does it work for the Portuguese Alentejo cuisine?

D. Guedes
*Institute of Social Sciences, University of Lisbon, Lisbon, Portugal*

V. Silva & R.V. Lucas
*CEFAGE – Center for Advanced Studies in Management and Economics, University of Évora, Évora, Portugal*

S. Tavares
*CIEP – Research Center in Education and Psychology, Department of Psychology, University of Évora, Évora, Portugal*

P. Infante
*CIMA – Research Centre for Mathematics and Applications, University of Évora, Évora, Portugal*

C. Simões, C.C. Pinheiro, F. Capela-Silva & E. Lamy
*ICAAM – Institute of Mediterranean Agricultural and Environmental Sciences, University of Évora, Évora, Portugal*

ABSTRACT: Restaurant menus have been shown to be important communicating and selling tools. In this online experimental study, we focused on the role of descriptive menus in influencing food choice and shaping customers' perception of a traditional restaurant. Participants were randomly assigned to one of two menu conditions. In the intervention menu, five traditional dishes from the region of Alentejo (Portugal) were described using sensory (e.g., "fresh") and authenticity (e.g., "genuine") labels, while in the control condition, the dish name and its ingredients were presented with no further description. No significant differences were found regarding hedonic expectations, choice intention or willingness-to-pay for any of the individual dishes. However, participants in the intervention condition imagined the restaurant to have better service and ambience and serving tastier and fresher dishes. This study adds to the evidence suggesting the potential impact of menus in shaping consumers' expectations of restaurants' service quality, which in turn may affect how people perceive and assess their dining experience.

## 1 INTRODUCTION

Traditional gastronomy has a major impact in the definition of a region's identity (e.g., Lin, Pearson, & Cai, 2011) and is becoming increasingly attractive to tourists, who actively search for a broad range of cultural and sensory experiences (Chang, Kivela, & Mak, 2010). The promotion of traditional recipes may also be strategic in promoting sustainability, for instance, by encouraging the use of local products. This is particularly evident in Mediterranean countries, where typical recipes rely heavily on local vegetables and cereals.

Despite Portugal's modest size, each of the country's regions has its particular and well-defined gastronomical identity. The Alentejo gastronomy is amongst Portugal's most widely recognized and internationally acclaimed cuisines. Due to the region's location and geography, traditionally linked to agricultural and cereal production (mainly wheat), dishes are predominantly based on the use of bread, vegetables, legumes and, to a lesser extent, meat (including local handmade

sausages) and river fish. Moreover, and similarly to other Portuguese regions, the Alentejo gastronomy makes considerable use of regional wine and olive oil, which are highly valued by national and international consumers (Amaral, Saraiva, Rocha, & Serra, 2015).

In the context of the "experience economy", however, the technical quality of food products is no longer the lead driver of customer satisfaction. In affluent societies, food has gone beyond its role in fulfilling basic survival needs and has primarily become a medium for experiences (Jacobsen, 2008). From this perspective, understanding what shapes consumer perception of food products has become of paramount importance.

In restaurant settings, customers construe their experience by systematically collecting information and organizing their perceptions into a set of feelings about the service (Berry, Wall, & Carbone, 2006). Restaurant menus are amongst the most influential environmental cues, as they convey material and immaterial meanings. Material meaning refers to the presentation of the products themselves (i.e., the available offer of food and beverage), while immaterial meaning relates to the role of menus in shaping customers' perceptions of the restaurant experience (Ozdemir & Caliskan, 2014).

Previous research has presented convincing evidence that the naming and description of food products may change consumers' perception of different attributes. For instance, naming food-items using "geographic", "nostalgic" or "sensory" labels (e.g., "succulent Italian seafood filet") positively influenced sensory expectations and changed customer's calorie estimation, comparatively to its regularly named counterparts (i.e., "seafood filet") (Wansink, van Ittersum, & Painter, 2005). "Family" and "tradition" labels have been shown to have a positive effect on sales (Guéguen & Jacob, 2012), while attractively named vegetables have been observed to be preferred by children (Wansink, Just, Payne, & Klinger, 2012).

As these studies seem to suggest, prior expectations towards food products may have significant effects on decision making and subsequent post-consumption evaluations. Despite the growing evidence on the effects of food-item labeling on domains such as sales, value perception or sensory profiling, less attention has been paid to perceived authenticity and consumer experience with traditional gastronomy.

In the present study, we explored the influence of a descriptive menu, using "authenticity" and "sensory" labels, on the perception of traditional dishes from the region of Alentejo and in the formation of expectations towards a traditional restaurant.

## 2 MATERIALS AND METHODS

Participants were recruited via email and social media networks. A total of 564 adults were enrolled and 493 completed the entire survey. 255 subjects were assigned to the intervention group and 238 to the control group.

The study was conducted online, using the Limesurvey platform. Informed consent was obtained for all participants before data collection. After agreeing with the terms of participation, each participant was randomly assigned a number of "0" or "1", which led to the intervention or control branch. Despite this randomization scheme, the higher dropout rate in the Control condition caused the two experimental groups to be mildly uneven.

The first section of the survey was common to both conditions and included items of sociodemographic characterization (e.g., age, gender, place of birth and place of residence). Frequency of restaurant use was assessed with a 9-point scale (1 = "Five times per week or more" to 9 = "Once a year or less") and self-perceived knowledge of the Alentejo gastronomy was assessed using a 5-point scale (1 = "None" to 5 = "Very Good"). For assessing participant's perception and attitudes towards the regional gastronomy of Alentejo, a 12-item questionnaire was developed,

using a 7-point Likert scale (1 = "totally disagree" to 7 = "totally agree"). Items were related to the dimensions of healthiness (e.g., energy-density, salt and fat content), hedonic appeal (e.g., taste, overall liking and positive impression), and authenticity (e.g., being traditional, use of local products and ingredients' traceability).

In the second block of the experiment, participants were presented with one of two restaurant menus. Both menus included traditional dishes from the region of Alentejo, including meat, fish and vegetarian foods. These dishes were selected from an official publication, issued by the Regional Office of Tourism (*Carta Gastronómica do Alentejo;* Confraria Gastronómica do Alentejo, 2013), and were assessed based on the use of local ingredients and traditional cooking methods. The final menu comprised five highly popular recipes, that were deemed to be iconic of the region's gastronomy. In the control menu, dishes were presented by their most common name (in bold), followed by the main ingredients, listed immediately below (e.g., "Açorda Alentejana" – Alentejo bread, garlic, olive oil, water, coriander and egg). In the intervention menu, dish names were presented with the same wording and formatting, followed by a description using sensory (e.g., "creamy egg") and authenticity labels (e.g., "genuine Alentejo bread"). Attention was paid so that the mentioned ingredients would be equivalent in both conditions, thus differing solely in the way they were described. The menus were presented as pictures in portrait format, with a neutral design (black font over white background) and prices were omitted, in an effort to avoid any confounding effects.

For each dish, participants were asked to rate their hedonic expectations ("Please, indicate how much you'd expect to like this dish") and choice intention ("Please, indicate how likely you'd be to choose this dish for your meal"), using a 7-point scale (1 = "extremely unlikely" to 7 = "extremely likely"). Willingness-to-pay was assessed with one item ("Please, indicate how much you'd be willing to pay for this dish"), using a scale of €6 to €35.

After the food-item assessment, participants were asked to imagine the restaurant to which the menu pertained and answer 10 additional questions. One item was used for assessing overall perceived restaurant quality, using a 5-star system. This choice of scale is justified by the Portuguese consumers' familiarity with the system for the hotel and restaurant sector. Nine additional items were developed for assessing more specific aspects of participants' attitudes and expectations towards the restaurant, comprising desirability, ambience, service quality and healthiness and authenticity of products served, using a 7-point Likert scale (1 = "totally disagree" to 7 = "totally agree").

Data analysis was conducted with IBM SPSS Statistics (version 24.0.). All data were analyzed using descriptive statistics and normality and homoscedasticity were evaluated with Kolmogorov-Smirnoff and Levene tests, respectively. Since data did not conform to these presupposes, non-parametric Mann-Whitney test was used to compare control and intervention groups for each evaluated parameter. Statistical significance was considered for p < .05.

## 3 RESULTS

Basic sample demographics are presented in Table 1. In the total study sample, 70.1% were female and mean age was 40.8 (SD = 12.4). Most participants (85%) held an academic degree and their knowledge of the Alentejo gastronomy was high (60.9% "good" or "very good" vs. only 8,3% "scarce" and 0% "none"). No significant differences were found between intervention and control groups regarding Age (p = .84), Gender (p = .08), Education (p = .97), Frequency of restaurant use (p = .56) or Knowledge of the Alentejo gastronomy (p = .64).

Table 1. Sociodemographic statistics for Control and Intervention groups.

|  | Control (n = 238) | Intervention (n = 255) | Total Sample (n = 493) |
|---|---|---|---|
| Gender (% Female) | 66,4% | 73,6% | 70,1% |
| Age (mean) (SD) | 40,66 (12,13) | 40,89 (12,66) | 40,78 (12,39) |
| Education (% higher education) | 82,4% | 87,4% | 85% |

At the food-item level, results of Mann-Whitney U test revealed no significant differences regarding hedonic expectations, choice intention or willingness-to-pay for any of the five dishes. In this context, descriptive menus, using sensory and authenticity labels, were ineffective in influencing participants' intended behavior towards food.

The overall quality assessment of the fictitious restaurant, using the 5-star rating system, did not differ significantly between the two experimental conditions. However, 4 out of the 9 items assessing attitudes and expectations towards the restaurant resulted in significant differences (see Table 2). The restaurant associated with the intervention menu was considered to offer a higher-quality service ($U = 26223,50$, p = .009, $Mdn_c = 5$ vs. $Mdn_i = 6$), serve tastier food ($U = 26810,00$, p = .023, $Mdn_c = 6$ vs. $Mdn_i = 6$), use fresher ingredients ($U = 26622,50$, p = .019, $Mdn_c = 5$ vs. $Mdn_i = 6$), and have a more pleasant ambience ($U = 26555,00$, p = .016, $Mdn_c = 5$ vs. $Mdn_i = 6$). No significant differences were found on items more directly related to the experimental manipulation, namely, perceived authenticity and tradition, use of regional products or employment of traditional cooking methods.

## 4 DISCUSSION

In this experimental online study, we tested the hypothesis that a descriptive menu could shape participants'

Table 2. Mann-Whitney U test results for experimental and control groups' ratings of the restaurant's attributes.

|  |  | n | Mdn | U | p-value |
|---|---|---|---|---|---|
| 1. Authenticity/ Tradition | C | 238 | 6 | 30203,00 | .924 |
|  | I | 255 | 6 |  |  |
| 2. Use of regional products | C | 238 | 6 | 28546,50 | .228 |
|  | I | 255 | 6 |  |  |
| 3. Service quality | C | 238 | 5 | 26223,50 | .009** |
|  | I | 255 | 6 |  |  |
| 4. Use of typical recipes | C | 238 | 6 | 29104,00 | .451 |
|  | I | 255 | 6 |  |  |
| 5. Extremely desirable | C | 238 | 6 | 28268,50 | .199 |
|  | I | 255 | 6 |  |  |
| 6. Tasty food | C | 238 | 6 | 26810,00 | .023* |
|  | I | 255 | 6 |  |  |
| 7. Healthy food | C | 238 | 4 | 28426,50 | .245 |
|  | I | 255 | 5 |  |  |
| 8. Fresh Ingredients | C | 238 | 5 | 26622,50 | .019* |
|  | I | 255 | 6 |  |  |
| 9. Pleasant ambience/ environment | C | 238 | 5 | 26555,00 | .016* |
|  | I | 255 | 6 |  |  |

*p < .05; **p < .01
C = Control Group; I = Intervention Group

perception of the Alentejo gastronomy and expectations towards a fictitious regional restaurant. Overall results did not support this hypothesis at the food-item level. However, participants in the descriptive menu condition had more favorable expectations towards the restaurant's service quality, ambience, and food taste and freshness.

One relevant factor in making sense of these results is the sample's high knowledge of the region's gastronomy. As previously mentioned, the dishes that composed the menus were considered "iconic" in the context of the Alentejo cuisine. Consequently, we may hypothesize that the dishes alone can elicit high perceived authenticity, regardless of the experimental manipulation. In fact, the median ratings of restaurant's authenticity and use of typical recipes is high in both conditions, suggesting that a "ceiling effect" could have taken place. Thereby, further research would be necessary in order to explore the possible mediator role of knowledge in shaping perceived authenticity of regional gastronomy. This distinction would be particularly relevant for the local industry, in face of a recent upsurge in tourist interest requiring adaptations to a new, less knowledgeable consumer profile (INE, 2019).

Despite the extensive research on the influence of restaurant menus on consumer behavior (e.g., Ozmedir & Caliskan, 2015), the evidence is still scarce on the influence of item description on perceived authenticity and traditionality. One of the few studies in this area showed that using traditional labels may influence choice for some food-items (e.g., fish and dessert) but not others (e.g., salad and meat) (Guéguen & Jacob, 2012). Likewise, it is not known whether such a labeling strategy could be generalizable to different cuisines and, particularly, to highly traditional gastronomies.

While labeling strategies mostly target consumers' affective response and food choice, manipulating the complexity of food-item has been predominantly associated with quality perception, price expectation (McCall & Lynn, 2008) and value assignment (Shoemaker, Dawson, & Johnson, 2005). As consumers seem to expect more information from higher-range restaurants (e.g., Mills & Thomas, 2008), descriptive complexity is more likely to be associated with a concept of fine dining than with regional or traditional gastronomy. This may help explain the present study's paradoxical results, in which the fictitious restaurant was perceived as having a higher quality service, but not as being more authentic or traditional, despite the employment of "sensory" and "tradition" labels.

Another important limitation of the present study is that it was conducted online, using a simulated menu. Extending menu research to restaurant settings could allow for a better understanding of "real world" decision making and to an improvement in ecological validity.

## 5 CONCLUSIONS

Consistent with previous research, the present study showed that manipulating menu description can have a positive effect on consumers' perception. The evidence in this regard is, however, often mixed or inconsistent. Future research should help elucidate the potential use of different descriptive strategies for enhancing customers' perception at the food-item level and its generalizability to different types of food.

In conclusion, the words by which food is presented and described may convey more meaning than what meets the eye. They can elicit memories, feelings and thoughts that influence expectations and, consequently, shape subsequent experience. While food quality, from a sensory perspective, is of paramount importance in the context of traditional gastronomy, it should be regarded that consumer experience is a holistic and multilayered phenomenon, resulting from the integration of numerous different cues.

Menus convey highly relevant information for customers' decision making and provide important cues for impression formation. Thereby, research on menu engineering may have important practical implications, most notably in assisting managers in designing more consistent and pleasant experiences for customers.

## ACKNOWLEDGEMENTS

This paper was funded by National funds through FCT under the project UID/AGR/00115/2013. Funding was additionally provided by POCTEP under the project Sabor Sur – and by FCT – Portuguese Science Foundation through the research contract CEECIND/04397/2017 of Elsa Lamy, while the foundation was not involved in carrying out this study or submitting it for publication.

## REFERENCES

Amaral, R., Saraiva, M., Rocha, S., & Serra, J. (2015). Gastronomy and wines in the Alentejo Portuguese region: Motivation and satisfaction of tourists from Évora. In *Wine and Tourism: A Strategic Segment for Sustainable Economic Development.* https://doi.org/10.1007/978-3-319-18857-7_13

Berry, L. L., Wall, E. A., & Carbone, L. P. (2006). Service clues and customer assessment of the service experience: Lessons from marketing. *Academy of Management Perspectives, 20*, 43–57.

Chang, R. C. Y., Kivela, J., & Mak, A. H. N. (2010). Food preferences of Chinese tourists. *Annals of Tourism Research.* https://doi.org/10.1016/j.annals.2010.03.007

Confraria Gastronómica do Alentejo (2013). *Carta Gastronómica do Alentejo.* Beja: Entidade Regional de Turismo do Alentejo

Guéguen, N., & Jacob, C. (2012). The effect of menu labels associated with affect, tradition and patriotism on sales. *Food Quality and Preference.* https://doi.org/10.1016/j.foodqual.2011.07.001

Instituto Nacional de Estatística (2018). *Estatísticas do Turismo 2018.* Lisboa: INE

Jacobsen, J. K. (2008). The food and eating experience. In J. Sundbo, & P. Darmer (eds.), *Creating Experiences in the Experience Economy* (pp. 13–32). Cheltenham, UK: Edward Elgar Publishing

Lin, Y. C., Pearson, T. E., & Cai, L. A. (2011). Food as a form of Destination Identity: A Tourism Destination Brand Perspective. *Tourism and Hospitality Research.* https://doi.org/10.1057/thr.2010.22

McCall, M., & Lynn, A. (2008) The Effects of Restaurant Menu Item Descriptions on Perceptions of Quality, Price, and Purchase Intention. *Journal of Foodservice Business Research*, 11(4), 439–445. doi: 10.1080/15378020802519850

Mills, J. E., & Thomas, L. (2008). Assessing customer expectations of information provided on restaurant menus: A Confirmatory Factor Analysis approach. *Journal of Hospitality & Tourism Research, 32*(1), 62–88. doi: 10.1177/1096348007309569

Ozdemir, B., & Caliskan, O. (2014). A review of literature on restaurant menus: Specifying the managerial issues. International Journal of Gastronomy and Food Science, 2, 3–13. http://dx.doi.org/10.1016/j.ijgfs.2013.12.001

Ozdemir, B., & Caliskan, O. (2015). Menu Design: A Review of Literature. *Journal of Foodservice Business Research, 18*(3), 189–206. https://doi.org/10.1080/15378020.2015.1051428

Shoemaker, S., Dawson, M., & Johnson, W. (2005). How to increase menu prices without alienating your customers. *International Journal of Contemporary Hospitality Management, 17*(7), 553–568. doi: 10.1108/09596110510620636

Wansink, B., Just, D. R., Payne, C. R., & Klinger, M. Z. (2012). Attractive names sustain increased vegetable intake in schools. *Preventive Medicine.* https://doi.org/10.1016/j.ypmed.2012.07.012

Wansink, B., van Ittersum, K., & Painter, J. E. (2005). How descriptive food names bias sensory perceptions in restaurants. *Food Quality and Preference.* https://do.org/10.1016/j.foodqual.2004.06.005

*Experiencing Food: Designing Sustainable and Social Practices – Bonacho, Pires & Lamy (Eds)*
*© 2021 Taylor & Francis Group, London, ISBN 978-0-367-49414-8*

# Seaweeds: An ingredient for a novel approach for artisanal dairy products

B. Campos, J.P. Noronha & P. Mata
*LAQV, REQUIMTE, Departamento de Química, Faculdade de Ciências e Tecnologia, Universidade Nova de Lisboa, Caparica, Portugal*

M. Diniz
*UCIBIO, REQUIMTE, Departamento de Química, Faculdade de Ciências e Tecnologia, Universidade Nova de Lisboa, Caparica, Portugal*

A. Henriques
*Granja dos Moinhos, Maçussa, Portugal*

ABSTRACT: Seaweeds are a food resource valued since early times. In recent years its global demand has grown significantly – food security is becoming a problem and the introduction of seaweeds in food is seen as being of major importance in economic, nutritional, health and environmental terms. This work describes the development, in a cheese factory, of dairy products enriched with seaweeds (*Palmaria palmata*, *Porphyra* spp. and *Ulva* spp.). Qualitative sensory evaluations of the dairy products were performed by a focus group. The cheese was evaluated as a moderately appealing product and suggestions were made for its improvement. Butter was extremely well accepted. A handmade packaging for butter, was developed using dry leaves of 'Palha de Tabugo' (*Typha domingensis*) resulting in an attractive and eco-friendly artisanal package. This work intends to contribute to increase the introduction of seaweeds in the Portuguese diet and to promote innovation in the artisanal sector.

*Keywords*: Seaweeds, Dairy Products, Cheese, Butter, Artisanal Food

## 1 INTRODUCTION

Seaweeds are thallophytes: plants lacking roots, stems and leaves (Lee, 2008). They are multicellular and photosynthetic algae, whose stipes reveal a high degree of complexity and tissue organization. They belong to Eukarya Domain, Plantae and Chromista Kingdoms, and are generally classified into three main phyla: Chlorophyta (green algae), Rhodophyta (red algae) and Heterokontophyta (brown algae) (Pereira, 2016).

Seaweeds have been part of the diet of coastal population since early times, as proven by archaeological discoveries from 14,000 yBP in southern Chile (Dillehay et al., 2008; Mouritsen, 2012; Wells et al., 2016). Many different species have been used as food all over the world, specially by Asian cultures (e.g. China, Japan and Korea), and also in the Pacific (e.g. Indonesia, Philippines, New Zealand and Hawai) (McHugh, 2003; Mouritsen, 2012; Mouritsen, 2013; Mouritsen et al., 2018; Yuan, 2007). In Europe (e.g. France, Iceland, Ireland and Wales) and America (e.g. Peru, Chile and Canadian Maritimes) exists a traditional, but not very intensive consumption of seaweeds (McHugh, 2003; Mouritsen, 2018; Yuan, 2007).

Recently the global demand of seaweeds for food purposes has been gradually increasing due to a growing awareness about well-being, sustainability and their general health benefits (Cardoso et al., 2015; del Olmo et al., 2018; Roohinejad et al., 2017). The popularity of sushi and Asian cuisine in western countries has also contributed to increase seaweeds consumption (Rioux et al., 2017).

Seaweeds are a good source of several key nutrients as minerals (e.g. Ca, Fe, K, Mg, Mn, Na and Zn), trace elements, vitamins (e.g. B-complex and A, D, E, K and C), proteins and essential amino acids (e.g. alanine, arginine, glycine and proline), soluble and insoluble dietary fibers, carotenoids, carbohydrates (e.g. cellulose, xylan and fucoidan), lipids ($\omega$-3 and $\omega$-6 polyunsaturated fatty acids) and antioxidant components (e.g. polyphenols and phlorotannins) (Cardoso et al., 2015; del Olmo et al., 2018; Mouritsen, 2012; Peng et al., 2015; Pereira, 2016; Rioux et al., 2017).

Human consumption of seaweeds can be part of the solution to the urgent need of finding additional sustainable ways to feed a hungry planet with a smaller carbon footprint (Mouritsen, 2013; Mouritsen et al., 2018). Several studies show that the addition of seaweeds to food products (e.g. meat, fish or plant-based products) can improve the shelf-life and nutritional, textural, organoleptic, sensory and health properties (Roohinejad et al., 2017).

Dairy products are widely consumed and rich in essential nutrients such as proteins (e.g. casein), lipids (e.g. triglycerides, cholesterol, monoacylglycerols and free fatty acids), minerals (Ca, K, P, Mg and Zn) and vitamins (A, D, $B_2$, $B_3$ and $B_{12}$),among others (Cifelli et al., 2011; Domínguez, 2013; Kwak et al., 2013). Seaweeds have already been added to dairy products (e.g. yogurt and cheese) to improve their functionality, and nutritional and organoleptic quality (del Olmo et al., 2018; Domínguez, 2013; Roohinejad et al., 2017).

Artisanal cheeses supplemented with seaweeds are currently offered in the market. Examples of these are: 'Le Ti Pavez', 'Tomme d'Iroise aux algues' and 'Embrun aux algues', from Brittany (France). 'Carrigaline Dillisk Seaweed Cheese' (a semisoft cheese) and some hard cheeses as 'Dilliskus', 'Beenoske' and 'Aran Goats Cheese with Dillisk' are produced in Ireland (Hell et al., 2017).

According to Hell et al. (2017) there is a lack of research about the impact of adding seaweeds to cheese. Nevertheless, recently a semi-hard cheese whose curd was supplemented with 1% dehydrated seaweed showed significant differences in pH value, dry matter and antioxidant activity, among other parameters, when compared to the control cheese (del Olmo et al., 2018).

In Ireland, in the 5th century, Dulse (*Palmaria palmata*) was used as a condiment in butter, and dried Dulse is still eaten between two pieces of buttered bread (Mouritsen et al., 2013). However, some authors consider that the first butter containing seaweeds was created by the butter and cheese craftsman Jean-Yves Bordier in 1986. 'Le Beurre Bordier' gained notability thanks to Eric Lecerf, a former head chef of Joël Robuchon (Bordier, 2018). Subsequently, in 2016, a seaweed butter with *Saccharina latissima*, was developed by gastronomist Mortan í Hamrabyrgi in collaboration with seaweeds producers and a supermarket chain of the Faroe Islands (Olavson, 2016).

Research suggest that the consumption of seaweed butter with a high iodine content is a good way to prevent iodine deficiency (Ochkolyas, 2015).

The main purpose of work described in this paper is the development of two artisanal dairy products (butter and goat milk cheese) supplemented with autochthonous seaweeds from the Portuguese coastline. Their quality, from sustainability, organoleptic, nutritional and health points of view, should contribute to the promotion, reinforcement of commercial strategies and competitiveness of a particular artisanal food sector, and valorize small producers and the local/regional economy.

## 2 MATERIALS AND METHODS

### 2.1 *Seaweeds*

Tok de Mar[®] 100% natural dehydrated edible seaweeds (produced through sustainable aquaculture practices by ALGA+[®] Production and Trading of Seaweed and Derived Products Ltd, Ílhavo, Portugal) (Tok de Mar, 2016) – *Palmaria palmata* Linnaeus F. Weber & D. Mohr (Dulse), *Porphyra* spp. (Nori) and *Ulva* spp. (Sea Lettuce).

Dehydrated seaweeds were partially grinded to small pieces (±1 cm) using a manual blender (Philips, HR7625/70/AC).

### 2.2 *Cheese manufacture*

Dairy products were developped at 'Granja dos Moinhos', a cheese factory based at Maçussa (39°11′37.7″N 8°51′47.5″W), Azambuja (NUTS III), Portugal, whose owner is a Slow Food member (Barbosa & Turaventur, 2015). This cheesemonger is the only artisanal producer of 'chèvre' cheese in Portugal – at 'Granja dos Moinhos' everything is handmade, unique, and high quality. The factory is certified as following all food safety (HACCP) requirements.

The milk is obtained from Saanen and Serrana goat breeds (*Capra aegagrus hircus*). The first one, native to the Saanen Valley of Switzerland, is widely recognized as the world's highest milk producing breed (Devendra & Haenlein, 2011; Solaiman, 2010). The second one, is the most representative of the Portuguese caprine breeds, constituting about 45% of the total goat population (Almendra 1994).

Cured cheese was manufactured using raw goat milk (pH 6.8). Coagulant (lamb rennet extract of 1:15,000 strength, 80% chymosin, 20% pepsin, Company Biostar S.A., Toledo, Spain) was added to the milk that coagulated at 32°C for 120 minutes. The curd was then cut into pieces, and hand pressed with a cloth to drain whey.

Subsequently, the curd was supplemented with each of the three previously selected seaweeds, salted with 1% of NaCl, mixed and shaped into 12 cm diameter steel moulds. The cheese was turned over every day and cured for 30 days at room temperature (Figure 1).

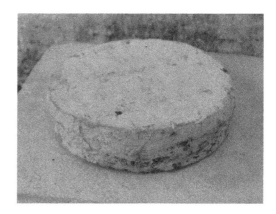

Figure 1. Cured goat milk cheese supplemented with seaweeds.

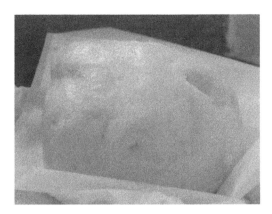

Figure 2. Traditional 'Granja dos Moinhos' goat butter.

### 2.3 Butter manufacture

Goat milk butter was obtained by following the traditional method until butter grains (fatty phase) and buttermilk (aqueous phase) were formed. The butter grains were hand pressed and running water was used to harden and control the size of the butter grains, as well as to remove the traces of buttermilk (Figure 2). Subsequently, butter was salted with 1.2% of NaCl and stored at ±5°C. Flavoured seaweed butter was made adding *P. palmata*, *Porphyra* spp. and *Ulva* spp. cuted into smal pieces (3 ± 1 mm).

### 2.4 Butter packaging

Seaweed flavoured goat butter was wrapped with dry leaves of *Typha domingensis* Pers. Steud. ('Palha de Tabugo'), tied with raffia (*Raphia* spp.) and stamped with 'Granja dos Moinhos' label.

### 2.5 Focus group discussion

A group of five participants (3 females and 2 males aged between 29 and 58 years old), without any taste disorders or food intolerances, and having similar backgrounds related to the research topic was selected (Hennink, 2014). All participants work at Faculdade de Ciências e Tecnologia, Universidade Nova de Lisboa (Portugal).

The focus group discussion lasted for about 60 min and was carried out in a comfortable circle seating, natural light and tape-recorded environment (Hennink, 2014; Kruger, 2002). The cheese was sliced, and the butter was provided in a single container. Slices of wheat bread and tap water were available.

The focus group was led by a single moderator. A brief introduction was made, followed by an overview of the topic and the main rules and characteristics of a focus group. Some pre-determined questions related to cheese and butter eating habits (frequence, occasion (meal), type, simple/cooked) and choice factors were asked. This was followed by a qualitative sensory evaluation of the products and a discussion about their positive and negative attributes, their compatibility with the Portuguese taste, and purchase intention.

### 3 RESULTS AND DISCUSSION

Two products were obtained from goat milk: (1) a ripened cheese supplemented with dehydrated seaweeds (*Palmaria palmata*, *Porphyra* spp. and *Ulva* spp.) and (2) a flavoured seaweed butter with the same dehydrated seaweeds.

According to Krueger (1998) and Guerrero et al. (2009), the most efficient way to get preliminary insights about food products, from a consumer's point of view is through qualitative research techniques, especially by using focus group discussions (Guerrero et al., 2009; Krueger, 1988). This was the selected method in this work.

When asked about their cheese consumption habits, a daily basis consumption was reported by two participants; other two participants eat cheese regularly, 2 to 3 times a week; one participant only eats cheese once every 2 weeks. Cow cheese (e.g. Flamengo) is the main cheese consumed, being complex cheeses such as 'Chèvre' or 'Brie' less consumed (once or twice a month). Cheese is consumed at all meals: breakfast, lunch, snack and before or after dinner, usually with bread or toasts.

Although cheese has been used as a cooking ingredient since Roman times in order to create an extensive array of dishes (Guinne & Kilcawley, 2004). Only one participant referred using cheese for this purpose ('Chèvre' wrapped in puff pastry baked in the oven, served with raspberry jam and also for lasagne').

Cheese preferences differed among participants. While some of them like salty cheeses, others prefer them with low-salt content or even without salt. Flavour and texture are the factors of choice most reported by participants. All the participants preferred lower intense cheeses on a day-to-day basis and highly intense cheeses at dinner, specially at special occasions.

When analysing the cheese supplemented with seaweeds (Figure 3), there was no consensus about the appearance of the cheese; most participants considered it attractive, although one of them strongly disliked it considering it too rustic.

Goat milk cheese is characterized by an intense smell which results from a relatively high proportion of short-chain fatty acids and medium-chain triglycerides (Amigo et al., 2011). According to Ha & Lindsay (1991), 4-ethyl-octanoic acid is the primary compound responsible for the goaty-type aromatic notes in goat milk cheese. Two participants referred that they do not like goat milk cheese due to its intense smell, and only one participant enumerated the cheese smell as a positive attribute.

Some negatives attributes were used to describe the cheese flavour as 'strange', 'unpleasant', 'smoky' and 'repulsive'. Some researchers agree that cheeses

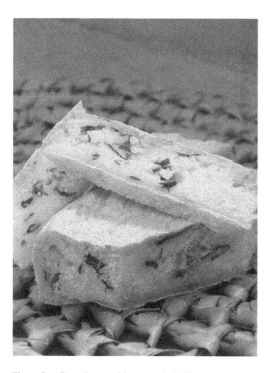

Figure 3.    Goat cheese with seaweeds in slices.

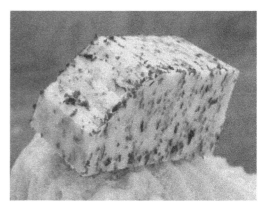

Figure 4.    Butter with three types of seaweeds (*Ulva* spp., *P. palmata* and *Porphyra* spp.).

made from raw milk develop a more intense flavour than those from pasteurized milk, because certain indigenous lactic acid bacteria of raw milk contribute positively to cheese flavour (Fox, 1993; Fox et al., 2017). However, it should be noticed that cheese is a dynamic product, and its flavour is constantly evolving during the stage of ripening and the range of cheese flavours varies from mild bland dairy notes to intensely putrid, overpowering and nauseous (Fox et al., 2017).

One of the participants referred a 'strange' or 'smoky' flavour which he considered the result of the combination between cheese and seaweeds. This participant confirmed this after tasting the same cheese without seaweeds addition. This can be attributed to the use of *P. palmata* seaweed, which according to Mouritsen et al. (2013) can be fried to a crisp and used as substitute for fried bacon, i.e., *P. palmata* could have developed a 'smoky' flavour when dehydrated.

Relative to the texture, participants considered that both cheeses (with and without seaweeds) were too dry, crumbling very easily. It is known that some cheeses made from raw milk ripen much quickly than pasteurized milk cheeses (Fox, 1993).

Concerning to butter, all the participants, except one, regularly consume cow butter. Two participants only consume butter without salt. Among the participants who eat butter, they all consume it at breakfast, usually with bread. Only one participant uses it in cooking preparations (e.g. chocolate cake). For the participants creaminess, low-salt content and flavour are the more important and decisive factors in the choice of butter.

After analysis of the butter attributes, all the participants appreciated its appearance (Figure 4). Butter flavour was very positively evaluated, however one participant mentioned a 'smoky' after-taste similar to that referred for the cheese.

Only one participant did not like the flavour of the butter. The participant who referred not consuming butter, made a positive evaluation saying: 'I like the jammy feeling that butter gives me'.

Since ancient times seaweeds have been used to replace salt in food. The sodium content of seaweeds is significantly lower than that of saltwater (Mouritsen, 2013) thus allowing to produce products with less sodium content without compromising their flavour. The saltiness of butter was considered balanced by the participants.

Regarding flavour compatibility of both dairy products with the Portuguese consumers habits, all participants defended a dual position: on the one hand, urban consumers will be the most prone to experience these types of products; on the other hand, the traditional consumers would be reluctant to accept them. According to Almli et al. (2011), tradition and innovation can be difficult to combine, because consumers tend to reject innovations that affect the traditional foods characteristics. Their degree of acceptance is dependent on the product and the type of innovation (Almli et al., 2011; Guerrero et al., 2009). In the case of cheeses, well accepted innovations in traditional products are those that reinforce the traditional and authentic character of them (Almli et al., 2011).

Participants were also questioned about their purchase intentions relatively to these two products. All the participants said that they would buy the butter, but not to use every day, just for special occasions, events and meetings. The participant that usually do not consume butter said that he would buy it to consume regularly, about twice a week. With respect to the cheese, only three participants would buy it to eat with

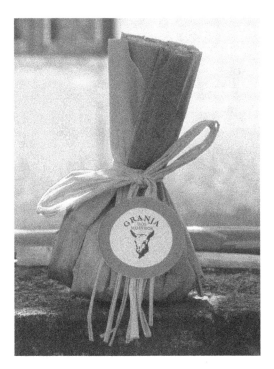

Figure 5. Flavoured butter packaged with *Typha domingensis* ('Palha de Tabugo').

friends on special occasions. However, they considered that an improvement of the texture is required.

The handmade butter packaging was based in a craft way common to preserve several food products. Currently, rigid and semi-rigid plastic packages are the most common commercial structures to contain foods (Brody & Lord, 2000), but in recent years the interest in the recycling of packaging materials has increased (Davis & Song 2006), as the amount of packaging waste became a serious environmental problem (Markowicz et al., 2019). In order to avoid these problems and to confer a distinct and attractive look to the seaweed butter, a handmade packaging, based on tradition, was developed at 'Granja dos Moinhos' (Figure 5). It is made from a spontaneous helophyte plant used by the population at Maçussa to seal wine barrels, and the result is an eco-friendly artisanal package.

## 4 CONCLUSIONS

Food acceptance depends on cultural aspects, habits and lifestyles, and innovation can cause a certain resistance. Introducing new food products enriched with seaweeds can be a challenge and strategies are being developed to overcome resistance. Introducing seaweeds in products usually consumed by the Portuguese – butter and cheese – is part of this strategy.

Artisanal production of cheese can be a difficult and long process that involves trial and error. The prototype cheese developed was moderately accepted by the focus group and requires further development. Comments and suggestions resulting from the focus group discussion will be used to optimize the final product. Other seaweeds will be tested, not only in mixtures but also using a single seaweed. Moreover, tests with other types of cheeses will also be made.

The high acceptance of the seaweed butter can lead to its production in a larger scale and to the development of similar products with different organoleptic characteristics, using different types of seaweeds or butters.

The results obtained show the potential of these new products to achieve the main purposes of the study. Finally, this work can also contribute to promote the introduction of seaweeds in the Portuguese diet, as well as innovation in the artisanal food sector and the valorisation of small producers, important aspects for the development of the local/regional economy.

## ACKNOWLEDGEMENTS

The authors gratefully acknowledge the financial support provided by the project "MAR-01.03.01-FEAMP-0016 – Alga4Food". This project has the financial support of the European Maritime and Fisheries Fund and is co-financed by the Operational Program MAR2020 in the field of Sustainable Development of Aquaculture in the domains of Innovation, Advice and Productive Investment – Innovation and knowledge Action.

This work was also supported by the Associate Laboratory for Green Chemistry – LAQV and UCIBIO – Applied Molecular Biosciences Unit funded by national funds from FCT/MCTES (UID/QUI/50006/2013 and UID/Multi/04378/2019 respectively) and co-financed by the ERDF under the PT2020 Partnership Agreement (POCI-01-0145-FEDER-007265).

## REFERENCES

Almendra, L. 1994. Agricultura Transmontana. ANCRAS (Associação Nacional de Caprinicultores da Raça Serrana).

Almli, V.L., Næs, T., Enderli, G., Sulmont-Rossé, C., Issanchou, S. & Hersleth, M. 2011. Consumers' acceptance of innovations in traditional cheese. A comparative study in France and Norway. *Appetite* 57(1): 110–120.

Amigo, L. & Fontecha, J. Goat Milk. 2011. In Fuquay, J.W., Fox, P.F. & McSweeney, P.L.H. (Eds.). *Encyclopedia of Dairy Sciences*. London: Academic Press.

Barbosa, A. & Turaventur. 2015. Roteiros Enogastronómicos do Ribatejo. Évora: Caminho das Palavras.

Bordier, J.-Y. 2018. Le Beurre aux Algues. *La Fromagee Jean-Yves Bordier*. Retrieved (http://www.lebeurrebordier.com/).

Brody, A.L. & Lord, J.B. 2000. *Developing New Food Products for a Changing Marketplace*. Florida: CRC Press.

Cardoso, S.M., Pereira, O.R., Seca, A.M., Pinto, D.C. & Silva, A.M. 2015. Seaweeds as Preventive Agents for Cardiovascular Diseases: From Nutrients to Functional Foods. *Marine drugs* 13(11): 6838–6865.

Cifelli, C.J., German, J.B. & O'Donnell, J.A. 2011. Nutritional and Health-Promoting Properties of Dairy Products: Contribution of Dairy Foods to Nutrient Intake. In Fuquay, J.W., Fox, P.F. & McSweeney, P.L.H. (Eds.). *Encyclopedia of Dairy Sciences*. London: Academic Press.

Davis, G. & Song, J.H. 2006. Biodegradable packaging based on raw materials from crops and their impact on waste management. *Industrial Crops and Products* 23(2): 147–161.

del Olmo, A., Picon, A. & Nuñez, M. 2018. Cheese supplementation with five species of edible seaweeds: Effect on microbiota, antioxidant activity, colour, texture and sensory characteristics. *International Dairy Journal* 84: 36–45.

Devendra, C. & Haenlein, G.F. 2011. Goat Breeds. *In* Fuquay, J.W., Fox, P.F. & McSweeney, P.L. (Eds.). *Encyclopedia of Dairy Sciences*. London: Academic Press.

Dillehay, T.D., Ramírez, C., Pino M., Collins M.B., Rossen, J. & Pino-Navarro, J.D. 2008. Monte Verde: Seaweed, food, medicine, and the peopling of South America. *Science* 320(5877): 784–786.

Domínguez, H. (Ed.). 2013. *Functional ingredients from algae for foods and nutraceuticals*. Cambridge: Woodhead Publishing.

Fox, P.F. 1993. Cheese: An Overview. *In* Fox, P.F & McSweeney, P.L.H. (Eds.). *Cheese: Chemistry, Physics & Microbiology*. Volume1, General Aspects. London: Elsevier Academic Press.

Fox, P.F., Guinee, T.P., Cogan, T.M. & McSweeney, P.L.H. 2017. *Fundamentals of Cheese Science*. New York: Springer.

Guerrero, L., Guàrdia, M.D., Xicola, J., Verbeke, W., Vanhoncker, F., Zahowska-Biemans, S., Sadjakowska, M., Sulmont-Rossé, C., Issanchou, S., Contel, M., Scalvedi, M.L., Granli, B.S. & Hersleth, M. 2009. Consumer-driven definition of traditional food products and innovation in traditional foods. A qualitative cross-cultural study. *Appetite* 52(2): 345–354.

Guinee, T.P. & Kilcawley, K.N. 2004. Cheese as an Ingredient. *In* Fox, P.F, McSweeney, P.L.H., Cogan, T.M. & Guinee, T.P. (Eds.). 2004. *Cheese: Chemistry, Physics & Microbiology*. Volume 2, Major Cheese Groups. London: Elsevier Academic Press.

Ha, J.K. & Lindsay, R.C. Contributions of Cow, Sheep, and Goat Milks to Characterizing Branched-Chain Fatty Acid and Phenolic Flavors in Varietal Cheeses. *Journal of Dairy Sciences* 74(10): 3267–3274.

Hell, A., Labrie, L. & Beaulieu, L. 2017. Effect of seaweed flakes addition on the development of bioactivities in functional Camembert-type cheese. *International Journal of Food Science and Technology* 53(4): 1054–1064.

Hennink, M.M. 2014. *Focus Group Discussions (Understanding qualitative Research)*. Oxford: University Press.

Krueger, R.A. 2014. *Designing and Conducting Focus Group Interviews*. St. Paul: University of Minnesota.

Kwak, H.-S., Ganesan, P. & Mijan, M.A. 2013. Butter, Ghee and Cream Products. *In* Park, Y.W. & Haenlein, G.F.W. (Eds.). *Milk and Dairy Products in Human Nutrition*. Oxford: Wiley-Blackwell Publishers.

Lee, R.E. 2008. *Phycology*. New York: Cambridge University Press.

Markowicz, F., Król, G. & Szymańska-Pulikowska, A. 2019. Biodegradable Package – Innovative Purpose or Source of the Problem. *Journal of Ecological Engineering* 20(1): 228–237.

McHugh, D.J. 2003. *A guide to the seaweed industry*. Rome: FAO.

Mouritsen, O.G. 2012. The emerging science of gastrophysics and its application to the algal cuisine. *Flavour* 1(6): 1–9.

Mouritsen, O.G. 2013. *Seaweeds: edible, available & sustainable*. Chicago & London: University of Chicago Press.

Mouritsen, O.G., Dawczynski, C., Duelund, L., Jahreis, G., Vetter, W. & Schröder, M. 2013. On the human consumption of the red seaweed dulse (*Palmaria palmata* (L.) Weber & Mohr). *Journal of Applied Phycology* 25(6): 1777–1791.

Mouritsen, O.G., Rhatigan, P. & Pérez-Lloréns, J.L. 2018. World cuisine of seaweeds: Science meets gastronomy. *International Journal of Gastronomy and Food Science* 14: 55–65.

Ochkolyas, O. 2015. The biological value of seaweed butter dressing. *Food Industry of Agroindustrial Complex* 1–44(6):45–47.

Olavson, R. 2016. Seaweed butter! *FAROEISLAND.FO. The Official Gateway to the Faroe Islands*. Retrieved (https://www.faroeislands.fo/).

Peng, Y., Hu, J., Yang, B., Lin, X.-P., Zhou, X.-F., Yang, X.-W. & Liu, Y. 2015. Chemical composition of seaweeds. *In* Tiwari, B.K. & Troy, D.J. (Eds.). *Seaweeds sustainability*. San Diego: Academic Press.

Pereira, L. 2016. *Edible Seaweeds of the World*. London: CRC Press.

Rioux, L-E, Beaulieu, L. & Turgeon, S.L. 2017. Seaweeds: A traditional ingredients for new gastronomic sensation. *Food Hydrocolloids* 68: 255–265.

Roohinejad, S., Koubaa, M., Barba, F.J., Saljoughian, S., Amid, M. & Greiner, R. 2017. Application of seaweeds to develop new food products with enhanced shelf-life, quality and health-related beneficial properties. *Food Research International* 99(Pt 3): 1066–1083.

Solaiman, S.G. 2010. *Goat Science and Production*. Iowa: Wiley-Blackwell.

Wells, M.L., Potin, P., Craigie, J.S., Raven, J.A., Merchant, S.S., Helliwell, K.E., Smith, A.G., Camire, M.E. & Brawley, S.H. 2017. Algae as nutritional and functional food sources: revisiting our understanding. *Journal of Applied Phycology* 29(2): 949–982.

Yuan, Y.V. 2007. Marine algal constituents. *In* Barrow, C. & Shahidi, F. (Eds.). *Marine nutraceuticals and functional foods*. Boca Raton, FL.

# Introduction of seaweeds in desserts: The design of a sea lettuce ice cream

B. Moreira-Leite, J.P. Noronha & P. Mata
*LAQV, REQUIMTE, Departamento de Química, Faculdade de Ciências e Tecnologia, Universidade Nova de Lisboa (FCT/UNL), Caparica, Portugal*

ABSTRACT: Marine macroalgae are complete foods through a nutritional point of view, however studies in the context of phycogastronomy are scarce. The present work intends to discuss the design and validation process of a novel food product made using the seaweed "sea lettuce" (*Ulva* sp.). First instrumental and sensory analyses of the seaweed were carried out to build a flavor profile. Then, an ice cream was formulated, evaluated by a focus group, and finally it was applied in high gastronomy dessert. Results of the analyses show that some algae, if properly processed and worked in the best way, have a potential to be introduced into various food products and recipes, including pastry formulations.

## 1 INTRODUCTION

### 1.1 *Seaweeds*

Algae are unicellular or pluricellular, photoautotrophic organisms that live in water or moist environments, with chlorophyll as the primary photosynthetic pigment. Unlike plants, there is no sterile cover in its reproductive cells (Lee, 2008). Algae form a diverse group of organisms that are differentiated by their size, color and morphology (Pereira, 2009).

Seaweeds are marine macroalgae consumed as vegetables in Japan and China for more than fifteen centuries. Its regular consumption occurs mainly in East Asia and island regions located in the Pacific Ocean. In a less extent, they are also consumed in Chile, some Northern European and Nordic countries (Pereira, 2016).

Nowadays it is possible to observe an increasing interest of the Western World – for example, North America, Iberian Peninsula and some of the European countries previously mentioned – in seaweed consumption mainly due to its alleged health benefits (Buschmann et al., 2017; Mouritsen, 2013). Another plausible explanation is the emergent use of seaweeds by chefs, which have the power of influencing people to adopt this ingredient as a food source (Mouritsen, 2012; Rioux et al., 2017).

Due to its high nutritional features, seaweeds have a great potential to be applied in food formulations: they are rich in proteins and dietary fibers, an excellent source of vitamins, minerals and trace elements, and are poor in sugars and lipids – having mainly polyunsaturated fatty acids (PUFAs), ω-3 (EPA and DHA) and ω-6 (AA) 3, in balance – which results in a low caloric intake (Mišurcová, 2012; Mouritsen, 2012).

Some of the advantages of seaweeds over other possible dietary sources are high protein levels (dry weight), rapid growth and productivity, onshore or offshore (which makes up about 70% of the earth surface) production, either alone or together with other marine organisms, in integrated multi-trophic aquaculture (IMTA) systems. Unlike livestock, one of the activities that most contributes to global warming, aquaculture of algae allows to convert carbon dioxide into biomass through photosynthesis, releasing oxygen into the atmosphere, with the advantage of not competing with other food crops for land or water (Buschmann et al., 2017).

### 1.2 *Phycogastronomy*

Phycogastronomy is a term that derives from the Greek suffix "*phukos*"[1] (φύκος) which means seaweed; and the word "gastronomy"[2], used to refer to the "study of the laws of the stomach" and that nowadays should be interpreted as the "art or science of choosing, cooking, and eating good food" (Rentería, 2007). Thus, it can be inferred that "phycogastronomy" is the art of preparing and cooking seaweed in the best way, taking advantage of its nutritional potential and enhancing or improving its organoleptic properties.

---

[1] "phyco-" in *Oxford Living Dictionaries* [online]. Oxford: Oxford University Press. Available at: https://en.oxforddictionaries.com/definition/phyco- (accessed in: 05/05/2019).

[2] "gastronomy" in *Oxford Living Dictionaries* [online]. Oxford: Oxford University Press. Available at: https://en.oxforddictionaries.com/definition/gastronomy (accessed in: 05/05/2019).

According to algaeBASE[3] there are around 10,500 catalogued species of which approximately 1500 are green, 7000 are red and 2000 are brown. However, only a small part (± 221 species) of these are considered edible and only 145 species are directly used in culinary preparations. Many edible seaweeds are also used for industrial purposes such as hydrocolloids extraction (Pereira & Correia, 2015).

Seaweeds (or sea vegetables) are highly versatile ingredients, allowing to make all sorts of preparations: drinks (specially teas), snacks, pastries, breads, salads, omelets, soups, stews and desserts, among others. They may also be used as seasoning, garnish or main ingredient (Pereira, 2016).

The seaweed "sea lettuce" (*Ulva* sp.) is characterized by the intense aroma of sea with some green notes, and should be consumed fresh, only hydrated or quickly cooked. It replaces very well leafy vegetables in salads, soups, stir fries and stews. In the Azores, this species is used in the confection of soups and "*tortas*", a sort of omelet (Mouritsen, 2013; Pereira, 2016).

### 1.3  *Ice cream*

The term "ice cream" can be applied to many different types of frozen dessert. These desserts have in common the fact that they contain ice crystals and are sweet, flavored, and usually eaten in the frozen state. Ice cream is frequently classified as premium, standard or economy. Premium ice cream is typically made from good quality ingredients, having a high amount of dairy fat and a low overrun (amount of air incorporated), whereas economy ice cream is made from low cost ingredients (for example, vegetable fat or oils) and up to 50% of the volume in air (Clarke, 2004).

The ice cream is a complex colloidal system comprised of a disperse phase of ice crystals (sol), air bubbles (foam) and fat droplets (ranging from 1 μm to 0.1 mm and forming an emulsion) and a continuous phase, also known as the matrix, made of a viscous solution of dissolved sugars, polysaccharides and milk proteins. The science of ice cream consists of understanding its ingredients, methods of preparation, microstructure and texture (as well as how these are connected). The ingredients and processing methodology create the microstructure that has a huge impact on the perceived texture. The solution coats the numerous ice crystals allowing them to bind smoothly to each other. The size of the ice crystals defines the creaminess of the ice cream, with larger crystals imparting a coarse or grainy texture, for example. The air bubbles dispersed in the ice cream weaken the matrix, making the ice cream lighter and allowing it to be eaten at low temperatures. In order to understand "one of the most complex food colloid of all" it is necessary to resort to many scientific disciplines (Clarke, 2004; Mcgee, 2004).

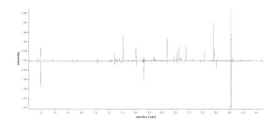

Figure 1.  Chromatograms of the fresh (above) and dried (below) "sea lettuce".

## 2   SEA LETTUCE FLAVOR PROFILE

### 2.1   *Seaweed sensory analysis*

A focus group with trained tasters, carried out in the context of a previous work (Moreira Leite, 2017), associated the flavor of the fresh "sea lettuce" with the aroma profile of fresh cut grass, green tea, seashore air and cooked cabbage or canned corn. Through sensory analysis tests of a cooked semolina pasta enriched with dried "sea lettuce", done by untrained tasters and using the "Check-All-That-Apply" (CATA) methodology, the following attributes were associated with the developed product: seaweed flavor and aroma, sea flavor and seashore aroma (Moreira Leite, 2017).

These similar, but distinct, results show how sensitive are the volatile organic compounds (VOCs) present in the "sea lettuce". In fact, a series of chemical reactions start taking place the moment the macroalgae are removed from its natural environment (Maarse, 1991). This makes seaweeds very delicate ingredients that can be easily affected by storage conditions, preserving and cooking methods (Le Pape et al., 2002; Shu & Shen, 2012).

### 2.2   *GC–MS analysis*

Analysis by gas chromatography coupled to mass spectrometry (GC–MS) showed that the volatiles profile changes with the conservation technique applied to the seaweed as emphasized in the previous section (Moreira Leite, 2017).

In Figure 1, a mirrored chromatogram of the fresh (above) and dried (below) "sea lettuce" is presented. It can be clearly seen that the seaweed loses some aromatic complexity when undergoing heat treatment[4], especially regarding to the presence of ketones and alcohols. In terms of aroma profile, this means that the samples changed from fresh, green, fatty and earthy notes to a more marine (sulfuric) and citric scent (Moreira Leite, 2017). These changes are the result of chemical reactions induced by thermal, autoxidation or enzymatic activities in which compounds as Dimethyl sulfide (DMS) and Nonanal are produced (Fujimura & Kawai, 2000; Maarse, 1991).

---

[3] *algaeBASE*. Available at: http://www.algaebase.org/ (accessed in: 05/05/2019).

[4] 25 VOCs (fresh seaweed) against 14 VOCs (dried seaweed) were identified.

### 2.3 Sea lettuce vs. green tea

Results of studies about volatile components in green tea reveals that it shares many VOCs with the "sea lettuce" (Ho et al., 2015; Maarse, 1991; Yang et al., 2018): 12 of the 14 VOCs identified in the dried sample[5] and 17 of the 25 VOCs identified in the fresh seaweed[6]. Except for the presence of some aliphatic acids, not identified in the GC–MS analysis due to extraction characteristics and methodology, in general the aroma of tea is related to the abundance of aldehydes, ketones, and alcohols presents. The key compounds for the characterization of the green tea seem to be (*E,E*)-2,4-Heptadienal, Nonanal and β-Ionone. The last two chemical compounds are possibly, along with DMS, primarily responsible for the aroma of the dried "sea lettuce" (Moreira Leite, 2017).

### 2.4 Food pairing

"Food pairing" theory is based on the following premise: the positive match of distinct foods is directly related to the amount of VOCs they share (Ahn et al., 2011). As a scientific theory, "food pairing" is the subject of several criticisms (de Klepper et al., 2011). However, food pairing has become a very useful tool for chefs and food companies when developing new dishes and novel products (Castells, 2016).

Based in the "matcha" aroma descriptor for the dried "sea lettuce"[7], and the correspondences in the main volatile compounds responsible for the aroma in both ingredients, it was decided to incorporate the dried seaweed in a sweet formulation that usually takes advantage of green tea as flavoring. This finding was the embryo for the development of the "sea lettuce" ice cream.

## 3 SEAWEED ICE CREAM DESIGN

Seaweeds are unique ingredients, adding color, texture and flavor to culinary preparations. For this reason, they are a great resource in culinary innovations (Rioux et al., 2017). Their pigments allow coloring savory and sweet dishes without resorting to synthetic dyes and some substances, such as phycobiliproteins, are endowed with fluorescence properties. Some of their hydrocolloids allow to create new textures in dishes and food formulations. Glutamic acid and the synergistic nucleosides present in macroalgae boost umami taste and enhance the overall taste of the food, allowing the reduction of salt, sugars and fats. Seaweeds can produce specific aromas, according to the type of preparation desired, because they are rich in aromatic substances (Mouritsen, 2013). The first and last highlights are relevant for the work that will be described in this paper.

### 3.1 Ice cream formulation and techniques

This section aims to detail the process of making the "sea lettuce" ice cream. The recipe for "*crème anglaise glacée*" (frozen English custard), by chef Alain Ducasse, was used as a base for the preparation of the ice cream base (Ducasse & Robert, 2005).

Instead of cooking on low heat until the custard reaches the right temperature, which has the property of pasteurizing the base and thickening through the denaturation of egg proteins, the *sous-vide* cooking method, suggested by the ChefSteps team[8], was chosen. This method involves heating the liquid ingredients, gently incorporating the liquid in the egg yolks and sugar mixture, vacuum packing the ice cream base and cooking for 45 minutes at 83°C. It is also important to sake the bag, from time to time, to ensure even cooking and to break the gel structure.

Compared to the traditional cooking techniques like *bain-marie*, *sous-vide* allows perfect temperature control and distribution, which leads to a creamy and lumps-free custard texture, prevents volatiles losses during heating and also an eggy flavor due to overcooking. Another concern regarding to ice creams is the proper pasteurization, ensuring that the preparation is safe for consumption (Myhrvold et al., 2011).

Although the use of disposable plastic for the *sous-vide* cooking embodies a sustainability dilemma, it should be empathized that this was the feasible technique to make a product with better qualities, using lab or restaurant equipment.

Stabilizers are any ingredients used to thicken the ice cream mixture, also slowing up the melting process. They make ice cream smoother, by retarding the growth of ice crystals and consequently their size. Many sugars may be added in order to lower the melting point and avoid ice recrystallization. These mechanisms are important because they can improve the texture and extend the shelf-life of the ice cream (Clarke, 2004). It was decided not to add other ingredients, such as hydrocolloids and many types of sugars (replacing part of the sucrose) based on the fact that the aim was to get an artisanal ice cream and also because of the characteristics of the equipment used to process it.

Tests were also made using the technique of extracting compounds by ultrasound as proposed by Myhrvold et al. (2011) in his encyclopedia "Modernist

---

[5] Dimethyl sulfide; Hexanal; Heptanal; Benzaldehyde; Octanal; (*E,E*)-2,4-Heptadienal; 2,2,6-Trimethylcyclohexanone; Nonanal; Decanal; β-Cyclocitral; β-Ionone; Pentadecane.

[6] Dimethyl sulfide; Hexanal; (*E*)-2-Hexenal [leaf aldehyde]; (*Z*)-4-Heptenal; Heptanal; 1-Octen-3-ol [matsutake alcohol]; (*E,E*)-2,4-Heptadienal; 2,2,6-Trimethylcyclohexanone; (*E,E*)-3,5-Octadien-2-one; Nonanal; (*E,Z*)-2,6-Nonadienal [cucumber aldehyde]; (*E*)-2-Nonenal; Decanal; β-Cyclocitral; 2,4-Decadienal; α-Ionone; β-Ionone.

[7] Obtained from a previous work (Moreira Leite, 2017).

[8] "Vanilla bean ice cream recipe" in *ChefSteps*. Available at: https://www.chefsteps.com/activities/vanilla-bean-ice-cream (accessed in: 05/05/2019).

Cuisine". High-frequency vibrations eventually accelerate the extraction because of the cell degradation, which makes particles size much smaller. The compounds present inside the cells are released to the outside, thus facilitating the extractive process (Chemat et al., 2017; Hielscher, 2018). According to the literature, the results reveal solutions much richer in aromatic compounds (volatiles or not) when compared to the traditional or *sous-vide* cooking methods. The extraction procedure consisted of packing the seaweed (2%) together with the milk and cream of the recipe – i.e., 20 g of dried seaweed per liter – and extracting the volatile compounds in the ultrasonic bath with the following settings: 60°C for 45 minutes, 100% power, 37 kHz frequency and sweep modulation.

Finally, the ice cream was frozen using 2 different techniques, i.e. the Swiss ice cream maker Pacojet[9] and with liquid nitrogen. The Pacojet has the property of making ice crystals around 5 μm by scraping, using the blades at high speed and a beaker under pressure, the surface of the frozen dessert base. The equipment also helps incorporating air (30%) and emulsifying the mixture, resulting in a very light and smooth ice cream (Mouritsen & Styrbæk, 2017; Myhrvold et al., 2011). Blumenthal (2009) was the pioneer in the use of liquid nitrogen for confectionery in "high gastronomy", such as the "Bacon and Egg Ice Cream" that was made in the presence of the customers. The great advantage of the use of liquid nitrogen (−196°C) for the preparation of ice creams is that, once the freezing is done very quickly, the formation of large ice crystals (>1 μm) and the incorporation of too much air is avoided, resulting in a dense, but with a soft texture, ice cream. This technique also allows ice creams to be made with bases with low freezing point such as alcoholic beverages (Mouritsen & Styrbæk, 2017; Myhrvold et al., 2011).

### 3.2 Ice cream preparation tests

The ice cream base was prepared according to the *sous-vide* technique. However, 3 different tests were performed, using dry seaweed and the milk and cream in the recipe as solvent, in order to test the volatile extraction: infusion, extraction with ultrasounds and cold mixing (during ice cream processing).

Infusion and the use of ultrasound did not result as expected – this can be justified by changes in the aromatic profile of the "sea lettuce" due to heating involved in both processes. For this reason, it was chosen not to apply heat and to incorporate the seaweed in the end of the preparation, which led to better results in terms of flavor.

Both freezing techniques worked well, providing very creamy and slightly aerated textures. However, Pacojet was chosen due to practical reasons and logistical aspects.

[9] "Pacojet Junior" in *Pacojet*. Available at: https://pacojet.com/en/pacojet_product/pacojet-junior-en/ (accessed in: 05/05/2019).

Table 1. Sensory analysis – affective acceptance test.

| | Appearance | Aroma | Flavor | Texture | Overall impression | Intention of consumption |
|---|---|---|---|---|---|---|
| MODE | 4 | 4 | 5 | 5 | 5 | 4 |
| MEDIAN | 4 | 4 | 4 | 5 | 4 | 4 |
| MEAN | 4.45 | 3.64 | 4.18 | 4.64 | 4.27 | 3.91 |
| STD. DEV. | 0.52 | 0.67 | 1.17 | 0.50 | 0.90 | 1.30 |

### 3.3 Ice cream focus group and sensory analysis

A focus group can be defined as a discussion panel for the purpose of obtaining qualitative information in depth. Exploratory focus groups are focused on the production of contents and can also be used to generate the knowledge necessary for the construction of measurement instruments. Its emphasis is on what makes possible to identify the relevant aspects of a target product (Hennink, 2014).

A focus group was performed to evaluate the formulation of "sea lettuce" ice cream. A script with all the relevant questions was formulated to help characterizing the developed product.

A further sensory analysis, in order to obtain some quantitative data, was performed using the "affective acceptance test" methodology (Meilgaard et al., 1999). The hedonic evaluation of the tasters regarding to aspects such as appearance, aroma, flavor, texture, overall impression and intention of consumption were obtained.

The elaborated ice cream was served in average portions of 60 g at the temperature of −9°C, along with mineral water for palate cleansing. The 11 participants completed both recruitment and evaluation forms. The assessment was made through a structured hedonic scale of 5 points, the extremes being (1) "Dislike very much" and (5) "Like very much" to qualify attributes regarding appearance, aroma, texture, taste and overall impression. In order to evaluate the intention of consumption and purchase, the "action scale", structured with 5 points, the extremes being the categories (1) "Would never consume" and (5) "Would certainly consume" (Lawless & Heimann, 2010).

The group consisted of 5 males and 6 females, of which 5 of the participants were older than 50 years old, 5 were between 36 and 50 years old and only one element was between 26 and 35 years old.

Most participants of the focus group associated the sample's flavor to seaweed and a smaller group to green tea. According to the sensory evaluation (Table 1), the positive aspects were the appearance, the texture and the flavor. Only 2 participants said they would not consume the ice cream, none remained indifferent and most of them would certainly (4) or possibly (5) consume it. One of the negatives point highlighted was the mild aroma. Despite of the good evaluation in terms of texture, 2 participants noticed the presence of small grains, perhaps by the precipitation of lactose crystals. In the future, to correct the grainy texture, it would be possible to increase the temperature of service, test a formulation with lactose-free milk or use hydrocolloids (lambda carrageenan, locust bean gum, etc.). Regarding the aroma, a higher concentration of dried "sea lettuce" (3%) should be tested. There was no consensus regarding sweetness, but most of the panel praised the fact that it was balanced and less sweet than in conventional ice cream. Almost everyone said that there was a more pronounced seaweed flavor in the end (aftertaste).

### 3.4 Application of the ice cream in a high gastronomy dessert

A dessert based in the periodic table was requested to an event, by the Portuguese Chemical Society (SPQ, from Portuguese "Sociedade Portuguesa de Química"), in order to celebrate the International Year of the Periodic Table. The four more abundant elements of the organic matter were used as a source of inspiration – i.e. carbon (C), hydrogen (H), oxygen (O) and nitrogen (N). Based on the symbols of the elements, the anagram "OH-C-N" was created. When the acronym is read it creates a sound that alludes to the word "ocean". Thus, it was decided to use the ocean as a source of inspiration and to employ the "sea lettuce" ice cream as the main element of the dish.

Because of the resemblance of the preparation with "matcha" (Japanese powdered green tea) ice cream, it was decided to join this ingredient with some ingredients that empirically create a good pairing with this frozen dessert. It is common in Japanese culture to pair matcha with "okashi" (sweet confections and dried or preserved fruits) in order to overcome the bitterness and astringency of the tea (Hosking, 2015). Seaweeds are also known for having some bitter aftertaste and astringency due to the presence of free amino acids and tannins, respectively (Mouritsen et al., 2019). Because of this, it was decided to work with some sweet elements – such as white chocolate, coconut and mango – balanced with sour notes – especially from the Greek yogurt, passion fruit and raspberry.

Two dishes from famous chefs were also a source of inspiration for the conception of the dessert (Figure 2). Blumenthal's (2009) savory dish "Sound of the Sea" is inspired by the seashore with all its main elements. This became one of the most famous dishes of "The Fat Duck" restaurant, especially because it was served with an iPod where the guests could listen to a seashore soundtrack while eating. The earphones were used to enhance the taste of the sea by the stimulation of hearing, an idea that emerged from dialogues with the experimental psychologist Charles Spence, one of the pioneers in the field of multisensoriality[10] (Blumenthal, 2009). Blumenthal was one of the first chefs to adopt the "multisensory kitchen", that

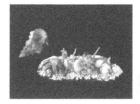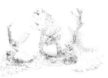

Figure 2. Left picture: Heston Blumenthal – Sound of the Sea; Right picture: Albert Adrià – Algas.

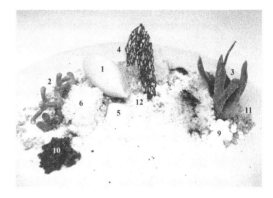

Figure 3. Dish created – OH-C-N (Ocean).

is a culinary style or "new science of eating" that considers the influence of physical stimuli, external to the food itself, as well as the emotional and mental factors, in the perception of the taste (Spence & Piqueras-Fiszman, 2014).

Mimicry is a word that comes from the Greek "mimikos" ($\mu\iota\mu\iota\kappa o\sigma$) which means "to imitate". As a culinary style, it refers to the art of creating dishes that are a faithful copy of elements or scenes from the nature. Albert and his brother, Ferran Adrià, had been exploring this concept in elBulli's kitchen for many years. However, it was only in the year of 2008, with the publication of the book "Natura", that "culinary mimicry" was materialized as a new creative style (Adrià et al., 2011).

Albert Adrià (2008) has created a dessert entitled "Algas" (seaweeds), composed of more than 10 elements, that tried to mimicry the seabed. Many of the employed techniques and dish plating were adapted from Adrià's dish.

In Figure 3 it is possible to see the final version of the "high gastronomy" dessert created, consisting of 12 preparations[11] that also try to mimetic the seabed and its elements:

1. 3% "sea lettuce" ice cream;
2. White chocolate coral covered with matcha;

---

[10] The multisensoriality, formerly Gastrophysics, is: "the combination of gastronomy and psychophysics: gastronomy being the knowledge and understanding of all that relates to man as he eats, and psychophysics being the branch of psychology that deals with the relations between physical stimuli and mental phenomena" (Spence, 2017).

[11] The items 7 and 8 cannot been seen because they are under the other elements of the dish.

3. "Chlorella" and yogurt crispy caramel (made in the dehydrator for 48 hours);
4. Raspberry coral reef (a *dentelle* covered with freeze-dried raspberry);
5. Bonbon shell (made with white chocolate and filled with mango and passion fruit);
6. Coconut sponge cake (made using a siphon and cooked in the microwave oven);
7. Greek yogurt with vanilla foam (made using hydrocolloids, a siphon and nitrous oxide charges);
8. Mango fluid gel (made with gellan gum);
9. Ginger pearls (made using the direct spherification technique and colored with potassium aluminum silicate and titanium dioxide);
10. Passion fruit roe (made with basil seeds infused in juice) and freeze-dried nibs;
11. Oats crumble;
12. Coconut powder (made with dried coconut and tapioca maltodextrin).

The service of the dish itself was again inspired by Blumenthal with the ice cream being done in front of the guests, using liquid nitrogen, some elements having pigments which glow in the dark under black light (riboflavin and phycocyanin), and a soundtrack was chosen to be played during the tasting of the dish. It was intended to create a context in which it was possible to explore the multisensory perception.

### 3.5 Health claims

A portion of 100 g of ice cream with 3% "sea lettuce" promotes a supplementation up to 8 times the daily reference intake of folic acid (vitamin $B_9$). In terms of minerals, this amount of seaweed (3 g) is able to supply the daily reference intake of: 28,19% of magnesium (Mg), 18,37% of iron (Fe) and 10,26% of manganese (Mn), among other elements in a lesser extent (FDA, 2016; Neto et al., 2018; Taboada et al., 2010).

## 4  CONCLUSIONS

Analytical chemistry (GC–MS) can be a tool, not only for compounds screening or quality control, but also for introducing new ingredients and creating new flavor pairings. This was the case in the development of the "sea lettuce" ice cream described in this paper, in which this technique was used together with sensory analysis.

The results of a focus group showed that the formulation was well accepted by the panel and some tasters associated the flavor, conferred by the seaweed "sea lettuce", with the Japanese green tea.

The introduction of the "sea lettuce" ice cream, along with *Chlorella* sp. micro-alga, in a high gastronomy shows new possibilities for the use of seaweeds in pastry.

Seaweeds are not only a sustainable ingredient; they can also be used as resource to promote health benefits in sweet products formulations.

## ACKNOWLEDGMENTS

This work was supported by Associate Laboratory for Green Chemistry – LAQV which is financed by national funds from FCT/MCTES (UID/QUI/50006/2013) and co-financed by the ERDF under the PT2020 Partnership Agreement (POCI-01-0145-FEDER-007265).

The authors would also like to thank Alga4Food Project (MAR-01.03.01-FEAMP-0016) for the research support and funds; Abigail Lopes Salgado for helping with the organization of the focus group and the members of the FCT Chemistry Department who volunteered to participate in the sensory analysis panel.

## REFERENCES

Adrià, A. (2008). *Natura*, 1st edn, Barcelona: RBA Libros.

Adrià, F., Adrià, A., & Soler, J. (2011). *La Historia de elBulli – Toda nuestra historia desde 1961 hasta 2011*, Roses, Espanha. Retrieved from http://www.elbulli.com/historia/version_imprimible/1961-2011_es.pdf

Ahn, Y.-Y., Ahnert, S. E., Bagrow, J. P., & Barabási, A.-L. (2011). Flavor Network and the Principles of food pairing. *Scientific Reports*, 1(196). doi:10.1038/srep00196

Blumenthal, H. (2009). *The Fat Duck Cookbook*, 1st edn, Loondon: Bloomsbury Publishing.

Buschmann, A. H., Camus, C., Infante, J., ...Critchley, A. T. (2017). Seaweed production: overview of the global state of exploitation, farming and emerging research activity. *European Journal of Phycology*, **52**(4), 391–406.

Castells, P. (2016, January). Maridaje de Alimentos: ¿Arte o ciencia? *Investigación y Ciencia*, (472), 51.

Chemat, F., Rombaut, N., Sicaire, A.-G., Meullemiestre, A., Fabiano-Tixier, A.-S., & Abert-Vian, M. (2017). Ultrasound Assisted Extraction of Food and Natural Products. Mechanisms, techniques, combinations, protocols and applications. A review. *Ultrasonics Sonochemistry*, **34**, 540–560.

Clarke, C. (2004). *The Science of Ice Cream*, 1st edn, Cambridge: Royal Society of Chemistry.

de Klepper, M., Klepper, M. de, & de Klepper, M. (2011). Food Pairing Theory: A european fad. *Gastronomica: The Journal of Critical Food Studies*, 11(4), 55–58.

Ducasse, A., & Robert, F. (2005). *Grand Livre de Cuisine d'Alain Ducasse: Desserts and Pâtisserie*, 1st edn, Paris: Les Éditions d'Alain Ducasse.

FDA. (2016). *FDA Vitamins and Minerals Chart*. Retrieved from https://www.accessdata.fda.gov/scripts/Interactive NutritionFactsLabel / factsheets / Vitamin _ and_Mineral_ Chart.pdf

Fujimura, T., & Kawai, T. (2000). Enzymes and Seaweed Flavor. In N. F. Haard & B. K. Simpson, eds., *Seafood Enzymes: Utilization and influence on postharvest seafood quality*, 1st edn, New York: CRC Press, pp. 385–409.

Hennink, M. M. (2014). *Focus Group Discussions*, 1st edn, New York: Oxford University Press.

Hielscher. (2018). Ultrasonic Extraction and Preservation. Retrieved May 5, 2019, from https://www.hielscher.com/extraction_01.htm

Ho, C.-T., Zheng, X., & Li, S. (2015). Tea Aroma Formation. *Food Science and Human Wellness*, **4**(1), 9–27.

Hosking, R. (2015). *Dictionary of Japanese Food: Ingredients and culture*, 1st edn, North Clarendon: Tuttle Publishing.

Lawless, H. T., & Heimann, H. (2010). *Sensory Evaluation of Food. Science*, 2nd edn. doi:10.1007/978-1-4419-6488-5

Le Pape, M.-A., Grua-Priol, J., Demaimay, M., & Crua-Priol, J. (2002). Effect of Two Storage Conditions on the Odor of an Edible Seaweed, Palmaria palmata, and Optimization of an Extraction Procedure Preserving its Odor Characteristics. *Journal of Food Science*, **67**(1996), 3135.

Lee, R. E. (2008). *Phycology*, 4ª, Cambridge: Cambridge University Press.

Maarse, H. (Ed.). (1991). *Volatile Compounds in Foods and Beverages*, 1st edn, New York: Marcel Dekker, Inc.

Mcgee, H. (2004). *On Food and Cooking – The science and lore of the kitchen*, Rev. Upd., New York: Scribner.

Meilgaard, M., Vance Civille, G., & Thomas Carr, B. (1999). *Sensory Evaluation Techniques*, 3rd edn, Boca Raton: CRC Press. doi:10.1201/9781439832271

Mišurcová, L. (2012). Chemical Composition of Seaweeds. In S.-K. Kim, ed., *Handbook of Marine Macroalgae: Biotechnology and Applied Phycology*, 1st edn, John Wiley & Sons, pp. 173–192.

Moreira Leite, B. S. (2017). *Novas Alternativas para o Uso de Macroalgas da Costa Portuguesa em Alimentação*, FCT/UNL, Caparica. Retrieved from https://run.unl.pt/bitstream/10362/23801/1/Leite_2017.pdf

Mouritsen, O. G. (2012). The emerging science of gastrophysics and its application to the algal cuisine. *Flavour*, **1**(1), 6.

Mouritsen, O. G. (2013). *Seaweeds: Edible, available & sustainable. The University of Chicago Press*, 1st edn, Vol. 1, Chicago: University of Chicago Press. doi:10.1017/CBO9781107415324.004

Mouritsen, O. G., Duelund, L., Petersen, M. A., Hartmann, A. L., & Frøst, M. B. (2019). Umami taste, free amino acid composition, and volatile compounds of brown seaweeds. *Journal of Applied Phycology*, **31**(2), 1213–1232.

Mouritsen, O. G., & Styrbæk, K. (2017). *Mouthfeel: How texture makes taste*, 1st edn, New York: Columbia University Press.

Myhrvold, N., Young, C., & Bilet, M. (2011). Volume 2 – Techniques and Equipment. In *Modernist Cuisine – The Art and Science of Cooking*, 1st edn, Bellevue: Cooking Lab, p. 477.

Neto, R. T., Marçal, C., Queirós, A. S., Abreu, H., Silva, A. M. S., & Cardoso, S. M. (2018). Screening of ulva rigida, gracilaria sp., fucus vesiculosus and saccharina latissima as functional ingredients. *International Journal of Molecular Sciences*, **19**(10). doi:10.3390/ijms19102987

Pereira, L. (2009). *Guia Ilustrado das Macroalgas. Biologia*, 1st edn, Coimbra: Imprensa da Univ. de Coimbra. Retrieved from http://hdl.handle.net/10316.2/2867

Pereira, L. (2016). *Edible Seaweeds of the World*, 1st edn, Boca Raton: CRC Press. doi:10.1201/b19970

Pereira, L., & Correia, F. (2015). *Macroalgas Marinhas da Costa Portuguesa: Biodiversidade, ecologia e utilizações*, 1st edn, Paris: Nota de Rodapé.

Rentería, E. (2007). *O Sabor Moderno – Da Europa ao Rio de Janeiro na República Velha*, 1st edn, Rio de Janeiro: Forense Universitaria.

Rioux, L.-E., Beaulieu, L., & Turgeon, S. L. (2017). Seaweeds: A traditional ingredients for new gastronomic sensation. *Food Hydrocolloids*, **68**, 255–265.

Shu, N., & Shen, H. (2012). Identification of odour-active compounds in dried and roasted nori (Porphyra yezoensis) using a simplified gas chromatography-SNIF technique. *Flavour and Fragrance Journal*, **27**(2), 157–164.

Spence, C. (2017). *Gastrophysics: The new science of eating*, 1st edn, London: Penguin.

Spence, C., & Piqueras-Fiszman, B. (2014). *The Perfect Meal: The multisensory science of food and dining*, 1st edn, Hoboken: John Wiley & Sons.

Taboada, C., Millán, R., & Míguez, I. (2010). Composition, nutritional aspects and effect on serum parameters of marine algae Ulva rigida. *Journal of the Science of Food and Agriculture*, **90**(3), 445–449.

Yang, Y.-Q., Yin, H.-X., Yuan, H.-B., Jiang, Y.-W., Dong, C.-W., & Deng, Y.-L. (2018). Characterization of the volatile components in green tea by IRAE-HS-SPME/GC–MS combined with multivariate analysis. *PLOS ONE*, **13**(3), 1–19.

*Experiencing Food: Designing Sustainable and Social Practices – Bonacho, Pires & Lamy (Eds)*
*© 2021 Taylor & Francis Group, London, ISBN 978-0-367-49414-8*

# From industry to the table: The tableware sector in Portugal

L. Guerreiro, F. Venâncio, L. Gomes & J. Frade
*LIDA, Laboratório de Investigação em Design e Artes, ESAD.CR, Instituto Politécnico de Leiria, Leiria, Portugal*

ABSTRACT: This article aims in the first place to contextualize historically the appearance of the ceramic tableware in Portugal and its evolution and industrialization. In second place (from the investigation work that has been done in the past seventeen months) by the researchers that did this article aims to present what the position of the tableware industry today in relation to the markets, public, sustainability, ecology, design, production methods and raw materials for production, regulation and laws in the sector and growth perspective. The article as some case studies to illustrate the addressed subjects.

## 1 INTRODUCTION

The genesis of the ceramic production in Portugal is very antique and difficult to set in time, once there's no documents that indicate when it begins. It's a fact that in XV and XVI centuries Portugal already had several pottery centers spreaded in all the Portuguese territory especially in areas that have clay in the soil. This centers evolve and in some cases where transformed in factories, some of them are working till today.

The EU is the leader of import and export in the food sector at the moment. This factor leaded to the development of new methods and concepts of production, management, security and quality in the industry, so this makes tableware sector a great example of that evolution.

Portuguese ceramic industry reflects that growth, in particularly tableware sector where the technologic advance, green thinking and the bet in creativity have been contributing for the affirmation of the industrial Portuguese products in this sector.

If in one time the competitiveness use to sit in low prices of the products, now it sits at the quality. When we talk about quality we have to associate various factors: production costs, resources used and its reutilization, raw material, environmental impact and design. All this concepts can be understood as ecology and sustainability in design practice (Ecodesign).

To this we can join other issues to have in mind: the security in the utilization and the non-contamination of the food present in de regulation R 1935:2004 de 27 de outubro (Artigo 5° e 23°), no Decreto de Lei DL 190:2007 de 11 de Maio and more recently by the rule NP 4555-1:2018.

## 2 DISCUSSION

### 2.1 *Historical review*

The oldest ceramic artifact known was found where is Chez Republic nowadays and it's dated of 28.000 aC (the end of the Paleolithic period). The first fragments of utility utensils in the shape of a vase are dated of 18.000 a 17.000 aC and were found in China. The use of ceramics spreaded successively to Japan and to the region of east Russia were the archaeologists found ceramic fragments from 14.000 aC. The use of ceramic increased in Neolithic period, when the communities connect to agriculture and shepherding were established. Starting approximately in 9.000 aC, ceramics turned popular as recipients for water and food and its utilization spread in to Asia, Middle East and Europe. In the beginning of the Bronze Age the grazed ceramic was produced in Mesopotamia. One of the first advances in production of ceramics was the invention of the wheel in 3.500 aC. It's introduction turned possible the utilization of the pottery wheel to produce very symmetric pieces. The Chinese were the firsts introducing high temperature muffles able to reach 1350°C and around 600 dC they developed porcelain (material with less than 1% of porosity) from caulim clay. During de Meddle Age, the trade through de Silk Route let the introduction and diffusion of porcelain in every Islamic countries first and then to Europe largely due to Marco Polo's travels. Throughout the 16th century, crockery continued to be the main class of ceramic products manufactured in Europe and the Middle East. During the industrial revolution, developments that broadened the range of utilitarian ceramic products were improved, as did their functional characteristics, turning pottery products into common goods.

The origin of ceramic production in Portugal is quite old and difficult to determine, since there are no documents that indicate the beginning of this event, although there are archaeological fragments that demonstrate this. It is true that in the fifteenth and sixteenth centuries, Portugal already had several oil centers, which spread throughout the country mainly in areas where the raw material was abundant, namely Prado (Vila Verde/Barcelos), Coimbrões (Vila Nova de Gaia), Molelos (Tondela), Ovar, Aveiro, Coimbra,

Leiria, and Flor da Rosa (Crato) (Rodrigues et al., 1999). These centers have developed and in some cases have led to the creation of centers of commercial activity that have given rise to factories, some of which have remained to this day.

Two factories that no longer exist, but that marked the history of the manufacture of ceramic china in Portugal were as follows:

– The Real Fábrica da Louça, located in Lisbon, in the Rato, appears on August 1, 1767.
– The Fábrica de Loiça de Sacavém was a fast industrial ceramic production unit founded in 1850.

Two other companies that still work and that also marked this story are:

– Vista Alegre, founded in 1824, located in Ilhavo.
– The Fábrica de Faianças Artísticas, by Raphael Bordallo Pinheiro, founded in 1884 and located in Caldas da Rainha.

Today, the subsector of Portuguese utilitarian and decorative dishes has more than 800 companies, 8000 workers and had a turnover of around 280 million euros in 2014 (data from APICER).

## 2.2 Regulamentation in Portuguese ceramic industry

The Portuguese ceramic industry has made notable improvements in its environmental performance in the last decades, in particular regarding the use of the best available technologies (BATs) that lead to lower energy consumption and emissions of pollutants in water, soil and up in the air. These changes are favorably reflected in the environmental impact of the companies, being a positive factor for a strategic positioning in this industrial sector, in particular in the most demanding markets from the environmental point of view.

With regard to food safety, it is imperative to take into account the materials used when producing this dish. Whatever the object or surface in contact with food should not have a negative impact on their cooking. Thus, any object to fulfill this purpose will have to be governed by the one described in the Normative Guide DL 190: 2007 of May 11 – Environment and Food Safety and more recently by the norm NP 4555-1: 2018 – Ceramic Utility. Specifications. This norm is an attempt to eliminate gaps by clearly defining the characteristics of the different types of ceramic pastes used for the production of utilityware and how these materials should behave in different contexts (performance attributes).

It is also important to mention that in 2012 the European Commission proposed the possibility of revising Directive 84/500/EEC 1 with regard to the reduction of the limits of Lead (Pb) and Cadmium (Cd) to significantly lower values, 400 and 60 times, respectively. As this is the priority issue in this directive, the possibility of inclusion of limits of release of other heavy metals considered dangerous in utility utilities because they exist in many ceramic raw materials and additives (color agents) such as Cobalt (Co), Copper (Cu), Manganese (Mn), among others.

## 2.3 CP2S – ceramics, heritage and sustainable products – from teaching to industry

The CP2S Research Project – Ceramics, Heritage and Sustainable Products – from teaching to industry; of the Laboratory of Research in Design and Art (LIDA) of the Superior School of Arts and Design of Caldas da Rainha of the Polytechnic Institute of Leiria, has as one of the objectives the dissemination of information about the state of the art of ceramic industrialization, proposing in particular the discussion the potential of the Design of industrial ceramic products on the general issues related to environmental, sustainability and innovation.

In this context, visits were made to companies from the utilitarian ceramic sector to investigate practices that would meet the issues of ecology and sustainability in the design practice associated with the Portuguese ceramic industry, and thus catalog the diversity in innovation and sustainability, applied in the various products of this industry. These visits made it possible to gauge the impact of the raw materials and production processes used and also to understand the importance of the role of design in this area.

From these visits, it is possible to observe that in these utilitarian dishes in particular these concerns are not so evident (for the user), and the strategies, as far as ecology and sustainability are concerned, are applied mainly in the production process, even increasing the mechanical and chemical resistance of the dishes (taking care of the pastes and also the glazes). However, in spite of the growing concern with design in these companies, there are few cases where the creation of own brand and consequently the definition of identity, etc. are pressing objectives. Most domestic manufacturers produce crockery according to the design and brand of customers, so in this context, these factories play an active role only in production.

## 2.4 Cases of study

From the set of products collected during the several visits it was decided to select for the present article some cases of study that show the most observed strategies in this ceramic sector. One of the strategies widely used in the crockery sector is the valorization of the ceramic products by the conjugation with other materials (wood, cork, metal, etc). This strategy allows adding some characteristics to the use of crockery, for example cork reinforces the thermal insulation of the set, creates a damping interface between the ceramic and the surfaces where it is placed, increases sustainability replacement of ceramic with other materials more "friends" "And opens up new opportunities for the ceramicware industry to partner with other sectors of industry and crafts in the creation and development of innovative and sustainable projects (Figure 1); the creation of crockery to enable its stacking, facilitating

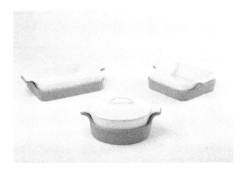

Figure 1. Grestel Company – the Ensemble project is the perfect combination between Stoneware and Cork. For home protection, transporting hot parts from the kiln to the table has become safer with this practical and simple solution through the use of environmentally friendly material.

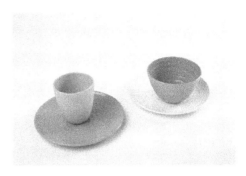

Figure 4. SPAL Company – Porcelain paste reuse Designer: SPAL Studio The production of parts is made through the use of sludge from ETARI (Wastewater Treatment Plants Industrial). The fact that these parts are glazed enlarges their use spectrum, such as the possibility of food use, among others.

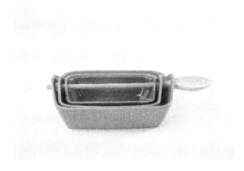

Figure 2. Grestel Company – Through the fit between them, these roasters allow an efficient storage, saving enough space in cabinets. With the addition of the wooden spoon as utensil, its transport was also facilitated.

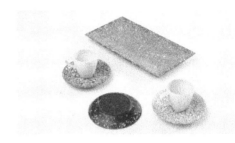

Figure 5. SPAL Company – Valorization of recycled ceramic materials (porcelain ground chips), epoxy resin and color additives. In the case of the cup, it is used as decoration, recalling its origin echo.

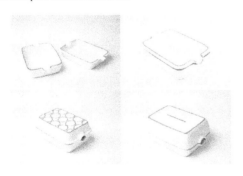

Figure 3. Val do Sol Company – Product with double functionality, the two platters also functioning as a baking sheet, when overlapping.

Figure 6. Empresa Vista Alegre – Porcelain glazed and of reduced thickness, with design inspired by Art Deco.

its transportation, distribution and storage (Figure 2); multifunctionality as a characteristic of the object (Figure 3); the use of industrial waste such as the use of sludge from sewage treatment plants as a component of pastes (Figure 4); recycling of nonconforming products – dishware that is discarded in quality control and used as a feedstock for polymer matrix composites (Figure 5); expressive reduction in the thickness of the objects (Figure 6).

If on the one hand there are several types of ceramic materials that can be used as utilitarian dishes (red clay, earthenware, stoneware, porcelain, sometimes combined with materials of other classes, such as cork, wood, etc.) However, the conformation and decorative methods have not undergone major changes over the years, the most common of which are: plastic pressing; conformation by roller; filling of gypsum molds by liquid route; reliefs and sub-reliefs; glazed; decals; serigraphy; tampography; hand painting; decorations (on glaze and in glaze) etc; (2 firings) and an

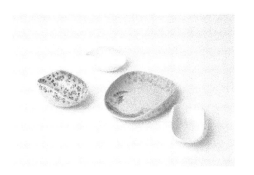

Figure 7. Empresa Vista Alegre (Fabrica Cerexport) – Grés The CASA project aims to establish the limits of acceptance of the properties of the final product, in development in the project, suitable for food contact.

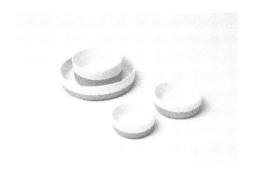

Figure 8. Company Val do Sol – Collection whit just white glaze in the interior and in the lip of the objects, having parts without glaze.

additional heat treatment when the products are subjected to decoration by the application of paints or other ways of direct and indirect application of ceramic pigments (third fire). However, it is important to add that during the visits, it was possible to observe cases where more recent and productive technologies are applied, such as: isostatic pressing; pressure filling; single-fired cycles; decoration in digital printing.

As regards decoration, taking into account the disposal of materials which did not comply with the requirements laid down by law for the constituents they held (such as lead and cadmium glazing) or the imposition of limits on use (the case of cobalt) and with the need to continue to use colors associated with these components, gives rise to a complex issue: the development of more sustainable solutions, although it is not a strategy present in most of the sector. If the tightness and texture conferred by glazing are essential in most ceramic products (for reasons of durability and food safety) there are other decorative methods such as the use of transparent glazes with low environmental impact (thus communicating the color of the pigmented paste) (Figure 7); and the application of glazes to the dishes where it is only strictly necessary, (Figure 8).

## 3 CONCLUSIONS

The niche markets of the utilitarian dinnerware industry are extremely demanding, leaving little room for new product creation or experimental designs. Trends continue to dictate what is produced in these companies. This is the biggest risk for this sector, the non-identity of the companies makes them equal to many others, thus being the price factor that dictates the rules in the growth of them. However, there is a growing need to focus on other virtues, such as quality, identity, innovation, sustainability, etc. There are more and more companies in Portugal that certify their processes, products and services through accredited standards that in a way guarantee good practices in terms of quality, social responsibility, environmental issues, sustainability, energy efficiency, etc.

The proximity to the European markets and consequently the recognition of the Portuguese product is a great advantage for the export, facilitating the creation of chains of supply of a fragile product.

The capacity of innovation, flexibility and adaptation of the ceramic industry in Portugal is also one of its strengths, allowing a wide range of solutions to the customer.

It is also important to mention that this industry meets specific standards: technical, environmental, energy efficiency, food safety, still combining the social responsibility of organizations and the appropriate response to the product life cycle and qualification of labor.

## REFERENCES

Ribeiro, A. P. – *A nova cerâmica das Caldas : Sec. XX.* [S.l.]: Edição do autor, 1989.

Queirós, J. – *Cerâmica Portuguesa e Outros Estudos.* Lisboa: Peres-Artes Gráfica, 1987. 514 p.

Singer, F.; Singer, S. S. – *Ceramica Industrial: Productos ceramicos* [sic]. Bilbao: Urmo, 1979.

Sampaio, A. F. – *Arte portuguesa: Cerâmica Portuguesa.* Ilustrações de Saavedra Machado; capa de Jorge Barradas. Lisboa: Empreza do Diario de Noticias, 1931. [16] p. (Collecção Patricia)

Sampaio, A. F. – *Arte portuguesa: A cerâmica.* Ilustrações de Saavedra Machado; capa de Jorge Barradas. Lisboa: Empreza do Diario de Noticias, 1926. [16] p. (Collecção Patricia)

## WEB

https://sites.ipleiria.pt/projetocp2s/
https://sites.ipleiria.pt/projetocp2s/quem-somos/
https://www.compete2020.gov.pt/admin/images/CERAMICA_DE_MESA_PORTUGUESA_Contributo_para_a_sustentabilidade.pdf
https://sites.ipleiria.pt/projetocp2s/2018/10/12/caldas-da-rainha-a-cidade-ceramica-depois-da-crise/
https://sites.ipleiria.pt/projetocp2s/201806/04/catalogo-exposicao-produtos-ceramicos-industriais-sustentaveis-em-portugal/

*Experiencing Food: Designing Sustainable and Social Practices – Bonacho, Pires & Lamy (Eds)*
*© 2021 Taylor & Francis Group, London, ISBN 978-0-367-49414-8*

# Designing grassroots food recovery circuits in urban Romania

I. Ionita

*FSAS, Doctoral School of Sociology, University of Bucharest, Bucharest, Romania*

ABSTRACT: Using a qualitative approach and the theoretical tools of Food Studies, under a Cultural Anthropology umbrella, this paper focuses on two instances of the burgeoning food-saving phenomenon in Romania with the aim of outlining processes whereby NGOs redirect food surplus to those in need in the absence of a local-level regulatory framework specifically setting out the path of recoverable edibles from retailers to food-insecure people. The findings herein are based on in-depth semi-structured interviews with the heads of two third sector organizations – one focusing on the social and professional reinsertion of vulnerable individuals, the other on the nutritional needs of those living below the poverty line – which are aiming to seek a formal regulatory recognition of "last resort" sorting and redistribution as methods to reduce waste and feed the hungry.

## 1 INTRODUCTION

### 1.1 *A bottom-up approach to food saving*

This paper proposes a discussion of the way in which soft, grassroots food-saving initiatives in the Romanian capital city (as opposed to the radical variants from geographic areas with a longstanding food-saving and food activism tradition) trigger changes in practical approaches to surplus/waste-food management and propose formal food saving models/mechanisms that might take the form of State-level regulations/laws governing the relationship between the retail and the third sector in matters related to surplus food redistribution.

Following a brief overview of the more general food waste theoretical background, this piece of research also takes a snapshot of theoretical discussions related to the perceived changes in status (waste versus food; commodity versus freely available food matter) that happen as food goes in and out of the traditional commercial circuit during recovery and redistribution. Finally, the ethnographic findings included herein point out the practical steps taken by two Romanian non-profit entities which aim to offer a more predictable and reliable future to the food recovery systems they employ in order to feed people at hunger risk.

### 1.2 *Food waste under the anthropological lens*

Food waste is a relatively new research theme for sociologists, the first formal attempt to define an approach that is specific to this category being the special issue dedicated to waste matters by The Sociological Review in 2013. The editors of this issue motivated their interest in this topic by the fact that there was a certain lack of interest among sociologists towards waste, in general, doubled by a relative indifference towards categories of objects taken for granted (Evans et al., 2013:6), such as food. They pointed out that, despite the appearance of a "sociology of everyday life" ever since the 70s, thanks to contributions by Jack Douglas and Michel de Certau, a "sociology of food" would only start to differentiate itself a decade later, with the studies conducted, for instance, by Murcott (1983). The three editors therefore argued that there was a need for a monograph of food waste to appear so that objects formerly categorized as waste, thus rendered "culturally invisible", would be brought back to the surface (Evans et al., 2013:6).

Having found that, until then, waste had only been perceived as the "redundant afterwards of social life" to be engaged with only when the need to do something about them arose (Evans et al., 2013:7), Evans et al. suggested a shift from waste as absence or void to waste existing in a specific social, economic and historical context, within which it moves as part of identifiable relationships and it generates meanings (Evans et al., 2013:8). Thus, a distinctive element of their new approach to waste would be that these remnants are no longer considered to stand outside the limits of social life, but to be part of their handlers' identities (Evans et al., 2013:8).

An important contribution which offers a structured way of understanding food waste is that of Zsuzsa Gille, who, coining the phrase "waste regimes" (Gille, 2013:27), proposes that an understanding of the way in which waste is generated and managed depends on the analysis of the social institutions and conventions that have a say in defining the waste status, as well as of the power relations that influence the production, representation and regulation of waste (Gille, 2013:29). Starting from the concrete example of how waste is generated during agricultural production, at farms, Gille seeks to explain global, trans-national waste production by outlining its close connection to social and institutional systems that support the production of various commodities.

On the subject of the perishability of food items and of the mechanisms whereby they reach the waste status, it is also worth mentioning Richard Milne's brief history of food safety in Great Britain, which sheds light on the various labelling systems and messages they were to convey to consumers: degree of freshness of the products on display, then the nutritional content of the food items they were applied on (ingredients, calorie content) and, finally, food safety parameters, empowering consumers to check, on their own, whether the food items were still fit for consumption, according to official standards (Milne, 2013). Thus, Milne opens a discussion about the trustworthiness of mentions such as "expiry date" and "best before", namely whether they match evaluations of the state of food items that consumers make based on their senses (sight/smell/touch) (Milne, 2013:91) as well as whether the authority of official food safety institutions should prevail over consumers' own practical experience in managing the risks associated with consuming perishable food (Milne, 2013:98).

## 1.3 *The social value of food surplus*

To better frame the findings reflected in this paper, mention should also be made of Midgley's article on the mechanisms at work in the redistribution of food surplus in response to food insecurity in England and which emphasizes the need to clearly distinguish between recoverable waste and redistributable food as a mandatory condition of a judicious use of food resources (Midgley, 2013). Midgley aims to complete the food waste production and use picture that had, until then, followed two separate lines of inquiry: why food waste exists in the first place and how appropriate it is to use it for welfare and what are the tensions and power relations at work between food waste middlemen. The author uses the "economy of qualities" concept, as defined by Michael Callon et al., which purports that objects undergo a permanent process of requalification, as they turn from prime matter to commodity and that this transformation affects both perceived, physical qualities and perceived values, depending on the context, handlers, etc., while also generating social distinctions (Callon et al., 2002 in Midgley, 2018:1876). Midgley also discusses at length how the food surplus category is defined as against the "normal" flow of goods on the market, the actual/perceived low(er) quality of surplus food, issues related to the dignity of food surplus redistribution and the ethics of the food aid "industry". Having set out to identify, in her own empirical study, "what subjective qualities enable a food product's transition to surplus from the market, its subsequent redistribution to non-buying consumers, and what relations are made visible

through this flow" (Midgley, 2018:1878), the author concludes that "the same logics that have given rise to the problems of food poverty and food waste are also the basis upon which surplus food redistribution is rationalized" and that there is a need for "greater understandings of the values and qualities associated with surplus food and how the tensions surrounding these are managed" (Midgley, 2018:1889).

Poppendieck's "secondary market", which includes "brokers who buy salvaged goods and manufacturers' rejects and resell them at flea markets, discount stores, roadside stands, and increasingly in Eastern Europe" (Poppendieck, 1998:168), is another excellent theoretical tool for the understanding of the two case studies included in this paper in so far as this concept encapsulates the reality of recovering otherwise discardable goods and of placing them within a more affordable and flexible economic circuit. It also gives rise to discussions around the way in which acceptability, standards and choice get a different meaning within this alternate circuit.

Finally, O'Brien's discussion of who, by what criteria and what authority decides what constitutes waste in the EU (O'Brien, 2013) might be used as a basis for understanding the problematic nature of establishing a point of no return for price-bearing food items, an aspect which is highly relevant especially for the second ethnographic data discussed in this paper.

These theoretical considerations are closely connected to my own reflections on the mechanisms at work in the identification of food that is fit for consumption despite its having reached it "best before" date. A less detailed approach (as compared to the quoted works) must be acknowledged here, and this is due both to the particular circumstance of Romania being just at the beginning of it food saving journey (lack of a food redistribution infrastructure, lack of a clear policy connecting food surplus and hunger combating efforts) and to the analyzed non-profit actors being less inclined to openly adopt more radical forms of opposition to the capitalist modes of production.

## 2 THE CASE OF THE VANISHING PRODUCE

### 2.1 *Creating a food saving model from scratch*

The association whose produce recovery activity is reflected in this section mainly focuses on the social and professional re-insertion of indivduals who are living in precarious conditions. These are people belonging to vulnerable social categories (former convicts, homeless, single parents, etc.) who, by lack of a specific professional specialization, cannot find employment and who, under the Association's guidance, learn to dismantle electronic equipment for the recovery and appropriate use of parts that have a high pollution potential. As a side activity, the Association runs a bio vegetable farm (located in the rural area, approximately 80 km away from Bucharest) which uses as fertilizer the compost obtained from donated produce (the so-called "ugly fruit and vegetables"). The interview with the head of the Association (referred to hereinafter as H.A) took place in autumn 2017, at a time when there was still hope for the first anti-food waste law to be adopted by the Romanian Parliament in a form that would place businesses under some kind of obligation to discard food unfit for commercial purposes in a responsible manner, both from an ecology and a humanitarian point of view. Having taken a very sinuous legislative path, now this law only sets an option, not an obligation, for businesses to adopt food saving measures as part of their stock management plans.

Given the initial context of the interview, the purpose of my inquiries was that of finding out whether and how the Association could afford to take over food that was about to expire and to redirect it to those in need. The disconnection between the Romanian legal framework and the Association's food saving and hunger combating actions was made clear from the start: "The Association's activity has nothing to do with the legal framework. Of course, we observe the legislation in force and all of the current norms, but we have a project, currently in its pilot phase […] we have been collecting, for a year now, waste produce from hypermarkets, we sort it every day, here, and we donate it […] under a partnership agreement with the General Social Assistance Direction and a social center close by, which provides cooked meals to those in need, social daycare services, and which also supports some emergency shelters for the homeless. […] Obviously, a legal framework would have helped develop some overall dynamics, at national level and, maybe, it would have led to the appearance of other structures that could do this sort of thing as well. But those who do food recovery and redistribution, before food becomes waste, are already into it even in the absence of a law to this effect. The law does not forbid this activity, at the moment, but it does not promote it either". (H.A.)

As it became apparent that the Association was in the process of building a produce recovery model that was lacking a proper regulatory context, the idea of the invisible fruit and vegetables sprung up as an expression of the difficulties in defining the legal status of the fruit and vegetables that the Association was saving and donating "under the radar" at the time: "We are operating outside of the scope of the anti-food waste law, outside of this legal framework that could have been created, that is missing, de facto, at the moment. […] We are an operator authorized by the Ministry of Environment, National Environment Agency to collect waste … this waste has a legal status in keeping, primarily, with the EU legislation, the community acquis. […] So, yes, we consider the produce we are sorting to be waste and we are re-sorting it – […] we still need to validate some steps to officially launch this activity – and the next step would be to build a model and to seek the approval of the National Animal Health and Food Safety Agency for the relevant safety norms". (H.A.)

With fuit and vegetables, the problem is complicated by the difficulty in establishing "best by" or expiry dates, the re-sorting process being based on the handler's non-specialized knowledge about optimal appearance and consistency. This is a painstaking effort, each item being inspected individually: "You don't get an apple with a "best by" stamp on it. In this case, we apply common sense and a set of rules that are not set in stone in any country …after all, if a potato is still good to eat, anyone can see it. Is it wilted, rotten, dehydrated, etc.? Then it's clear for anyone that it's not good anymore. But if it looks like an ordinary potato, why throw it away and waste it, when we can use it for the purpose it was created: human consumption?". (H.A.)

When asked about why this sorting is not done by the hypermarket itself, my interlocutor pointed out a regulatory loophole which actually promotes waste by virtue of very strict quality standards: "It all depends a lot on how economic operators are accredited: under a Ist category permit, a spotted banana is to be taken out of the commercial circuit immediately, even if it's still good on the inside, because these are the terms of their accreditation". (H.A.)

Therefore, the accelerated or the discount sale options are not universally available to all fruit and vegetable retailers because, paradoxically, a permit for the sale of a higher quality product does not include permission to sell its lower quality version as well. Under these circumstances, redirecting "ugly fruit and vegetables" to food recovery channels rather than to composting units is a matter of individual choice, rather than a general regulation to be observed by hypermarkets. My interlocutor confirmed that this is done as an act of benevolence towards third sector actors that take care of feeding those in need: "Yes, that's it: it's a favor. And this is exactly what the intended purpose of the [anti-food waste- my note] law initially was: to support general interest initiatives. There is a great difference between a social store, an association, a foundation or a social enterprise, on the one hand – even where there is an act of sale – and a business, on the other hand, based on capital, with a duty to distribute dividends to its shareholders and which is profit-driven. A huge difference. All countries favor general interest initiatives, and attribute a special status to associations, foundations and social enterprises. The latter are not placed in competition with profit-driven businesses". (H.A.)

My interlocutor then went on to decry the lack of a more coordinated view of the food waste issue in Romania. To her mind, there should have been two main directions to be developed in parallel: poverty combating policies and the national plan for the management and reduction of waste and pollution. Instead, the negotiations around the food-waste law had strongly leaned in favour of economic agents and of the retail industry representatives who had complained about the extra obligations and costs that food saving regulations would have imposed on them. As I pointed out the absurdity of a situation in which these food saving measures are not acceptable due to the potential for food poisoning outbreaks (a strong argument invoked by the food industry representatives) but in which people are left to eat from trash bins (my interlocutor confirmed having seen this frequently in her neighborhood), the question of absurdly strict safety regulations came up: "We are more Catholic than the Pope himself in certain contexts, and it is precisely those contexts of a general interest, that could bring about social innovation, that could help solve immediate problems, everything that pertains to how a community is organized, participation, direct democracy issues …. On the other hand, when it comes to activities strictly related to business and profit, we [the State – my note] will turn a blind eye to very many things and many things can happen. […] There's a great imbalance from this point of view". (H.A.)

With the price of food in mind, I mentioned to my interlocutor the type of action that other similar organizations were planning to implement, for instance the creation of community kitchens. When asked about her opinion on the feasibility of such a project, my interlocutor admitted to cooking being the less costly alternative from numerous points of view: "Obviously, by re-using food instead of throwing it away, you lower your costs a lot and of course you can produce even more food by relying on recovered waste […] clearly, putting together all of these mechanisms would greatly lower the level of resources required for the production of a new round of food items. Costs aside, there's also the use of natural resources and the pollution that ensues from food production, the packaging, etc". (H.A.)

Finally, my interlocutor pointed out that the Association was leaning towards a form of integrated support, while food aid resulting from food recovery was as just a small element of a wider picture with strong ecological and social hues: "We propose a complex form of intervention, meaning that we try, in everything that we do, to create paid jobs, tax-paying jobs, as a transition to the greater labor market, whereby we help those we employ here to rehabilitate themselves, to re-build themselves socially, professionally, emotionally and from a family point of view […]. On the one hand, we reduce waste and waste matters, and, on the other hand, those to whom we donate this food will get a hot meal – one that they really need – so it's a combination of needs and answers to those needs. A public policy framework might enable a wider application of these initiatives, at national level". (H.A.)

## 3 "BEST BEFORE": A RACE AGAINST THE COMMERCIAL CLOCK

### 3.1 *Creating a food saving model from scratch*

This section focuses on the case of a non-profit which struggles to keep food from crossing the border into waste category under very tight deadlines. In the presence of an absolute interdiction against feeding expired food (still fit for human consumption) to those in need, this organization's operating model under the Romanian law illustrates the extreme flexibility and time-consciousness required to redistribute food that is about to go to waste to human beneficiaries who count on it for their daily meals.

This is the case of a so-called social store, in fact a hypermarket with controlled prices which offers a limited range of food and non-food items to those living in precarious conditions in one of the Bucharest sectors. This is a closed-circuit store, with access granted based on specific criteria and where clients can make a limited number of purchases. The store operates in a space offered by the City Hall, in a back alley of a large peasant's market located near the main train station of the capital city. According to the FAQ section of its web site, the store has instated a few buying restrictions to prevent overcrowding and situations where the food is further resold by potential buyers. Clients can buy from the store a maxim of three times a week and they also have a total purchase value limit for each visit. Those entitled to purchase from the social store must not exceed a revenue of 500 RON per person per month, but there are other situations where buyers are accepted as well: unemployment, a large number of dependent minors, chronic conditions that require permanent treatment in the absence of which the patient's life would be at risk, homelessness, retirement, severe disability, being an only parent, having been a beneficiary of the State-administered foster home system, being a Roma ethnic, being a former prison convict (on condition that the respective person also attends a professional reinsertion program). The store clearly states that it does not benefit from any direct funding from the Romanian State, and that the status of its beneficiaries is monitored permanently, implying that access to this type of "protected" purchases can be withdrawn.

The interview with the store manager (referred to hereinafter as S.M.) took place during the autumn of 2017, when the Romanian anti-food waste law was still stuck in the legislative limbo of a suspended enforcement. The discussion focused on the non-profit's contribution, as part of a working committee made up of several similar organisations, in shaping the anti-food waste law. Thus, the discussion touched upon the value of the law as an environment protection and hunger combating tool, as well as on the specific way in which the social store works, namely the sale, at modic prices, of donated goods. As this lengthy interview helped outline the very complicated route that takes a non-profit's proposal to law status, it became apparent that the universe within which this store operates moves at a very fast pace, and that one day can make a significant difference in the legal status of a food item and in the type of actions that it can be used for. This permanent state of urgency requires a very complex balancing act on the part of the person who manages the store stocks in point of choosing sale versus donation, unconditional acceptance versus selection and expression of needs: "We don't really go out making donation proposals to companies. [...] For instance, we had a case last week [...] this is an importer, he gets butter from Ireland, as far as I remember. This is a high-end brand, quite expensive. He said ok, that he would put us on the negotiation list. This is how the system works: he imports the product with one month left before its "best before" date; the freshly imported product is the one at full price. If the butter remains in his warehouse for a week, this term is down by 25% and the price goes down as well. The importer negotiates prices with suppliers and he stands by a minimum price that he must obtain for each portion of the term up to the "best before" date. And that's where the difficulty arose: it took him quite some time to understand that we only want the butter after he has gone through the whole negotiation process and there's still some butter left to give". (S.M.)

Heavy limitations concerning the possibility of making specific requests (based on the store manager's information about client needs) or of suggesting categories of food that the store can receive (based on its available storage equipment) impact product range and variety: "We don't get to choose the type of products. [...] Obviously, we've gone and contacted specific producers, a dairy product manufacturer, for instance. Then again, we cannot go and say: "We don't want banana milk, we want another kind!". It doesn't work like that. We now know that we rarely get sugar, flour, maize flour and I try to reach out to companies I know to have them. With staple food items there's the issue of their long shelf life; these products don't really get close to expiry dates". (S.M.)

In fact, choice is an exceptional privilege, having to do with donors' benevolence and under no guarantees for long-term availability: "You saw those schnitzels that are now on sale in our store ...there's a factory in T. that makes them. They actually make them for us as part of each batch they turn out; with each batch, they make an extra couple of packs for us. This means that these products are there, in their warehouse and we can come and pick them up whenever we want. This is an exception, and these are not items that we seek in connection to food waste". (S.M.)

A discussion around the commercial status of donated items revealed a countercurrent of "social" food, where principles of acceptability are the opposite of the mainstream market logic, and that the store manager eloquently summarized as follows: "When people out there don't want any, we have a lot here; when there's a high demand on the market, we don't get any here". (S.M)

Therefore, it appears that the social store contributes to the saving of "ugly" merchandise, in a manner very similar to the "ugly fruit and vegetable" system: "These are "second-quality" products – strictly speaking about their appearance: [...] chocolate the color of which is non-standard, with some darker patches, which is perfectly fine qualitatively, but fails to meet the manufacturer's [aesthetic – my note] standards. Still in the sweets category: broken items – not the packaging, but the chocolate itself – if it's just some broken chocolate figures, but the chocolate is fine, the respective retailer can no longer sell it". (S.M.)

Commercial decisions related to temporary discount strategies are also likely to generate stock for the social store: "We've also got sampling items [...]. For instance, two 300 grams cans, plus an extra 150 gram can of food for free, all packed together; if they [the manufacturer – my note] keep this promotion on with a certain retailer for a month or two, they are not allowed to unpack those items and sell them separately beyond that date, so they all end up here". (S.M.)

Seasonal variations are also key, with availability influenced by holidays, on the one hand: "At the beginning of the year, once Christmas is over, even for those who celebrate it on January 6, according to the old Christian Orthodox calendar, we get a lot of Christmas sweets. Same story for Easter. Manufacturers can't help it; the products would be fit for consumption for another six months, but no one buys a chocolate Easter bunny in July" (S.M.) – and by a combination of cultural factors and the ebb and flow of natural resources, on the other hand: "There are companies that work with powder milk and which have somehow solved this problem, but there are companies that work with fresh milk only. For instance, during Lent, before Easter, dairy consumption is down; but they [manufacturers – my note] get the same quantity of milk and process it, there's no other way. Before Christmas and Easter, we get more [dairy – my note] than normally; on the other hand, dairy supply goes down in summer, as cows produce less milk then." (S.M.)

Despite the small size of donated batches, stock management is crucial for waste avoidance given the high time pressure the store operates under. Therefore, surplus redistribution happens even here, in a last man-standing type of effort to avoid throwing any food away. Several strategies are employed: (a) informal internal redistribution: "What might happen is for three-four pieces [of an item – my note] to be left, in the end, but they will go to the store employees. We have learnt, here, that shelf live is not something real."(S.M.); (b) formal redistribution: "If we are offered a specific quantity of a product, we know, from the start, that it would be too much for us to take on until the "best by" date. This means that we donate excess food, free of charge, to other charitable organizations."(S.M.); (c) redistribution to clients, where sale expectations endanger the chances of the food being consumed: "Take today, for instance: we received some yoghurt yesterday, and its "best by" date is tomorrow; [...] we donated a few boxes yesterday, and we're left with a few boxes that our clients can get for free, here, at the store." (S.M.); (d) sorting and full redistribution of fresh produce: "Just as any retailer, we are bound by law to have a contract with Protan [collector of non-dangerous animal and non-animal sub products that are not fir for human consumption – my note]; we pay for the services under that contract, but we have never delivered any food to them. From time to time, when we get vegetables, fruit, there might be a few moldy pieces. We'll just select those ourselves and throw them away." (S.M.)

These attempts at beating "best before" restrictions at their own game, are accompanied by a distrust in the ineluctable nature of official recommendations concerning the optimum consumption time frame. The relative nature of a manufacturer's quality guarantee was made apparent by my interlocutor, who swore by a sense-based principle of food state assessment even at home, with his children: "Take a strawberry flavored yoghurt: 90% of its initial quality may mean that the yoghurt has a slightly more liquid consistency, […] that the strawberry flavor is not as intense, […] that its pink color is lighter. From the content point of view, there is no change. Between 100% quality and a danger to health there is a very long timeframe that is not regulated, unfortunately." (S.M.) The alternative offered was a more hands-on decision-making process, with the consumer acting as the ultimate authority: "At the end of the warranty period, what do you do with your tv set at home? Do you throw it away or do you at least try to see if it still works, at least?" (S.M.)

Another line of inquiry which proved that the road to no food waste was lined with legal loopholes and policy shortcomings was the idea of selling food to those at hunger risk. The social store manager was responsible, together with the representative of the Romanian welfare workers association, for the successful negotiation of an exception to the "no sale" rule initially included in the anti-food waste law. To obtain this victory, they had fought a good amount of public pressure created by a few large international retailers which had signed a letter to the Romanian President pleading against the sale option, despite being among the biggest promoters of social economy abroad, in their home countries. Because of this victory, donated food was still off limits for re-sale in the social store, but when food was purchased from retailers at a high discount, it could be resold at a maximum of 25% of the purchase price. This was a crucial point for the operation of the social store, as it had to juggle with the uncertainty of its merchandise flows, while also covering the costs of full time employment – "It is very difficult for us to work with volunteers because anyone who touches the merchandise must be legally fit for work, must go to an annual health check, an occupational medicine check…there are criteria to be met whether you're a driver, a seller, etc." (S.M.) – and of the standard logistic apparatus required of any public caterer – "We must work very flexibly: yesterday evening they called N. to ask whether he could go [get donated food – my note] this morning, at eight. So, yesterday, at five in the afternoon, I found out that the car must be ready, that it must have enough fuel, and at eight o'clock in the morning I must have a driver who is fit for work and whom I should trust that he would not run the vehicle into the first streetlight. […] Everything costs. And it's cost upon cost upon cost." (S.M.)

Furthermore, it became apparent that under the anti-food waste law, the State intervened very late in the life of products and only regulated a small fraction of the food waste problem. This delay also influenced the relationship between retailers and the third sector beneficiaries, with the latter being practically left with no power of negotiation under this permanent last-minute salvaging scenario: "The main unsolved issue in the law: how would a company prove to have taken the necessary steps to go through the waste hierarchy? How does a store prove that it has attempted to donate for human consumption? We are talking about a short window of opportunity, these must be rapid steps, as it's a matter of days." (S.M.)

According to my interlocutor, despite the turbulent history of the anti-food waste law and the tremendous efforts that had been made by the non-profit sector to perfect it, an even vaster territory of corporate responsibility and non-profit empowerment was left completely unregulated: "Something else should be mentioned here: the second point in the [food saving – my note] hierarchy is accelerated sale, which now exists in stores. These are products that have three days or less until their "best before" date. […] If someone donates to us food that is four, five, six days away from its "due date", this law [the anti-food waste law – my note] does not apply; this means that we can continue to receive [it] free of charge, but sell it in our turn." (S.M.) Also, the store manager pointed out that a scenario in which the third sector organization would have a buyer status and the State would impose fines on food waste for retailers would empower NGOs to negotiate a less time-sensitive working mechanism for food transfer: "That's where we believe our force lies. […] A company offers us 5,000 cups of mayonnaise; I will buy 100; for the rest, "I'm sorry!", you [the retailer- my note] pay the fine for now, but, next time, let's strike a deal so you give me a call one or two days earlier…You get away without a fine, and I can continue doing what I have been doing with the products [ i.e. sell them – my note], under your control, and we won't even need to get into this [anti-waste – my note] legislation at all." (S.M.)

## 4    CONCLUSIONS

These interviews surfaced grassroots processes of policy creation – possible models of how the non-profit sector might apply presure for change on State structures and on the retail sector while testing and perfecting, of its own initiative, a waste recovery and hunger-combating model.

From this point of view, through its sorting and redistribution activity, the Association takes it upon itself to perform one stage in the food recovery process that the commercial entity is not willing to undertake and thus manages to make visible whole batches of "invisible" produce. This so-called invisibility relates to the legal status of the merchandise, which leaves the store as compostable waste, goes through a common-sense-based sorting process within the Association and then partly re-emerges as edible food to be donated. By taking on the task of seeing this process regulated, according to H.A.'s statements, the Association seeks to compensate a lack of State-level strategic coherence in connecting food waste and hunger combating efforts.

This curious case of food saving happens in between the production modes of a capitalist entity (the retailers that donate the produce) and a social enterprise (the bio farm that benefits from the compost). The question that arises in this context is why the supermarket does not sort the produce itself and whether the "last resort sorting" model that the Association seeks to regulate is likely to be applied by the commercial sector as well. The supermarket does not sort produce because it is under no legal obligation, just an option, to do so; in the absence of a penalty for wasting food in this way, sorting entails costs that cannot be recovered through the sale of the saved produce only, so it is economically illogical. Therefore, this type of sorting can only be done in a non-profit context. Also, given its unregulated nature, one might go as far as to say that the sorting work itself is doomed to remain invisible (unrecognised as working hours, unpaid, therefore not evaluated as worthwile according to market criteria). This is also due to the fact that, at the other end of the chain, the bio farm is only capable of covering 40% of its operating costs through the sale of its vegetables, so the sorting work remains unrecognized and unpaid there as well. As a consequence of that, unless the polutting potential of the sorted produce and the hunger-combating potential of the recovered food are translated into a form that makes sense in market terms (fines for economic agents not willing to do sorting, tax deductions or other facilities for those that do, a coherent sustainable development strategy that makes environment protection one of the top priorities at State level, etc.), there is no urgency in transforming the Association's individual efforts into a model applicable within the commercial sector as well.

The social store case surfaces the need to cross time barriers that can become crucial both for environmental and for hunger-combating reasons. The store manager swears by a more relaxed view of the "best before" date – which rings similar to a recommendation made to EU officials about EU-level food safety standards being excessively tight (Deloitte, 2014:57) – but he cannot apply this principle at work because it would be against the law.

On the other hand, impediments to the social store acquiring a buyer status in its relationship with the retail sector impairs its capacity to negotiate more predictable food transfer circuits and to share the logistic and financial burden of food saving with the latter. However, its ability to identify a different window of opportunity for its operations – food that is more than 3 days away from its "best by" date, more specifically food that is outside the scope of the current anti-food waste law – and its advocacy in strengthening food saving incentives/penalties opens the way for a more balanced participation in the food saving effort as the third sector entity would be empowered to ask that the retail sector draw up more extensive and predictable food-saving plans.

REFERENCES

Callon et al. 2002 in Midgley, J. 2018 'You Were a Life-saver': Encountering the Potentials of Vulnerability and Self-care in a Community Café *Ethics and Social Welfare* 12(1):1876.

Deloitte 2014. Comparative Study on EU Member States' legislation and practices on food donation, Final Report. *European Social and Economic Committee*. Retrieved from: https://www.eesc.europa.eu/resources/docs/comparative-study-on-eu-member-states-legislation-and-practices-on-food- donation_finalreport_010714.pdf

Evans, D., Campbell H., & Murcott, A. (ed) 2013. A brief pre-history of food waste and the social sciences. *The Sociological Review* 60(S2): 5–26.

Gille, Z. 2013. From risk to waste: global food waste regimes The Sociological Review 60(S2): 27– 46.

Midgley, J. 2013 The logics of surplus food redistribution, *Journal of Environmental Planning and Management* 57(12): 1872–1892.

Midgley, J. 2018 'You Were a Lifesaver': Encountering the Potentials of Vulnerability and Self-care in a Community Café *Ethics and Social Welfare* 12(1): 49–64.

Milne, R. 2013 Arbiters of waste: date labels, the consumer and knowing good, safe food *The Sociological Review* 60(S2): 84–101.

Murcott, A. (ed) 1983 The Sociology of food and eating: essays on the sociological significance of food. Aldershot, Hants: Gower.

O'Brien, M. 2013 A 'lasting transformation' of capitalist surplus: from food stocks to feedstocks *The Sociological Review* 60(S2): 192–211.

Poppendieck, J. 1998 *Sweet Charity? Emergency Food and the End of Entitlement*. London: Penguin Books.

*Experiencing Food: Designing Sustainable and Social Practices – Bonacho, Pires & Lamy (Eds)*
© 2021 Taylor & Francis Group, London, ISBN 978-0-367-49414-8

# Food Design Dates: Design-under-pressure activities in a cross-cultural and multidisciplinary online collaboration

D. Irkdas Dogu & K.N. Turhan
*IUE, Izmir University of Economics, İzmir, Turkey*

R. Pinto, T. Franqueira & C. Pereira
*University of Aveiro, Aveiro, Portugal*

ABSTRACT:  This paper describes how the online Food Design Dates initiative, which was planned as an exercise to explore the potentials of two different approaches of **design-under-pressure** activities in a **cross-cultural** and **multidisciplinary scenario** was structured and implemented. The two sessions of this exercise were constructed around the **co-creation** method and the contributions that Design can offer to other fields of knowledge in their **proof of concept phase**. Students from the Development of New Food Products (DNFP) course, of the Master in Biochemistry from the University of Aveiro, collaborated with Design students from the University of Aveiro and the Izmir University of Economics looking for a designerly approach to their research findings. The end products from these activities were prototyped and presented at Design Factory Aveiro's Food Design lab.

The outcomes reinforce the idea that by integrating design in an early stage of product development (being it food or other), helps building stronger results by anticipating problems, identifying solutions and mainly by adding narratives that enhance non tangible values. Form the Design perspective, we believe that this initiative reinforced the idea that designers need to have an *elastic mind* and that a concept can have multiple valid outcomes, which are symbiotic to context involved. In addition, it helped Design students to understand that problem solving processes in multidisciplinary working groups, are faster with a mediator and that negotiation must be corroborated with strong, grounded arguments.

## 1  INTRODUCTION

In the context of Globalization and the Anthropocene, new project-based learning education processes around multicultural and multidisciplinary learning approaches, challenge design education. In order to help manage the complexity that these realities generate, there is an increasing trend towards multi and interdisciplinary pedagogical approaches. Furthermore, virtual platforms help build cross-cultural learning experiences.

The Food Design Dates (FDD) initiative was organized to establish a multidisciplinary platform for collaboration between Biochemistry and Design students. The focus of FDD was to explore the potentials of a co-creative learning process in a multidisciplinary and multicultural virtual environment.

Rather than bringing together students from different disciplines to discuss a common given problem definition, we started off by introducing the Design students to the Biochemistry student's new food proposal, as condensed as possible – the recipe. This set of ingredients, acted as a (pre) brief, and no further information was given, for this reason this phase was called a Blind Date.

In the second moment, entitled as the Speed Date phase, that was held a week later, Design and Biochemistry students met online for the first time and during a 15 to 20-minute online videoconference got to pitch their ideas to each other. Each group was challenged to generate a unified solution, that kept its core ingredients, intended public and designations.

The groups then had one hour to prepare their Food Design proposals.

### 1.1  *Background*

Food Design Dates initiative is a joint initiative organized by Design Factory Aveiro, University of Aveiro and Izmir University of Economics. The workshop addresses issues of co-creation as well as multidisciplinary design approach in the proof of concept phase.

FDD workshop was inspired by the ongoing collaborations between the Design and Biochemistry departments of the University of Aveiro and by the *Biomaterials: Designing with Living Systems* elective course, which was taught collaboratively to Food Engineering and Industrial Design students as an elective course at Izmir University of Economics.

In a time where Artificial and Synthetic are no longer the opposite of natural, Food arose as the Common Ground media between Design and Biochemistry students. This workshop additionally intended to generate student's awareness of the advantages of bringing Design as a mediator as early as possible into change provoking process'. Contributing towards a better understanding of the role of Design, and designers in the construction of narratives, and as mediator of people and matter in this constantly shifting Globalized, Anthropocene age (Afreixo, 2017).

## 1.2   Co-creation and collaboration

Co-creation and/or collaboration are approaches that are increasing among industrial practice and in educational exercise, the two approaches are influencing each other in ways that promote acts of collective creativity.

There are different views about the role and level of involvement of the actors of this collective creativity in the design process. According to Sanders & Stappers (2008), any act of collective creativity shared between people is co-creation. The phases of a design process can be broken down to four phases as: pre-design, generative, evaluative and post-design (Sanders & Stappers, 2014). When these phases are overlapped with design research methods; tools, probes and generative toolkits, these are usually seen in the pre-design and generative phases. This revised version of design process developed by Sanders & Stappers (2014) introduces two mindsets: designing for and designing with, which correspond to the user as subject and as partner. In this new proposed model, the mindset areas are overlapping with each other expressing the changing role and participation of the user with the designer. This new designing approach are also called co-design.

However, existing practices to co-design projects in general, and in the field of food design are limited to probes, where the users share their stories and experiences while using the related artefacts. The challenge here is the designer's ability to understand the user's generative problems which may differ from technical to cultural challenges. The designer's role is then identified to develop products that are consciously integrated with the knowledge gathered from appropriate research methods.

According to Lee (2004), major attempts to cultural challenges are still limited to aesthetic stereotypes that lack solid theoretical and cultural frameworks. This is probably because it is not easy to develop a successful co-design process. Leading to the idea that the designer as a mediator, is key to set a common language and to help demystify the *status quo*.

## 1.3   Multidisciplinary and experiential learning

Traditional learning is focused on acquiring knowledge rather than fostering behaviors or viewpoints. Experiential learning on the other hand, is when students are taken out of their traditional-classroom or online-learning environments for a period of time, and are given the opportunity to experiment in context (Montana-Hoyos, Scharoun, & Poplin, 2015).

The term multidisciplinary is used when members of two or more disciplines cooperate using their own tools and knowledge to solve problems (Newell, 2001; Repko, 2005). Multidisciplinary in this context is project based, which means students from different disciplines come together to find a solution to a problem by using their own toolset.

Experiential learning is the structuring paradigm, where the balance between thinking and making is the format to stimulate learning (Stables, 2007), as Donald A. Schon describes in his book *The Reflective Practitioner: How Professionals Think In Action*, there is a synchrony between making and thinking, that can be referred to as a 'conversation' between the designer and the matter (1983). This "current trend [to] bring making into education to stimulate learning through making" (van der Poel, 2015), is not a new one, as Frayling argues while talking about the role of craft in design education when he affirms that the famous phrase "we must all return to the craft" by Walter Gropius in his characterization of the Program of the State Bauhaus in Weimar, was mistranslated. What Gropius really wrote was "we must all turn to the craft", and that Gropius didn't see Craft in its traditional definition but as a "research work for industrial production, speculative experiments in laboratory-workshops where the preparatory work of evolving and perfecting new type-forms will be done" (2011). This idea is reiterated by Otl Aicher in *Analogous and Digital*, stating that "we must move over from thinking to making and learn to think by making" (1994).

With the above assumptions in mind, the FDD initiative, was structured to promote activities as negotiations, tinkering, playing, gathering, sketching, experimenting and predicting instead of focusing on more conventional design activities of convergent thinking that narrow down options towards a final singular solution.

## 1.4   Design-under-pressure for online multidisciplinary collaboration

When collaboration is involved, the value of adopting design-under-pressure activities has shown to improve students' learning performance (Pinto, 2018). As Nassim Taleb explains in his book, *Antifragile: Things that Gain from Disorder,* "stress is knowledge" and "stressors are information"; he expands this thought by explaining that "nonliving-materials, when subjected to stress, typically, either undergo material fatigue or break", and that the opposite is what normally occurs when we are working with living-materials and people. Living materials when exposed to stressors (under a reasonable level), have the tendency to react, adapt and in most cases become "stronger". He also considers every constraint to be a stressor, and that we get "sharper and fitter in response to the stress of the constraint" (2013).

With this mindset, all elements that were considered to be enhancers of states of strain or tension, were not eliminated, they were simply managed by the instructors/mediators in order for things not to get out of control: stress can lead to self-doubt, making you rethink your ideas; first encounters with strangers can be paralyzing, this forces one to empathize and to get out of his/her comfort zone; language limitations force one to keep to the essential and to seek different forms of communication; fear is connected to social and cultural contexts, dogmas and personal experiences, requiring for all to negotiate and reason; and time limitations requires for one to be focused on results and follow their instincts.

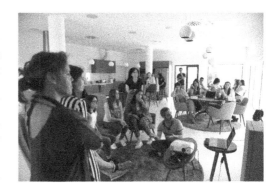

Figure 1. Online videoconference.

## 2 A STUDY FOR MULTIDISCIPLINARY PEDAGOGY IN CROSS-CULTURAL ENVIRONMENTS

### 2.1 Introduction

Food Design Dates initiative aims to reinforce basic design principles through a new media, and to broaden the students' understanding of design as a cross-disciplinary problem-solving process.

We consider a framework for Design and Biochemistry students to guide a couple of design activities to enable multidisciplinary activities and reinforce design thinking during the earlier phases of concept development.

This initiative was planned and implemented as a series of Design sessions of blind and speed "dating", intended to explore the potentials of two different approaches of design-under-pressure activities in a cross-cultural and multidisciplinary scenario.

The Food Design Dates initiative's phases were BLIND & SPEED [dating]. Where the dates in this context were not between people but between ideas.

Considering a blind date to be the first social engagement between strangers, commonly arranged by a mutual acquaintance, the analogy and the intended objectives matched the purpose – to grasp as fast as possible what was being presented, define an approach and present a seductive outcome. For the second phase, the speed date (15 to 20 minutes online video conference), each student *elevator-pitched* their proposal, then as a group, they discussed pros and cons, and defined the intended unified proposal.

The initiative ended with a workshop where the students cooked their redesigned recipes, and with a tasting session.

### 2.2 Content

Food Design Dates involved 27 college students from three different frameworks, without any cross-cultural online experiences. Of these students, 22 of them were from the University of Aveiro in Portugal and the remaining 5 from the Izmir University of Economics in Turkey. Of these 22 Portuguese students, 17 of them were enrolled in the elective course *Development of New Food Products* (DNFP), of the biochemistry master's degree, and 5 volunteered from the master's and undergrad Design courses. The Turkish students were from the senior year of Industrial Design undergrad, that were previously enrolled in a course called *Biomaterials: Designing with Living Systems* (2018).

Both Portuguese and Turkish students knew English but were not confident in communicating outside of their mother-tong. The majority of the online video-conference session was mediated by the course instructors, in order to avoid unclear aspects or misunderstandings during the conversations.

Contrary to many online learning experiences, that are based on continuous interactions, in this case no online meetings were conducted before starting the project. Only one final session via videoconference (Figure 1) was held to discuss each's perspectives and to obtain a group consensual product design proposition.

### 2.3 Method

The chosen method for this study focus group, included the following research stages:

**BLIND [dating]:** A summary of the research findings (in the form of short recipe card) (Figure 2) from the DNFP students' elective course exercise, was made available to the Industrial Design students from Izmir University of Economics and Design students from the University of Aveiro. Without any contact, the Design students were given a week to elaborate concepts and scenarios for applications of the given research findings into new market-focused products.

In order for the proposals to be considered market-focused, and not product-focused, students were requested to justify there options, based their forecast of consumer habits, and to take into account commercial, logistic and consumption aspects that my influence form-giving to a product.

Aspects like mistranslations, cultural clashes and subjectivity were not seen as obstacles, instead these aspects were cherished as opportunities to be explored.

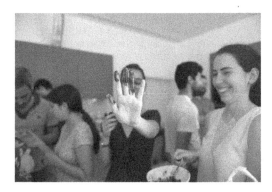

**CARACTERÍSTICAS DO SEU PRODUTO**

BOLACHA RECHEADA COM IOGURTE.
BASE FEITA COM:
AVEIA, MEL, BOLOTA, CANELA, (BANANA)

RECHEADA COM:
IOGURTE NATURAL E MEL LIOFILIZADOS.
CHOCOLATE DE LEITE

SEM FARINHAS REFINADAS
É NUTRITIVA, SAUDÁVEL E PRÁTICA.
FORMATO ORIGINAL

Figure 2.    Example of a short recipe card.

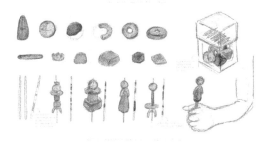

Figure 3.    Example of a concept board by one of the students.

The "recipes" given by DNFP students had no intervention or filtering by the lectures, and were presented as following:

- Aspheric cookie that is 100% vegan, with no sugar and all ingredients used have a Portuguese origin;
- Energy drink for snacks and breakfasts that is rich in spices, coffee and oats;
- Biscuit made with honey, oats, acorn and cinnamon filled with lyophilized natural yoghurt and honey;
- A Portuguese healthy version of a Petit Gateau;
- A lollipop with honey and fruit that has shapes that stimulate a child's cognitive abilities

The Design students were asked to interpreter the "design briefs" based on their empirical knowledge and subjectivity, for the second phase they should prepare presentations to explain their concepts (Figure 3).

Figure 4.    Prototyping.

**First Flirts:** After the first deadline the DNFP students presented their projects and were introduced for the first time to their Design dates (the Design students from both institutions that have been working on their projects).

**SPEED [dating]:** On the 31st May, DNFP and Design students operated during a 6-hour work session looking for common scenarios and unified objectives for the final proposals. The final projects were prototyped (Figure 4), and a final presentation took place at the Design Factory Aveiro.

### 2.4    Research questions

This research was done to better understand the issues regarding online cross-cultural and multidisciplinary collaboration. There were three research questions: (1) how to form an online multidisciplinary collaboration, (2) how to form an online cross-cultural collaboration, and (3) how to better design this learning experience?

For the first question, the study was interested in observing the communication between the multidisciplinary teams, and to assess the importance or not for the presence of a mediator. For the second question, the study evaluated the proposed designs and prototypes, as well as if aspect that are normally seen as obstacles, as are language and cultural differences, were actually approached as opportunities. For the third question, the study evaluated the students' feedback, and a compared the outcomes in a tasting session (Figure 5).

### 2.5    Technicalities

Researchers in this project, were also the instructors responsible for planning and observing the online workshop. Different to many online learning projects with several contact sessions, in this case students collaborated verbally and visually during an online, one-shot videoconference, were not only did they have to convey their ideas, they also had to end that session in unison. Instructors role as mediators was crucial in

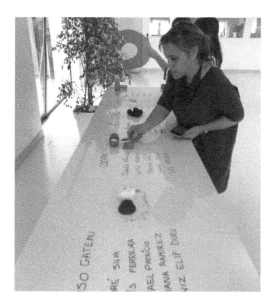

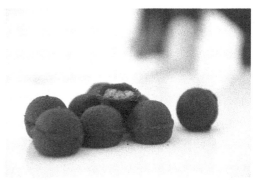

Figure 6. Vegan Aspheric cookie.

Figure 5. Setting up the outcome showcase.

of instructional design for online cross-cultural collaboration. The challenges of offering cross-cultural learning environments should not be underestimated (Braskamp, 2008). Given that the future world will be inevitably more globalized and "flat" (Friedman, 2005), promoting cross-cultural online collaboration for learning will definitely be a valuable and meaningful goal to pursue.

enforcing the rhythm, quickly clarifying mistranslations and filtering the clatter, that is common when working with big groups and online.

While there were several advantages on using an online video platform, some disadvantages were the sound quality and space restrictions. These aspects foreclosed a constant visual communication between all group elements during the entire session, and this was considered a drawback. The role of the instructors as mediators was fundamental in order to guarantee the flow and forcing the students into instinctive responses.

Moreover, students from different cultural backgrounds usually have different online collaborative behaviors, and the instructor needs to take these cultural differences into consideration when facilitating the online collaboration (Kim & Bonk, 2002). It is also demanding for the instructors, as they need to facilitate communication without contaminating the message with their own personal perspectives (Braskamp, 2008). Although some general tips for online cross-cultural collaboration were proposed (Saphiere, 2000) such as being mindful, being comfortable with silence, to encourage differing viewpoints, to avoid debates, to be observant, and to normalize diversity, more teaching strategies and suggestions for operating online cross-cultural collaboration in educational settings are needed.

The teacher is the key for the success of collaboration (Sammons, 2007), and except for complying with the capability of the technologies, teachers must develop a pedagogical framework that starts from "what it takes to learn" to challenge the development of technologies as well (Laurillard, 2009). However, there are few empirical studies that address the issues

## 3 FINDINGS: DESIGN OF CROSS-CULTURAL FOOD DESIGN

This intensive initiative was a 07-day collaboration where teams of Bioengineering students were assigned with 2 Design students, one from Portugal, and the other from Turkey, the main intent was to explore cross-cultural food design process.

As tangible outcomes, the following 5 projects incorporated the design students' ideas into the original food concept:

– *Aspheric cookie that is 100% vegan, with no sugar and all ingredients used have a Portuguese origin* – The idea of a festive cookie led the students to a *piñata* type of experience. A rigid outer crust that is crushed with a spoon, setting free colorful fruit particles (Figure 6);
– *Energy drink for snacks and breakfasts that is rich in spices, coffee and oats* – in this case the design students interpreted the beverage to be consumed on-the-go and suggested that the drink should be served in an edible spherical packaging. This idea was not explored by the group because it was considered to alter the initial concept (consumed at home) too much (Figure 7);
– *Biscuit made with honey, oats, acorn and cinnamon filled with lyophilized natural yoghurt and honey* – the proposal of a cookie that had a soft filling, that could be consumed in separate from the outer shell, led the students to develop a spoon-type artifact out of the same doe used in the cookie, to induce this form of its consumption (Figure 8);

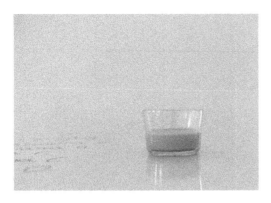

Figure 7. Vegan Aspheric cookie.

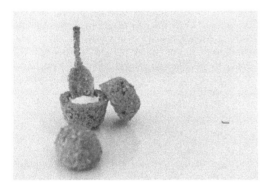

Figure 8. Vegan aspheric cookie.

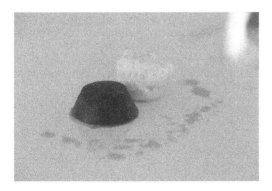

Figure 9. A Portuguese healthy version of a Petit Gateau.

- *A Portuguese healthy version of a Petit Gateau –* students here tried to propose a different serving experience to this well-known desert typology. Inspired by the traditional way of ice-cream making (mixed on top of an iced surface), here they to tried to explore the potentials of this hot and cold clash, introducing the iced platter as a part of the desert (Figure 9).
- A lollipop with honey and fruit that has shapes that stimulate a child's cognitive abilities (Figure 10); this product looked into how to stimulate children's

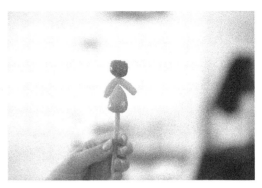

Figure 10. Lollipop.

cognitive capacities by giving each shape a different taste that could be assembled onto a beeswax stick that could then be used as a Mikado sticks or as a crayons.

## 4 DISCUSSION

Food has a symbolic dimension that is rooted into our cultural heritage, and language not only defines where we are from, it also expresses the form we perceive our surroundings.

This initiative offered students the opportunity to test their own skills in communicating their ideas in a multilanguage group. Their problem-solving abilities under social tension, that is both present due to cultural differences and to intense social interactions with strangers. In addition, teamwork and co-creation methods, helped students realize that a subjective concept, can be addressed as a "universal" proposal if it's elastic enough to incorporate external insights.

Within a multicultural and multidisciplinary approach, the strong cultural emphasis on local Portuguese food proposals, proved to be a big challenge for the Turkish students. This might seem to have been a setback, but it turned out to generate opportunities, not only did it bring forward the discussion to the basics, it forced the Portuguese students to question absolute truths and cultural dogmas.

The challenge here was for the designers to gain the ability to understand that the user's generative problems may differ from technical to cultural challenges. Most clashed did not result from cultural differences, they were the consequence of miscommunication: communicating in a foreign language, in which their lexicon was limited, under a stressful environment. This actually worked in favor of the groups, it helped each element to empathize with the others by sharing the same stress levels, making them more open to the suggestions of others.

We consider that the solutions to the given problems were constricted by the limitations of the actors, for this reason a conditioned workspace, where space/time for unfavorable judgment was extracted, that the approach shifted from a problem-based to a solution-based one.

As one of the most significant conclusions was that when a work environment is implemented (blind dates) where there is "no blockage of negative feedback", radical ideas flow easier. On the other hand, when the final proposal must be achieved under stressors (speed dates), the actors tend to negotiate instead of imposing their ideas. And that because this negotiation occurs inside their comfort zones, the final solution is stronger because the result outcomes as a unified group idea that is enriched by personal contributions.

## REFERENCES

Afreixo, L., Providência, F. & Rocha, S. (2017). *Food design symbolic dimension: contribution for a better, funnier and healthier life in the twenty-first century*. ETD'17 VI Ergotrip Design conference. Aveiro.

Aicher O. (1994). *Analogous and Digital*. Berlin Ernest & Sohn.

Donald A. Schon. (1983). *The Reflective Practitioner: How Professionals Think In Action*. New York: Basic Books.

Frayling C. (2014). *On Craftsmanship: Towards a New Bauhaus*. London, Oberon Books, pp. 88.

Janneke van der Poel, Iris Douma, Koen Scheltenaar, & Tilde Bekker. (2015). Maker Education – *Theory and Practice in the Netherlands: White paper for Platform Maker Education Netherlands*.

Montana-Hoyos, C., Scharoun, L., & Poplin, J. (2015). The importance of cross-cultural learning in the design disciplines: A case study reviewing a series of short term study tours designed to support cross-cultural exchange in the Asia-Pacific region. *International Journal of Arts and Sciences*, 8(5), pp. 435–442.

Newell, WH. (2001). 'A theory of interdisciplinary studies', Issues in Integrative Studies, vol. 19, pp. 1–25.

Pinto, R., Irkdas Dogu, D. et al. (2018). Neo-nature: Boundaries beyond Design with/in/for living systems. Twelfth International Conference on Design Principles & Practices. Barcelona, 2018 Special Focus: No Boundaries Design

Repko, A. (2005). Interdisciplinary practice: A student guide to research and writing, Preliminary edition, Pearson Custom, Boston.

Sanders, E.B.N. & Stappers, P.J. (2008). *Co-Creation and the New Landscapes of Design. CoDesign*, 4 (1), pp. 5–18.

Sanders, E.B.N. & Stappers, P.J. (2014). *Probes, toolkits and prototypes: Three approaches to making in codesigning*. CoDesign: International Journal of CoCreation in Design and the Arts.

Wrigley, C. & Ramsey, R. (2016). *Emotional food design: from designing food products to designing food systems*. International Journal of Food Design, 1(1), pp. 11–28.

*Experiencing Food: Designing Sustainable and Social Practices – Bonacho, Pires & Lamy (Eds)*
*© 2021 Taylor & Francis Group, London, ISBN 978-0-367-49414-8*

# Development of dishes free from the main food allergens – a case study

J. Sato, B. Moreira-Leite & P. Mata
*LAQV, REQUIMTE, Departamento de Química, Faculdade de Ciências e Tecnologia, Universidade Nova de Lisboa (FCT/UNL), Caparica, Portugal*

ABSTRACT: The necessity to develop alternatives for restaurant dishes containing allergens has led to the use of techniques in which cutting-edge scientific and technical knowledge are explored. This paper describes the development of a dessert free from the main food allergens, inspired by the dessert "Soup of Letters", created by chef Ferran Adrià and initially served at the El Bulli restaurant in 2004. All ingredients in the original recipe containing food allergens were identified and alternatives were selected. Finally, a new dessert was developed using a range of new cooking techniques. The work done was validated by a focus group and sensory analysis in which desserts prepared using the original recipe and the developed one were analyzed and discussed. It was concluded that in the proposed free from allergens dessert the main characteristics of the dish, particularly texture and flavor, were maintained or even improved.

*Keywords*: food allergy, allergens, dessert, aquafaba, hydrocolloids

## 1 INTRODUCTION

It is estimated that currently 17 million Europeans suffer from some form of food allergy. Studies analyzing the prevalence of food allergies show a significant increase in recent years (Panesar et al., 2013). These values emphasize the importance of the topic of this article.

Adverse reactions to food or intolerance derived from an immune mechanism are referred to as "food allergy", the non-immunological form is called "food intolerance". IgE-mediated food allergies are the most common and dangerous type of adverse food reactions (Ortolani & Pastorello, 2006).

Professionals working in restoration have yet limited knowledge about allergens and food allergies and intolerances. Particularly, about how to deal with demands from customers suffering from them, or to apply preventive methods of cross-contamination. Previous studies showed that in Portugal there is a lack of information not only related to the current legislation, but also about ways to deal with demands and to apply preventive methods. Training is required in order to raise awareness, help kitchen professionals to deal with this problem, and allow the development of quality and creative allergen-free dishes (Sato, 2018).

European Union Regulation (EU) No. 1169/2011, on the provision of information about food to consumers, requires hotels, restaurants, bakeries, bars and any establishment providing or selling food products to report the presence of any allergenic substance (EU, 2011). In Portugal, Decree-Law No. 26/2016 of 9th June ensures its execution and compliance with the obligations arising from the referred EU legislation (República Portuguesa, 2016).

The work here reported intends to illustrate the methodology, new ingredients and techniques that can be used to assist cooking professionals in the development of quality and creative dishes free from the main allergens.

Hydrophilic polymers (polysaccharides or proteins) which control moisture and provide structure, flow, stability and organoleptic qualities to food products are commonly referred by hydrocolloids. These food additives and ingredients may be obtained from a wide range of natural raw materials. They can be of animal origin (usually proteins such as gelatin, or egg proteins) or may be obtained from plants (from trees exudates, seeds, tubers, etc.), from seaweeds, produced by microorganisms or by chemical alteration of natural products such as cellulose or starch. Their approvals for food use are closely controlled by regulation (Moura, 2013).

Hydrocolloids have characteristics which allow them to be used as food stabilizers, emulsifiers, thickeners and gelling agents. Due to these capabilities, they are widely used in the food industry as food additives, having an important role also in food quality and safety (Imeson, 2010).

In the last decades hydrocolloids have been introduced in professional kitchens. The process started in *haute-cuisine* restaurants by creative and influential chefs such as Ferran Adrià and Heston Blumenthal. The work produced using hydrocolloids was considered a great innovation in cooking, as these ingredients were not common in restaurants (Moura et al., 2011).

The properties of hydrocolloids above referred, make them particularly convenient in the development of new food products compatible with a range of food restrictions. They were particularly useful as replacement ingredients in the work described in this paper, which consists in the development of a dessert free from the main food allergens, inspired by the dessert "Soup of Letters", a pop art homage to the well-known savory alphabet soup, created by chef Ferran Adrià and initially served at the El Bulli restaurant in 2004. It consists of a strawberry soup, a reduction of amaretto, a fresh cheese and Greek yogurt ice cream, and a dehydrated meringue shaped as letters, forming the words "THE SOUP", (Adrià et al., 2006).

## 2 MATERIALS AND METHODS

All elements and ingredients containing food allergens were initially identified in the original recipe, then possible replacements were selected. Subsequently, dish preparations using substitutes were made in order to identify the most satisfactory ones for all the dessert components. The method used, as well as references to the unaccomplished tests, will be presented in the next sections.

The final dessert was validated by a focus group in which desserts prepared using the original recipe and the developed one were analyzed, compared and discussed.

### 2.1 Materials

Ingredients used in the preparation of the dessert free form the main food allergens such as white sugar, light brown sugar, powdered sugar, frozen and freeze-dried raspberries, canned chickpeas, rice milk, rice cream, tigernuts, beetroot, rose and almond essences were purchased from a local market. Gelburguer, gellan gum, locust bean gum (LBG), guar gum, iota carrageenan, mono- and di-glycerides of fatty acids and glucose syrup were bought from Sosa®.

### 2.2 Identification of the main food allergens and its replacers

In order to produce a dish free from the main allergens, analysis of all ingredients of the original recipe of the "Soup of Letters" dessert (Adrià et al., 2006), was performed for identification of those containing allergens. There was the need to substitute several ingredients in order to get flavor and texture compatible with the characteristics of the original dessert. Results are presented in Table 1.

The main challenges encountered in the substitutions, and for which hydrocolloids were used, were the replacement of the ice cream base (cheese and Greek yoghurt) rich in lactose and milk proteins and

Table 1. The main identified ingredients containing food allergens in the original dessert "Soup of Letters", by Ferran Adrià and the selected substitutes.

| Dessert component | Ingredients containing allergens | Substitutes |
|---|---|---|
| Strawberry soup | Strawberry | Raspberry |
| Fresh cheese, yogurt and honey ice cream | Cheese, yogurt and ice cream stabilizer (that could contain milk proteins and/or lactose) | LBG gum, guar gum, iota carrageenan, mono- and diglycerides of fatty acids, tigernuts, rice beverage and cream |
| Meringue letters | Egg and strawberry | Aquafaba, Gelburguer, beetroot juice and freeze dried raspberry |
| Amaretto reduction | Almonds (bitter and sweet) | Almond artificial aroma and caramel syrup |

the development of egg-free meringues which could be dehydrated maintaining their shape.

### 2.3 Preparation of the raspberry soup

The original dessert "Soup of Letters" is composed of a soup of strawberries, in terms of replacement the option was another red fruit, in this case the raspberry (Table 2).

Table 2. Raspberry soup.

| Ingredients | Qty |
|---|---|
| Frozen raspberries | 500 g |
| Sugar | 60 g |
| Water | 40 g |
| Gellan gum (0,2% of the total juice weight) | 0.6 g |

PREPARATION:
1. Raspberries and sugar were vacuum packed and cooked in a thermostatic bath for 60 minutes at 65°C.
2. The mixture was strained, and 200 g of the juice were reserved.
3. The remain pulp was mixed with water and cooked in the microwave for about 3 minutes. It was transferred again to a sieve to remove the juices and allowed to cool.
4. Gellan gum was dispersed in 100 g of the liquid from the second extraction and this mixture was boiled to dissolve the hydrocolloid, which was then added to the reserved raspberry juice while mixing.
5. The mixture was left to set, the gel was passed through a tamis and the air was removed using a vacuum machine.

### 2.4 Preparation of the meringue

Egg white is an important element in the formation of meringues, since its proteins have excellent properties for the formation and stabilization of foams

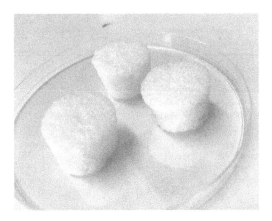

Figure 1.   Aquafaba meringue stabilized with Gelburguer.

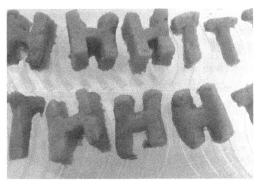

Figure 2.   Dehydrated aquafaba meringues letters stabilized with Gelburguer.

Table 3.   Meringue with aquafaba and Gelburguer.

| Ingredients | Qty |
|---|---|
| Aquafaba | 100 g |
| Sugar, powdered | 40 g |
| Gelburguer (2% of the aquafaba) | 2 g |
| Roses, essence | 15 drops |
| Beetroot, concentrated juice | 10 g |
| Raspberry, freeze-dried | Q.S. |

PREPARATION:

1. Aquafaba was whipped at low speed, using a Kitchen Aid® stand mixer, until a soft peaks foam, like the one obtained with egg whites, was achieved.
2. Sugar was added while whipping.
3. Finally, the Gelburguer, the essence of roses and the beetroot concentrated juice were previously mixed and then added, always whipping, until a stiff peak foam was achieved.
4. The preparation was spread in a tray, covered with parchment paper, in order to obtain a layer of 1 cm and was put in the refrigerator until it became solid (±3 hours).

(Alleoni & Antunes, 2004). For this purpose, in the preparation of the meringue, egg whites were replaced with aquafaba (canned chickpea water) and hydrocolloids in order to obtain a good foam which maintained its stability during dehydration, thus allowing to get the desired shape and texture for the letters (Shim et al., 2018).

Stability was attempted with the use of a range of hydrocolloids: Gelburguer (commercial name of a mixture of alginate and calcium salts marketed by the company Sosa®), agar and xanthan gum. The hydrocolloid which produced better results was Gelburguer (Figure 1). Ingredients and method are presented in Table 3.

Gelburguer stabilizes the foam through the formation of an alginate gel, which is thermo irreversible and allows the foam to maintain the shape during the dehydration process. For the preparation of the letters, the solid meringue preparation was shaped using a pastry letter-cutter. The letter-shaped meringues were sprinkled with dried raspberry powder and moved carefully to the dehydrator (Figure 2).

To dry the meringues and make a solid foam, the equipment, a Lacor® dehydrator, was programed to work overnight (minimum 8 hours) at a temperature of 55°C. The goal was to obtain a crispy product.

The letters were removed from the dehydrator and reserved in an airtight container at room temperature to be used latter.

### 2.5   Preparation of the ice cream

The structure of an ice cream can be described as a partially frozen foam (gas bubbles, ice crystals and fat droplets dispersed in a continuous aqueous concentrated solution of sugar, milk proteins, flavor molecules and other components).

An ice cream was created without the identified ingredients containing allergens. To achieve the desired results the development of a lactose-free stabilizer was required. This was composed of a combination of LBG, guar gum, iota carrageenan and mono- and di-glycerides of fatty acids (Table 4).

It was chosen to prepare an horchata ice cream, made with tigernuts, a tuber also known as chufa (original Spanish name), almond-of-the-earth or juniper nut because of its intriguing flavor. Horchata is a typical Spanish beverage made with tigernuts, water and sugar, which is already known as a substitute for cow's milk (Table 5).

### 2.6   Preparation of the almond scented caramel

The original dessert "Soup of Letters" is composed by a reduction of Amaretto. The Amaretto Disaronno is composed of apricot kernels, other fruits and mainly sweet and bitter almonds – the main component to be replaced.

In order to suppress the almonds, synthetic almond essence (benzaldehyde) was added to caramel to keep the flavor as close as possible to the original (Table 6).

Table 4.   Ice cream stabilizer base.

| Ingredients | Qty |
| --- | --- |
| Water | 200 g |
| Locust bean gum (0.4% of the base water) | 0.8 g |
| Guar gum (0.3% of the base water) | 0.6 g |
| Iota carrageenan (0.2% of the base water) | 0.4 g |
| Mono- and diglycerides of fatty acids (6% of the total ice cream fat) | 5 g |

PREPARATION:
1. All the ingredients, except the mono- and diglycerides, were mixed until complete dissolution.
2. The solution was vacuum pack and heated in a thermostatic bath for 30 minutes at 85°C.
3. While still hot, the gel was transferred to a bowl and the mono- and diglycerides were melted by the residual heat, being emulsified with a hand mixer.
4. The mixture was cooled for 12 hours before use.

Table 5.   Horchata ice cream free from lactose.

| Ingredients | Qty |
| --- | --- |
| Tigernuts, peeled | 200 g |
| Rice beverage | 100 g |
| Rice cream | 100 g |
| Stabilizer base (1 part : 2 parts of flavored liquid/puree) | 200 g |
| Sugar, white | 100 g |
| Glucose, atomized | 50 g |

PREPARATION:
1. The tigernuts were hydrated by covering them with a layer of 3 cm of water and letting them soak for 12 hours.
2. The water was drained and the tigernuts were powdered in a blender.
3. The powder was mixed with the rice beverage and cream. The puree was reserved again for 12 hours, covered inside the fridge, and then blended again.
4. The resulting tigernut and rice mixture was strained using a cheesecloth, and the fibers reserved for another preparation. If the yield is less than 400 g of the flavored liquid, then the required warm water should be added to the pulp, and the straining process repeated.
5. All the remaining ingredients were incorporated in the *horchata*, until fully dissolved, and transferred to a Pacojet beaker.
6. After being frozen for 24 hours, the *horchata* ice cream was ready to be processed in the Pacojet machine. An alternative solution could be using liquid nitrogen and a stand mixer to prepare the ice cream.

## 2.7   *Focus group and sensory analysis*

The validation of the free from allergens dessert was performed by a focus group followed by sensory analysis made with 8 experienced participants (aged from 26 to 42 years), having activities related with

Table 6.   Almond scented caramel.

| Ingredients | Qty |
| --- | --- |
| Sugar, light brown | 40 g |
| Glucose, syrup | 5 g |
| Water | 100 g |
| Almond, essence | 15 g |

PREPARATION:
1. The sugar and glucose were heated until they acquired a golden colour.
2. Water was added and the syrup was brought to boil until reaching the temperature of 105°C.
3. The caramel was removed from the heat and allowed to cool.
4. The essence was then added, and the preparation was transferred to a sauce bottle.

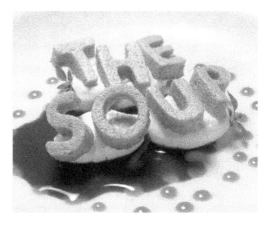

Figure 3.   Dessert "Soup of Letters", by Chef Ferran Adrià (Adrià et al., 2006).

gastronomy. The group was not previously trained, and the evaluation was made in one single session.

The main objective of the focus group analysis was the evaluation by tasters of aspects such as: texture, flavor, selection of ingredients, processing effects, storage stability, consumer reaction and acceptance (Teixeira, 2009).

The affective evaluation, the method used for sensory analysis, can describe the individual acceptance of the product in test (Leite, 2017).

The objective of the sensory analysis and focus group was to evaluate the acceptance of the dessert, to characterize it and to compare it with the original version. Recruitment and evaluation forms were distributed to the participants. Attributes flavor, texture and global impression were evaluated using a 5-points structured scale (from "I really liked it" to "I really disliked it").

Samples of a dessert based on the original recipe of the "Soup of Letters" by Ferran Adrià (Figure 3) and

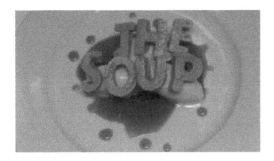

Figure 4. Free from allergens dessert inspired by "Soup of Letters". Photo: Luiz Coutinho.

Table 7. Sensory evaluation of the original dessert.

| Attributes | Number of participants | | |
| --- | --- | --- | --- |
| | I really liked it | I liked it | I liked it moderately |
| Flavor | 1 | 7 | |
| Texture | 1 | 6 | 1 |
| Global Impression | 3 | 5 | |

Table 8. Sensory evaluation of the dessert free from allergens.

| Attributes | Number of participants | | |
| --- | --- | --- | --- |
| | I really liked it | I liked it | I liked it moderately |
| Flavor | 6 | 2 | |
| Texture | 7 | 1 | |
| Global Impression | 8 | | |

the developed version of the dessert (Figure 4) were sequentially served to participants.

## 3 RESULTS AND DISCUSSIONS

A long process, involving several tests to evaluate different options of ingredients and quantities, allowed to reach a product with characteristics considered satisfactory. The developed version (Figure 4) had characteristics and quality compatibles with the original dessert.

Results from the affective test of acceptance are presented in Tables 7 and 8.

Opinions about the flavor were divided between "I really liked it" and "I liked it", however, the dessert developed had a much higher rating. The same happened to the texture attribute, nevertheless, for the original dessert, one of the tasters ranked it as "I liked it moderately", but the dessert developed had predominantly the classification of "I really liked it". For global impression, the opinions about the original dessert were divided between "I really like it" and "I like it", for the developed dessert the unanimous response was "I really liked it". Thus, based on the attributes analyzed, it can be concluded that the developed dessert achieved a better acceptance than the one prepared following the original recipe.

During the focus group discussion, it was referred that one of the main reasons for the better evaluation of the developed dessert was the crispiness of the meringue letters, which were considered as having a better texture than that of the original recipe.

The participants also praised the chosen set of flavors: the *horchata* ice cream was evaluated as having a better flavor, and the raspberry soup as having a better balance between the sweet and sour.

## 4 CONCLUSION

Food allergies are a relevant issue that should be considered in restaurants. Consumers are increasingly demanding quality and dishes compatible with their food restrictions.

In order to develop dishes for consumers suffering from food allergies, one good option is, as far as possible, to create dishes in which all food allergens are replaced, to cover multiple allergy situations and to reduce the risk of errors.

This requires the use of a range of ingredients and techniques which demand skills, working methodologies, and specialist knowledge. However, these are not mastered by all cooks, because they are unaware and/or lack the necessary experience. On the other hand, the product development process is long and requires many tests. Therefore, in this area, training and intervention are necessary.

After an extensive developing process, it was possible to produce a dessert, inspired by the "Soup of Letters" from El Bulli, free from allergen which was extremely well rated by experienced tasters.

We hope to contribute with this work, and others under development, to show that it is possible to cater for customers suffering from allergies, or other food restrictions, with the same quality as for customer without restriction. We expect also to make cooks aware of the fact that there are alternatives and illustrate the development methodology.

Urgent action is required for law enforcement and the development of new food alternatives to accompany the exponential growth of food allergies and intolerances in the world.

## REFERENCES

Adrià, F., Soler, J. & Adrià, A. 2006. *El Bulli 2003–2004*. 1ª ed. New York: HarperCollins.

Alleoni, A.C.C. & Antunes, A.J. 2004. Albumen foam stability and s-ovalbumin contents in eggs coated with whey protein concentrate. *Brazilian Journal of*

*Poultry Science* 6(2):105–110. DOI: 10.1590/S1516-635X2004000200006

EU. 2011. *Regulation No 1169/2011*. European Parliament and of the Council. 25 October 2011 on the provision of food information to consumers, amending Regulations (EC) No 1924/2006 and (EC) No 1925/ 2006 of the European Parliament and of the Council, and repealing Commission Directive 87/250/EEC, Council Directive 90/496/EEC, Commission Directive 1999/10/EC, Directive 2000/13/EC of the European Parliament and of the Council, Commission Directives 2002/67/EC and 2008/5/EC and Commission Regulation (EC) No 608/2004. Retrieved from: http://data.europa.eu/eli/reg/2011/1169/oj. Accessed in: 25/06/2019.

Imeson, A. 2010. *Food Stabilisers, Thickeners and Gelling Agents*. New Jersey: Blackwell Publishing.

Leite, B. 2017. *Novas Alternativas para o Uso de Macroalgas da Costa Portuguesa em Alimentação*. MSc dissertation, Faculdade de Ciências e Tecnologia, Universidade Nova de Lisboa. Retrieved from: http://hdl.handle.net/10362/23801. Accessed in: 25/06/2019.

Moura, J. 2013. *Cozinha com Ciência e Arte*. Lisboa: Bertand.

Moura, J., Viegas, J., Dias, S., Prista, S., Loureiro Dias, C. & Guerreiro, M. 2011. Cooking in the 21st Century: The role of hydrocolloids in the changing of process and attitudes. *in Proceedings from 4th Iberian Meeting on Colloids and Inter-faces*, E.F. Marques & M.J. Sottomayor (Eds.) 257–264.

Ortolani. C. & Pastorello E. 2006. Food allergies and food intolerances *Best Practice & Research Clinical Gastroenterology*. 20(3):467–83. DOI: 10.1016/j.bpg.2005.11.010

Panesar S.S., Javad S., De Silva D., Nwaru BI, L. Hickstein, A., Roberts, G., Worm, M., Bilò, M.B., Cardona, V., Dubois, A.E.J., Dunn, A., Eigenmann, P., Fernandez-Rivas, M., Halken, S., Lack, G., Niggemann, B., Santos, A.F., Vlieg–Boerstra, B., Zolkipli, Q. & Sheikh, A.(on behalf of the EAACI Food Allergy and Anaphylaxis Group). 2013. The epidemiology of anaphylaxis in Europe: a systematic review. *Allergy*. 68:1353–1361. DOI: 10.1111/all.12272

República Portuguesa. 2016. Decreto lei nº26/2016. *Diário da República* nº111/2016 Série I de 2016-06-09. Retrieved from: https://data.dre.pt/eli/dec-lei/26/2016/06/09/p/dre/pt/html. Accessed in: 25/06/2019.

Sato, J. 2018. *Alergias e Intolerâncias Alimentares e forma de lidar com elas na restauração portuguesa*. MSc Dissertation. Faculdade de Ciências e Tecnologia, Universidade Nova de Lisboa.

Shim, Y.Y., Mustafa R., Shen J., Ratanapariyanuch K. & Reaney M.J. 2018. Composition and Properties of Aquafaba: Water Recovered from Commercially Canned Chickpeas. *Journal of Visualized Experiments*. (132), e56305. DOI: 10.3791/56305.

Sosa Ingredients. 2018. *Gastronomic Ingredients*. Retrieved from: https://www.sosa.cat/gamas.php?lang=en. Accessed in: 25/06/2019.

Teixeira, L.V. 2013. Análise sensorial na indústria de alimentos. *Revista do Instituto de Laticínios Cândido Tostes*. 64(366): 12–21. Retrieved from: https://www.revistadoilct.com.br/rilct/article/view/70/76. Accessed in: 25/06/2019.

*Experiencing Food: Designing Sustainable and Social Practices – Bonacho, Pires & Lamy (Eds)*
*© 2021 Taylor & Francis Group, London, ISBN 978-0-367-49414-8*

# Integrating and innovating food design and sociology – healthy eating

M. Hedegaard Larsen
*Aalborg University Copenhagen, Copenhagen, Denmark*

ABSTRACT:   The aim of this paper is to discuss how food design as a discipline can strengthen its contribution to solutions that increase healthy eating patterns and environments, through a fuller and more innovative integration with food sociology and food studies perspectives in both the problem definition as well as the actual solutions.

This aim is tried achieved through a brief presentation and critical discussion of general orientations within food design and food sociology/food studies in relation to the current use of social theory exemplified and contextualized through a non-exhaustive literature review of current health and nutrition initiatives and concepts. This is done, firstly, to critically, assess the usefulness of applying food design approaches to socio-health-related problems, and, secondly, to present and discuss the possible innovative benefits of increased integration between food design and food sociology both theoretically and in possible various (future) applications.

## 1   INTRODUCTION

Healthy eating is dependent on many socio-economic and cultural factors beyond the influence of the individual consumer or citizen. This influence of, often, large societal structures on how healthily we eat, can be hard to integrate at an end-user-design-level. To many food designers such structures can, justifiably, seem both superfluous and hard to integrate if you are looking to improve specific food environments and/or products with assumedly quite specific commercial end-users. However, as food design grows into a more mature field of research, it will, invariably, need to deal – even more – with social and societal issues, as has also been proposed by Parasecoli (2017): *'the social function of food design: Will it limit itself to being a useful and creative tool in the experience economy, or will it also contribute to increase citizens' involvement in crucial decisions about what and how they eat?'*

Parasecoli (2017), also, suggest that food studies (including sociology) can aid the prospering, but still quite young discipline of food design – here illustrated using food design education as a focus: *'The acquisition of critical thinking tools and analytical skills borrowed from history, anthropology, sociology, politics, economics and media – just to mention some of the areas explored in food studies – can provide food design students and practitioners with fresh perspectives and more refined tools to develop their projects and interventions'.*

This is an original and relevant statement, but also a statement that could do with some contextualization and elaboration. It has for many years been in vogue, within academia, to highlight the power and

potentials of multi and interdisciplinarity, but successful real-life application of interdisciplinary thinking can seem harder to accomplish. So besides describing and discussing the possible strengths of further integration and alignment between food design and food sociology and food studies in relation to health and nutrition initiatives, it seems pertinent to illustrate some of the main differences between how (food) sociology/food studies and (food) design differ in their approach to the study of the social – both theoretically and in relevant health eating contextualizations. Thus, this paper will use the framework of a non-exhaustive literature review to achieve such ends, with the obvious limitations in generalizability this might entail.

## 2   UNDERSTANDING THE SOCIAL

Food design has proven to contribute, positively, to many aspects of healthy eating including (but not exclusive of): Food environments (both in production and consumption), Promotion, products, packaging, shopping, cooking, storing and even in broader food systems/infrastructure and new ways of 'thinking' food etc. You can, therefore, argue that food design, by default, incorporates social needs and wants, as the use-values of design changes are directly correlated to the increased utility of the people who engage with these products and environments.

However, the social perspectives in many design studies seem, often, only there to serve as background information on themes like obesity, health etc. Rarely do the broader social mechanisms (Larsen, 2015) affecting unhealthy eating, for instance, seem to influence the actual design-solutions even when the problems being addressed are undeniably social in nature. Designers frequently use sociological knowledge on citizens and consumers as short cuts in order to provide inputs into the "black-box" that is "ideation" or "creativity", from where most final design solutions seemingly arise. To social scientists such "creative" solutions can seem too far removed from the original social contextualization and description, and at times so heavily reduced (in order to accommodate commercial or policy aims) that the solutions no longer makes sense for the groups in society that need them the most; or they are executed in ways that manipulate environments but do little to empower actors living in those environments.

The reasons for these preferences could be that many food designers naturally tend to prefer "social theory" that invokes causality over complexity, as is evident in various nudging approaches to foodscapes. Such approaches are heavily promoted by researchers like Brian Wansink (Wansink & Sobal, 2007) for instance, in order to improve the healthy eating practices of various public and private food environments and its users. Charles Spence (Spence et al., 2014) provides similar attractive but reductive conceptualizations of the social, albeit from a cognitive psychological perspective, but still focusing – like Wansink – on the manipulation of food environments and objects, and rarely emphasizing the socio-cultural or socio-economic status of the research participants as being of significant importance. Within these environments, participants are considered to be easy subjects to the manipulative whims of the designer/researcher, and their responses to various (naturally occurring) stimuli are explained solely from apparently inherent causal cognitive traits – "How does noise from an airplane affect the sense of umami?"

Trouble is – from a sociological perspective – that most food design solutions, ultimately, have to work in environments where actors/participants can, and will, resist manipulation – sometimes they will even try and manipulate the manipulators! We should always remind ourselves that the world is not a lab, and the design-lab is not necessarily representative of the world at large.

Nudging is both noble and naive. The reason for its current popularity is probably, also, that it offers authorities and politicians, especially, simplistic and reductive tools to approach socially complex issues like obesity, for instance. Surely nudging can be part of remedying the effects of obesity, but does it address the underlying reasons for obesity or indeed other health related structures and factors beyond the individual consumer? Or does it merely quell, or even hide, these reasons, while simultaneously ascribing (even) more personal responsibility to consumers and citizens who are already buried in guilt-messages from the media? (Holm, 2003) Research shows that most people know what is healthy and unhealthy food anyway (Kearney & McElhone, 1999), but most people, nevertheless, continue to engage in unhealthy eating

practices; what is otherwise known as the conundrum: "knowledge-action-gap".

It can be alluring for designers to adhere closely to causality-ridden conceptualizations of food environments and their actors in their design efforts. They offer clear and simple ways to understand object/subject interaction that are easily transferrable to a more visual template. For instance, it is assumed that the color red induces certain emotions and thus also particular consumption preferences, and that designing smaller plates and heavier cutlery apparently reduce serving sizes and thus intake of food etc.

These conceptualizations of the foodscape and its actors might prove valuable in small incremental innovations within food design – especially food products or services. But they tend to reduce complexity rather than to explicate it. Also, by focusing on a singular "how" in design solutions before understanding, properly, from a sociological point of view, the many "why's" behind health and nutritional choices made by multiple and varied users – there are inherent limits to the uses of design. The most important factor to explain health and nutritional choices lies perhaps less in the object/subject interaction as with the subject-to-subject interaction, where food habits and choices are shaped primarily through continuous social negotiations and frequently opaque questions of identity, social-economic status etc.

In the following paragraph I have provided some concrete examples to help clarify my points:

## 2.1  *Healthy meals in schools*

If you want to decrease obesity rates among elementary school children, manipulation, or re-design, of their eating environment and utensils might provide small and, most likely, temporary improvements. Furthermore, these do little to address if the meals being served are inherently unhealthy or unappetizing due to low budgets, low level of skills and indifference of staff or other factors that are outside of the "plate-scape-problem" tried solved through food or gastronomy design measures. As a designer you can end up mitigating downstream symptoms rather than addressing the upstream factors and reasons. Reducing the complexity behind the factors behind unhealthy eating might enhance, positively, the public or political perception of applied design solutions in the short-term, but this reduction comes at a price of then not being able to address the long-term, or permanent, upstream causes.

Nudging school children towards the fruit bowl rather than the fries do not address the root of the problem – rather it can, and not necessarily intentionally, make the problem seem like one that is reduceable to good or bad individual choices. This, ultimately, can have the opposite effect of accelerating poor health choices as is also indicated by food sociology literature.

## 2.2 The obesity epidemic

The "obesity epidemic" is not infrequently positioned and explained as the result of aggressive and successful marketing and related product design of attractive but unhealthy food products, and/or manipulative food environments. Consumers are seen as willing slaves to these well-designed environments. But could this development not also have root in decreasing agricultural prices? Low prices that have been brought about as a result of increasing growth of mono-crops that can be grown cheaply and used as feed to animals, often to the detriment of the environment in many places. Or could the obesity epidemic not also be explained by political unwill to tax sugar and fat?

Design efforts to fix downstream symptoms to larger societal problems are applaudable and necessary – trying to reduce overeating through nudging designs, for instance. But attention must, also, be given to upstream causes like food production, manufacturing and promotion for instance if food design as a discipline is to contribute to positive systemic changes that encompass the complexity of contemporary food systems (culturally, economically, socially etc.) and its eaters, while also addressing the power relations that are inherent in these systems.

Within communication theory – that share some similarities to design theory – the concept of the 3 E's is utilized, by communicators in order to evaluate if a problem or challenge is indeed a communication problem entirely – often it is not. The 3 E's stand for: Education, Engineering and Enforcement. And if one, or more, of those three are the likely main causes of the problem sought fixed by communicative efforts solely, then even the most creative, well-thought out and executed health promotion/communication campaign will fail; or its success will be short-lived, as the structural or societal set-up is not changed, addressed or integrated.

## 2.3 Foodscape as a bridging conceptualization?

Within food studies the concept of foodscapes has come into fashion over the last two decades.

*'Consider the places and spaces where you acquire food, prepare food, talk about food, or generally gather some sort of meaning from food. This is your foodscape. The concept originated in the field of geography and is widely used in urban studies and public health to refer to urban food environments. Sociologists have extended the concept to include the institutional arrangements, cultural spaces, and discourses that mediate our relationship with our food.'* (MacKendrick, 2014: 1)

Foodscapes can thus be utilized as both a conceptual and a mapping tool to frame and help us better understand, how specific environments and its actors are mutually affecting each other, and what general structures/discourses seem to affect different actors and their environments the most. This could be regarding health promotion in schools (Ruge, 2015),

or institutional change in relation to food (Hansen & Kristensen, 2012), or local food systems (Sonnino, 2013), for instance. Now some of these texts might seem quite removed from food design perspectives in general. However, if the strength of food designers is their ability for holistic thinking, as suggested by Schifferstein (2016), then such broad, albeit also quite specific, framework of conceptualization, could be a way to innovate food design thinking, invoking the social (both environment and user) in both a more stringent and complex fashion. Within design and social innovation for instance, the conundrum of social complexity is recognized: *'This complexity, however, has been largely misunderstood, with the idea that the mere involvement of users in setting ideas and understanding their needs would correspond to the introduction of design and its practices in SI development.'* (Deserti et al., p. 69)

Involvement of representative actors does not guarantee representation in the final solutions.

Admittedly, much research and literature within the social sciences and humanities that explore the human experience of unhealthy eating in "real life", like food sociology, anthropology along with the vast and, at times, multidisciplinary food studies literature, can themselves seem to "get lost" in complexity. This might be explained by the fact, that the purpose of much food studies research is not necessarily to come up with solutions, but to point out problems (both structural and individually) and/or dilemmas in relation to various aspects of, and reasons for, unhealthy eating. Some of this research do contain prescriptive solutions to improve conditions, but these can, at times, seem biased or unhinged from the actual governing structures or societal context. Sometimes the idealism inherent in such studies distorts the actual situations explored as pointed out by critics of parts of the food movement (Zilberman, 2017). However, sociology – and perhaps particularly applied sociology in food studies – share a crucial aim with designers, namely the wish and ambition to better the current health status of citizens and consumers. This could happen through "civic agriculture" (Lyson, 2012), school and community gardens attendance (McVey et al., 2018), new/alternative food systems and a return to more "traditional" food ways (Pollan, 2006), or different ways of addressing, communicating and critiquing public health initiatives (Nestle, 2007) among many other, seemingly, ever expanding small and large sub-categories. This utopian streak inherent in design (both theory and application), is a believe that design can "save the world" or just make it a little better both aesthetically, socially and culturally, is shared by many sociologists and food studies researchers.

The work of the perhaps most well-known sociologist Pierre Bourdieu is, traditionally, interpreted as being quite deterministic and leaving little room for individual agency or choice within the organizing structures of society. Most individuals just reproduce (food) habits and general behavioural patterns of peers and parents – to put it somewhat crudely. His seminal work 'Distinction' (1984) on habitus and capital has had a great influence beyond sociology. His work has informed work on segmentation and consumer preferences in relation to users/consumers' place in the different distinction "hierarchies" of culture, economy etc. For instance, food consumers with much cultural capital but not much economic capital might distinguish/reproduce themselves by consuming heirloom tomatoes for instance. This is a product that might require more knowledge to appreciate (history, production etc.) than standard 'industrial' tomatoes but is still not too expensive. Whereas, food consumers with both high cultural and economic capital might also purchase heirlooms tomatoes, but they might also purchase vintage wines or organic cocktails – things that require both plenty of knowledge as well as plenty expenditure of available capital. These categories can be replicated and applied on almost anything and anyone in various societies, cementing its success as a practical research tool, also beyond sociology.

However, it is, also, recognized that Bourdiean thinking acknowledges that existing structures can generate (positive) social change – but often fails to do so. The point is, if you know how societal structures operate and are reproduced through individual action, your chances of designing solutions to aid change and positive social development is far greater than if you are not too aware – awareness (of the hidden governing structures), also, being one of the main learning points derived from Marxism. In order to change societal structures you must first understand them, their interconnections and, possibly, exploitative nature. Acknowledging these structures hold particular risks for (food) designers in particular. Firstly, it would mean acknowledging the spaces and places that we – as people – engage with objects and each other are not neutral or universal, but largely dependent on sociocultural status and the guiding political structures – there is no "tabula rasa". This might mean that food designers will have to become political with all the risks of losing income that this might entail. However, different environments should be approached differently. Designing new food experiences and products for an amusement park is probably less political than working with healthy school meals in underprivileged communities – and who is not to say that the former cannot enrich the latter or vice versa? Integrating sociological thought into food design is not about removing creativity, as much as it is about making designers aware of the "hidden" effects of their creative solutions, in order for them to heighten the utility and innovation of their solutions. Thus, hopefully, further integration can help fuel creativity by opening up new perspectives and interconnections rather than just inventing new pillars and "boxes" of thought. The strong commercial tradition and collaboration with industry within food design might also compliment and challenge some of the more implicit anti-capitalist sentiments that, at times, can seem inherent to, and thus unquestioned, in much food studies literature.

## 3 DISCUSSION

### 3.1 The great potential for further integration

The great potential inherent in food design – and design in generally – is that it has the potentials to transcend and integrate different disciplines and approaches. Therefore, it might be advisable to look for truths and less so *the* truth in singular, searching less for fixed and static socio-environmental causalities and rather exploring complexity; looking less for universal solutions and more for contextualized solutions that invariably will vary depending on the socio-economic and cultural dimensions of the environments explored. The social is rarely static or simple by nature, but that does not mean that you cannot generalize or convert complex knowledge of the social into relevant food-design solutions – products and/or environments.

Solutions to healthy eating challenges – in whatever form they make take ultimately – are full of conundrums, "wicked" problems and knowledge-action gaps that have deep seated roots in social practices, societal discourses, community values among many other important factors to be included if one is to understand the "landscape of unhealthy eating" and its actors.

It is not only food design that could benefit from further integration of sociological theory and applications, but also the other way around. Over the last two decades the theories of the aestheticization of everyday life has arisen (originally coined by Mike Featherstone) enriching and explaining societal tendencies. *'The aestheticization of everyday life refers to the growing significance of aesthetic perception in processes of consumption and consuming. It points to the observations that increasingly more aspects of everyday activity are subject to the principles of aesthetics (the appreciation of beauty and art) and that even the most mundane forms of consumption can be expressive and playful.'* (May, 2011).

Food design could help bring these theories of everyday experience of the aesthetic forward. Design could help test them, and thus help innovate and expand the boundaries of much sociological thinking. Such a development could help position design and aesthetics as more than appendices to society to be addressed in the arts and related cultural spheres, or as tools of the manipulating market forces selling desires in an increasingly unequal experience/aesthetic economy.

Maybe food designers will not have to choose between working within the commercially lucrative experience economy and the more socially conscious, but less well paid, citizen's health area. Integrating thoughts and tools from sociology and food studies, design could be seen as complimentary albeit also more political and complex than at present – without resorting to complete political activism. Indeed, it is the ability of designers to break down boundaries and think in new broader perspectives that, ultimately, will have to be renewed. And this should be done without necessarily dividing the world into endless subcategories (as is often found within food studies) or position capitalism as opposite forces to citizenship. Such a renewal could be fueled by further integration and experimentation, in order to innovate both food design and food sociology, respectively.

It would require some work to be able to better position and utilize food design and sociology as integrated and explanatory forces for positive societal change – and many of the mentioned integration possibilities are still in the abstract. However, the concept of foodscapes, for instance, might, provide one form of testing ground for such endeavors of the aesthetics and design matters that influences the social and vice versa.

## 4 CONCLUSION

Food design as a discipline has a lot to gain through further integration with sociological and food studies perspectives. Especially so if this integration is achieved all through the design-process (and not just as background information). It could help generate more innovative and societally relevant solutions within the areas of health and nutrition. But, also, solutions that can seem more complex and political than at present.

Also, sociology and food studies researchers might be positively aided by incorporating design approaches in their work, in order to better illustrate (in a literal sense too) – or make explicit – possible practical solutions and new theoretical frameworks arising from their research.

Despite its limitations the hope is that this paper have contributed to see even more ways to integrate and innovate both food sociology and design within health and nutrition initiatives and beyond.

## REFERENCES

Bourdieu, P. (1984). *Distinction: a social critique of the judgement of taste.* London: Routledge & Kegan Paul.
Deserti, A., Rizzo, R., Cobanli, O. *"From Social Design To Design For Social Innovation"* https://www.socialinnovationatlas.net/fileadmin/PDF/einzeln/01_SI-Landscape_Global_Trends/01_14_From-Social-Design_Deserti-Rizzo-Cobanli.pdf

Hansen, M. W. & Kristensen, N. H. (2012). The Institutional foodscapes: potentials for changes in a school food context. In *Proceedings from NCCR 2012.*
Holm, K. L. (2003). 'Blaming the consumer: on the free choice of consumers and the decline in food quality in Denmark' *Critical Public Health,* vol. 13, no. 2, pp. 139–154.
Kearney, J. M., & McElhone, S. (1999). Perceived barriers in trying to eat healthier. Results of a pan-EU consumer attitudinal survey. *British Journal of Nutrition,* 81(Suppl. 2), S133–S137.
Larsen. M. (2015). Nutritional advice from George Orwell. Exploring the social mechanisms behind the overconsumption of unhealthy foods by people with low socioeconomic status. *Appetite,* Volume 91, 1 August 2015, Pages 150–156.
Lyson, T. A. (2012). *Civic agriculture: Reconnecting farm, food, and community.* Tufts University Press Medford Massachusetts.
MacKendrick, N. (2014). 'Foodscape', *Contexts,* 13(3), pp. 16–18.
May, H., (2011). Aestheticization of Everyday Life (Chapter in) *Encyclopedia of Consumer Culture* ed. Dale Southerton Sage Publications.
McVey, D., Robert Nash, Paul Stansbie (2018) The motivations and experiences of community garden participants in Edinburgh, Scotland Regional Studies, Regional Science, January 2018.
Nestle, M. (2007). Food politics: how the food industry influences nutrition and health. Berkeley, University of California Press.
Parasecoli, F. (2017). Food, research, design: What can food studies bring to food design education? International Journal of Food Design. 2. 15–25.
Pollan, M. (2006). The omnivore's dilemma: a natural history of four meals. New York, Penguin Press.
Ruge, Dorte, Nielsen, Morten Kromann, Mikkelsen, B. E. & Jensen, B. B (2015). Examining participation in relation to students' development of health-related action competence in a whole school food setting: Insights from the 'LOMA' case study. Health Education.
Schifferstein, Rick. (2016). What design can bring to the food industry. International Journal of Food Design. 1. 103–134(32). 10.1386/ijfd.1.2.103_1.
Sonnino, R. (2013). *Local Foodscapes: Place and Power in the Agri-Food System.* Acta Agriculturae Scandinavica, Section B – Soil & Plant Science 63 (S1), pp. 2–7.
Spence, Charles & Smith, Barry & Michel, Charles. (2014). Airplane Noise and the Taste of Umami. Flavour. 3. 10.1186/2044-7248-3-2.
Wansink, Brian & Sobal, Jeffery. (2007). Mindless Eating: The 200 Daily Food Decisions We Overlook. Environment & Behavior. 39. 106–123.
Zilberman, D., (2017). The innovations behind the new food revolutions. http://blogs.berkeley.edu/2017/05/23/the-innovations-behind-the-new-food-revolutions/ (Links to an external site.)

*Experiencing Food: Designing Sustainable and Social Practices – Bonacho, Pires & Lamy (Eds)*
© *2021 Taylor & Francis Group, London, ISBN 978-0-367-49414-8*

# Design, short food supply chain and conscious consumption in Rio de Janeiro

E. Gonzalez
*Pontifícia Universidade Católica do Rio de Janeiro, PUC-Rio, Rio de Janeiro, RJ, Brazil*

C. Cipolla
*COPPE, Universidade Federal do Rio de Janeiro UFRJ, Rio de Janeiro, RJ, Brazil*

ABSTRACT: This study on food supply chain addresses the way upper-scale chefs from Rio de Janeiro can influence and encourage conscious consumption of food, thus changing the way food is perceived and consumed and the relationships between the end-user and producer. Design thinking is adopted as a methodology to bring out ongoing actions to augment farm-to-table in Rio. The methodology required an immersive and empathetic process in the issue under analysis which was empowered in this study by the personal experience of the first author, with over ten years of experience as a restaurant chef de cuisine. The study also presents the impediments faced by a chef to work with small scale agriculture. It suggests actions to surpass this hindrance by designing a service for chefs that relies on a network of small scale farmers to overcome the difficulties to interact with this kind of provider and to allow informed consumption.

## 1 FOOD FOR THOUGHT

The short food supply chain (SFSC) and the conscious consumption of food are deeply connected to the sustainability tripod. These food system topics directly address the economic, social and environmental concerns, being top listed in the UN Agenda for Sustainable Development Goals (UN, 2015) and the Paris Agreement (2016). "Food systems have the potential to nurture human health and support environmental sustainability; however, they are currently threatening both. Providing a growing global population with healthy diets from sustainable food systems is an immediate challenge". "Because much of the world's population is inadequately nourished and many environmental systems and processes are pushed beyond safe boundaries by food production, a global transformation of the food system is urgently needed." (EAT-Lancet Report, 2019). The way food is produced and consumed has to change in order to meet the planet's capacity.

"Over recent decades, agricultural productivity has risen, food trade has increased and the once ever-present threat of famine has receded in most parts of the world. This means many people have better diets than before." (FAO – Food and Agriculture Organization of the United Nations, 2018, p. 4). On the other hand, agribusiness crops grow in quantity as fast as they decline in diversity. This agricultural model produces commodities for the food industry, and the urban population consumption of highly processed foods increases rapidly.

Also according to FAO's Global Panel, it's about time we thought beyond agriculture and considered all the processes and activities involved in the food production chain, such as processing, storage, transportation, trade, transformation and retailing. The SFSCs connect directly to those premises. Consisting of a sequence of actors and actions, it ensures the least possible middlemen are present, and assures a fairer and cleaner trading system, for all involved, from land to final consumer. From this chain, three main characters will be featured on this exercise. The two edges are the most discernible, being the producer and the consumer. They are, sometimes, worlds apart, and still, get glimpses of each other every time the service is exchanged. The third actor on this stage is the restaurant chef, responsible for some of these touchpoints between the boundaries.

In 2016 agriculture covered a third of our planet's land area. Of that surface, Brazil is amongst the group of countries that take around 40%. According to FAO, coping with the food and agriculture challenge: smallholders' reports, most food in the world is produced by family farming, in less than a quarter of the planet's surface, with an astonishing figure of around 70% versus 30% from the agribusiness, which takes over 75% of the farming lands. What is also alarming is the fact that crops for biofuel production have grown at a faster rate than crops for food production in the past decade.

Another remarkable difference in the farming systems are the roles played by the contrasting agriculture structures: small-scale farmers perform economic, social, cultural, environmental and reproductive functions and are key to keeping agrobiodiversity, territories, landscapes, cultural heritage, and communities, within a rational and socially just food system. "As a result, the motivations of family farmers often go far beyond maximizing economic profit to encompass other social, cultural and ecological motives" (FAO Reports, 2018, p. 17).

On the further end of the chain lie the consumers, and the importance of instrumenting these individuals with the origins of the consumed food. "A conscious consumer is someone who looks beyond the label. When you opt to be a conscious consumer, you are putting yourself in the driver's seat of making a decision for which brand(s) you choose to support. It's about keeping your mind engaged and making sure that you understand just what you are choosing to support or not support." (Nature Hub, Conscious Consumer, 2018).

According to statements made on the Global Panel on Agriculture and Food Systems for Nutrition, 2016, the consumer, once embedded with knowledge and empowered, will demand better food, and this new approach will make the food supply system provide quality food for all, with a direct impact on the agriculture trade, which directly affects the environment and public health. To keep up, businesses will have to change or address certain policies to stand in the market.

This study on food supply chain focuses on how the restaurant chef de cuisine, which has the skills and capacity to source and modify food, can affect the demand on the production end. The aim is to ameliorate the farm-to-table stream in Rio de Janeiro, Brazil, to reach and influence as many final consumers as possible, thus changing the way food is perceived and consumed, and changing the social and economic relationships established between the end-user and producer.

During the MAD Symposium 2017, Carlo Petrini spoke about the importance of the food system on the world's general health, be it the environment or its people when he said, "it's not a food system, it's a criminal system". Petrini was bold about it: "Where's tomorrow cooking going? It has to go against this system". We need to forge an alliance between the kitchen, chefs, farmers, fishermen, producers, and citizens. "I won't call them consumers; I'll call them co-producers because consumerism is an illness" (Petrini, 2017). The MAD project, a parallel of the G-20 for the world's gastronomy, unites the cook's community from all over the globe since 2011, raising awareness on how the food system directly affects the global environment and its population. It proposes "remodeling our food system by giving chefs and restaurateurs the skills, community, time, and space to create real and sustainable change in their restaurants, in their communities, and across the world." (MAD, 2017).

Along the food consumption chain, the chef is an important element. As a qualified consumer, this professional has the knowledge to better source the ingredients, in terms of quality and origin. The chef is also responsible for, especially having a share in the business, determining where the products will come from, what labels the restaurant will carry, and transmit this image through the food served.

Being a more capable and skilled purchaser, the trained cook has the technical abilities to steer even through unknown ingredients and develop ways to prepare and present them. The chef is also a connection between the farm and the city, and in an optimal situation, links both worlds, fusing the two ends of the chain.

The Slow Food movement has a worldwide group named Chef's Alliance, engaged in perpetuating food traditions, biodiversity, local culture, and artisan food producers. They state chefs have a fundamental role to play in safeguarding the biological and cultural diversity of our food. They interpret the histories and ecosystems of their regions with skill and creativity, supporting local producers while awakening eaters to the role we all play as custodians of biodiversity.

On top of all the technical aspects, there's an ever-growing recognition of the importance of the profession. It is clearly seen in the amount of media showcasing chefs, to the point of having dedicated series being amongst the most-watched TV programs. Another touchable proof of that is the inclusion of Gastronomy courses in Universities worldwide (Adrià, 2017).

The food chains that supply consumers are growing longer, with global trade increasing the distance between production and consumption, as well as the diversity of foods available to consumers. Value and power in food systems are shifting towards the middle of these food chains, with agricultural produce becoming ingredients for processed products (FAO, 2012). To reverse this mechanism, individuals must be stimulated to eat more real, fresh food, either by cooking their own meals or eating them at the venues which offer the least processed quality food possible.

"Another thing cooking is, or can be, is a way to honor the things we're eating, the animals and plants and fungi that have been sacrificed to gratify our needs and desires, as well as the places and the people that produce them" (Pollan, 2006, p. 404). Urban life dictates a rhythm in people's lives in which cooking one's everyday meals can be a time-consuming task, and time must be spent in a different manner. Individuals need, then, to reach for this nurturing service. In comes the restaurant and its team, offering a convenient way of eating fairly well, without the trouble of elaborating and executing a daily menu.

Adding to this, the chef's career has also risen in the media spotlight and this had led to some influential power over clients' behavior and consumption habits. This media power adds on the responsibility, for this qualified cook can influence and shift the demands for more sustainable agriculture via the impact over end consumers. By modifying the way food is perceived and consumed, there will also be a transformation in the social and economic relationships established between the end-user and producer.

The way food is treated and offered has sensibly changed, and to an extent, so has the sourcing. By establishing direct contact with the farmers, the chef acts on preventing third parties and market traps, making the short supply chain an economic, cultural and social transformation mechanism.

How can the chef, as the leading character on this purchasing and transformation food system, be connected with a range of suppliers on a daily basis and raise the customer's interest not only on the food prepared but on what is it made from? Through the theoretical background and the processes used to understand and analyze the daily issues of the chef and the restaurant, the key is how to connect these actors and enhance the goods purchasing logistics.

## 2 METHODOLOGY

Design thinking is a strategy comprising techniques to address complex problems that are ill-defined or unknown, in human-centric ways, understanding the value and nature of human relationships, being them person to person, person and things or person and organization (Stickdorn & Schneider, 2014).

This study has followed a step by step guide by MJV, a Brazilian consulting agency, focused on Innovation, Strategy and Design Thinking (Vianna, 2018) and was developed through fieldwork aimed at identifying opportunities to develop an answer to the main question of this study: how can the restaurant chef de cuisine, who has the skills and capacity to source and modify food, affect the demand on the production end of the food chain?

The fieldwork aimed to identify anything that impairs or impedes experience (emotional, cognitive, aesthetic) and well-being in participants (Vianna, 2018, p. 13). The guide proposes five steps for problem-solving, employing a practical project as an example of the methodology presented. It is divided into Prototyping five iterative actions: Immersion, Analysis and Synthesis, Ideation, Prototyping, and Implementation.

The path followed in studying the chef and the small-scale food supply system beholds three out of the five above mentioned steps. Since this is an ongoing study, the last two steps were left out for the moment. The process starts uncertain of what the final product will be. It could come out as a product, a service, a user interface or something else (Stickdorn & Schneider, 2014). The procedure resulted in the outcome of a service concept, which required the identification of the most relevant contact points for service delivery which may result in an experience that is consistent across all of these contact points and responds to the chef de cuisine's needs (Sanders & Simons, 2009; Stickdorn & Schneider, 2014).

Design Thinking requires an empathetic process in the issue under analysis (Vianna, 2018), which was embellished in this study by the personal experience of the first author, which has over ten years of experience as a restaurant chef de cuisine. It is important to understand how every day of a chef involves particular challenges, being the one person responsible for all the food and team of a restaurant kitchen. The elaboration of a menu involves a series of decision-making processes, as of the origin, quality and value of the product chosen, and also as in the manners this food will be processed, presented and ultimately sold to a consumer. The chef has to consider, as well, technical restraints of both the kitchen and the brigade, food waste, client acceptance, and the restaurant revenue.

### 2.1 Immersion

#### 2.1.1 Preliminary immersion: desk and exploratory research

The subject has been under study since 2018, and the bibliographical review on the subject pointed out a couple of more meaningful sources. Writings by authors such as Michael Pollan, Dan Barber, Carolyn Steel, and Marion Nestlé, have set the canvas with reputable journalism; while NGOs such as the Fair Trade Foundation; Food, Agriculture and Environment related forums, the UN and FAO reports, along with their collaborator researchers articles have provided for a deeper and more comprehensive understanding of the issues surrounding food production chains.

In this phase, twelve chefs, mostly from Rio de Janeiro, but also from Brasilia and Curitiba were surveyed and interviewed to disclose their views and provenance of the foods used in their kitchens, as well as the factors influencing the choice and what this choice entails in the consumption chain. Based on this information it was possible to circumscribe the area to be researched with more focus.

In addition to reading and exploratory research, the personal experience of the first author, having worked in restaurant kitchens from different countries, has been added to bring out the important points in the process.

#### 2.1.2 In-depth immersion
##### 2.1.2.1 Interviews
The chosen chef's profiles follow analogous characteristics, the most important being the use of locally sourced or traceable origin ingredients, small-scale restaurants, and A/B consumer public. The questions were carried personally and focused on the routine of the kitchen, the development of menus, purchase/delivery of goods, client acceptance and financial issues.

From the carried interviews, the most relevant answers were selected and are presented by their authors:

I. Chef 01: works with a daily lunch menu. Has pointed out the following aspects: distribution logistics (quantity and quality), weekly elaboration of the menu, datasheet and cost control, constantly acquiring knowledge from the producer and the patrons.
II. Chef 02: practices a set menu for the dinner service and a daily menu for lunch service. Has brought out the need for a marketing strategy to value the local, recognized choice of merchandise, pedagogical function without fetishism, a plurality of suppliers and needs.
III. Chef 03: high end daily tasting menu, needs to rely on additional suppliers to meet the demand and standards of quantity and variety. Plans menu daily. Gets missing or less conventional supplies from a local produce shop nearby.
IV. Chef 04: functions with a daily tasting menu, elaborating the menu based on the available produce. Has an initial plan, but only finalizes after going personally to the local markets. The process demands chef and client flexibility of needs, the immediate economic impact on the producer, shared knowledge.
V. Chef 05: works with a set menu, seasonal specials and some "daily" items. In this way is thus able to circumvent most of the harvest oscillation. Formulated a compilation of preparations for the main vegetables, so the kitchen staff has the autonomy to prepare them the best possible way. Aside from working with small producers, runs an institute and several related projects.
VI. Chef 06: set seasonal menu of casual fine-dining, seeks to keep small producers close by, including cheese and sausage artisans. National visibility.
VII. Chef 07: comfort food cuisine, uses CSA products and regular fresh produce, has been promoting monthly dinners with small producers and crafters of various products, promoting their visibility and sales. The daily salad buffet gives out seasonal items, and the menu changes frequently, making use of weekly specials as well. In the specials, it unveils the origin of its merchandise.
VIII. Chef 08: runs two vegan vegetarian restaurants based on the same set of options, including a salad of the day. Uses most organic ingredients from family farms, with set suppliers and relies on a local crop shop nearby.
IX. Chef 09: menu focused on wine pairing, works with full usage of supplies, producing a minimum of daily waste. Menu items are very flexible, and once a week works with tapas, to make the best of everything in stock.
X. Chef 10: Other than flour, this baker uses most of the produce from local makers, also has the backup of the local vegetable market nearby. It

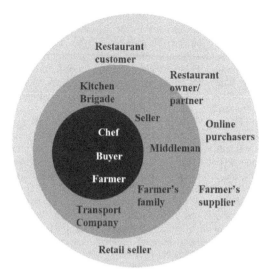

Figure 1. Actors map.

makes a point in supporting and endorsing its suppliers. It has great visibility in the local and national scenario.
XI. Chef 11: the high end daily tasting menu uses practically only local produce, with most plant-based preparations. Supports and conveys the work of small agriculturalists and trader, has a project of an urban garden on the outskirts of the city. Gives lectures and has good visibility in both national and international scenarios.

### 2.1.2.2 Actors

The short-chain of food consumption in restaurants directly involves and has the possibility to bond the producer, the chef, and the final consumer. Based on that, an actor's graphic was formulated, depicting the several layers of people involved (Figure 1).

### 2.1.2.3 Analysis and synthesis

How can kitchen chefs intervene in the consumer chain and boost conscious food consumption? This was the issue of the Immersion phase. The interviews and next steps have this inquiry as background, directing the exercise and trying to draw a picture of what is already happening towards this habit change.

### 2.1.2.4 Insight cards

After compiling and analyzing the information collected in the interviews, the data was placed in Cards, and the most recurrent topics could be grouped into three macro-areas: Logistics, Menu, and Consciousness.

### 2.1.2.5 A day in the life

Based on the knowledge acquired after years of cooking practice, the first author was able to synthesize a day in the life of a chef who works with small scale suppliers. Together with two of the interviewed chefs,

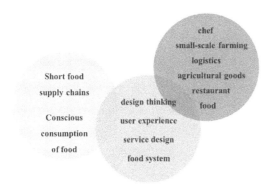

Figure 2. Conceptual map.

a pair of dinners were designed, in two different cities, with a menu entirely drawn on local products and small producers. The purpose of this exercise is to experience and have the possibility to analyze the whole process, from purchasing to fitting the ideas to preparing the products that will compose a preset menu.

#### 2.1.2.6 Generative sessions

During the interview days, it was possible to join together, in some of the sessions, kitchen chefs and other people related to them for small brainstorming sessions. For the brainstorming process, the aim was to raise the most relevant issues to the chain, particularly in the section that ranges from the producer to the chef. Initiatives like urban gardens, CSAs (Agricultural Supportive Community), agroforestry and sustainable management made on the scale of family farming were amongst the mentioned.

#### 2.1.2.7 Conceptual map

The intention of a Conceptual Map is to illustrate the connections between the data, enabling more linear reasoning and allowing new meanings to be extracted from the information. It is also a way of granting a visual organization at different levels of depth (Figure 2).

#### 2.1.2.8 Persona

The interviewees for this exercise made it possible to draw a user profile chef de cuisine. Scrutinizing the data and regrouping, a Persona has been drawn.

#### 2.1.2.9 User journey

Once the issues have been assessed and appointed as the object of the exercise, the actors were mapped and the persona was elaborated. The User Journey framework was then designed, trying to distinguish the most problematic or inspiring points of contact in the chain of purchase, producer to the chef.

#### 2.1.3 *Ideation*

Based on the data collected and on the analysis and synthesis of the problems pointed out in the previous phase, the Logistics issue was chosen as the object of this exercise. The focus will be on understanding and improving the purchase and delivery of goods, with the chef being the central user of this service. How can the process of production, purchase, and delivery of agricultural goods be facilitated so that the chef can work with the ideals of conscious consumption of food?

#### 2.1.3.1 Co-creation and ideas menu

Using the interview section as a base point, and having had the chance to work with Focus Groups at the same time, an initial idea menu has been designed mostly from the Generative Sessions above, synthesizing all the ideas generated in the project. Adding to that, co-creation has taken place when chefs ideas were merged with the experience of the first author, as a cook and researcher.

#### 2.1.4 *Prototyping and implementation*

Considering the small time-frame given for this research, the final two stages of MJV's proposed method will not be elaborated.

### 3 RESULTS

The study introduces the obstacles faced by a chef to work with small-scale agriculture. Upon analysis of the data collected, a scenario has emerged, showcasing actors and issues involved. The diagrams below display the actors involved between the two ends of the short food supply chain and a Conceptual map.

Based on the profile of the interviewed chefs and the current overall panorama of the local supply chain fed restaurants, both a Persona and a Customer Journey map have been drawn (Figures 3 and 4). This information will be used to develop a more suited solution for the questions proposed.

The motos presented by John Thackara are true to the interviewed chefs. Authenticity, local context, and local production are increasingly desirable attributes in the things we buy and the services we use. Local sells, and for that reason is a powerful antidote to mobility expansion. But design to enhance locality is easier said than done." (Thackara, 2005, p. 73).

By dividing the answers given in the Interview phase in three main areas, the most relevant issues in the process, from the point of view of the chefs were:

I. Logistics: drawbacks or matters related to the delivery of merchandise, both in quantity and variety. In some situations, it is necessary to have a multiplicity of suppliers so that the demand of the restaurant is met (according to the same delivery/quality/quantity criteria). Another aspect is the technical question of drawing up technical datasheets and controlling costs when the menu oscillates so frequently.

II. Menu: when there is a need for frequent preparation of new dishes and preparation, which can be an exhaustive exercise, and there is often no possibility of testing. The magnitude of the establishment also has great weight in this menu model.

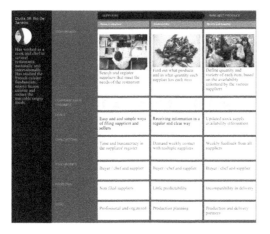

Figure 3(a).   Customer journey map.

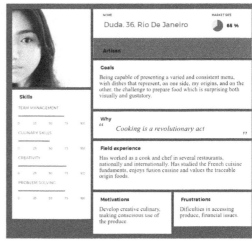

Figure 4.   Persona.

Figure 3(b).   Customer journey map.

III. Consciousness: when it is realized that this business model directly impacts the chain, in the economic, cultural and social spheres, it is possible to attribute to the chef the pedagogical role, access, preparation, and consumption; besides being able to directly connect the producer and final consumer. No fetish. The enterprise can also develop a strategy of valuing the option adopted, and attract customers

In regards to delivery logistics, the possibility of setting up a small-scale warehouse has been raised. There could also be some kind of online shopping network, with several registered producers, who update the goods weekly. This would make it possible to request a single central office and provide a more reliable and efficient distribution.

This set of actions is to overcome the hurdles of current commercial relationships, by designing a service for chefs that relies on a network of small scale farmers, taming the difficulties of interacting with this kind of commerce and to allow informed consumption.

A physical and online platform was appointed as a conceivable answer, one outcome of this process. A network of small-scale farmers, CSAs and urban farmers, connected online via an online shopping platform and a central physical store, which works as a market for both pre-acquired goods and over the counter purchases as well.

The chefs would be able to access a single website and/or mobile app, displaying a span of farmers and artisans and their certified goods. The shopping list could be made twice a week, meeting the chef's needs for freshness and stock capacity. The next step is simply choosing the amount and variety of products needed, and upon check out, deciding whether the purchase would be delivered at the physical store or at the restaurant.

Displayed on the online catalog would also be a brief profile of the producers, geographic coordinates and other relevant information. The service works as a bridge to directly connect the farmer and the chef. On the producer's end, it can be updated twice a week with the variety and quantity of the product available, which will display as sold out as the stock gets sold. On the chef's end, there's the chance of buying the necessary items from a range of producers but still on a single channel, minimizing the hassle of contacting several people. There's also the facility of planning the purchases twice weekly, to attend the space or budget restraints of the restaurant and ensure freshness.

This platform would work as a middleman but in a nonperverse, charging enough to cover operating expenses and fair profit. Figures could range from 15% to 25% of the price offered by the farmers. The target here isn't maximum profit, but paramount quality and ethics.

## 4 DISCUSSION

The experience of designing service for chefs, focusing on making tangible their intention to work with small-scale farmers and the possibility to source their agricultural goods has shown there's room for improvement, but also has signalized palpable efforts towards a more sustainable use of the food crops.

The chefs interviewed are aware of their role in making changes from their choices, and the effects these choices have in the long run. They also suffer from the market swings and the financial pressures of delivering the best possible food, with the least possible cost. On top of that, end consumers aren't always receptive to the chance of not having their favorite dish at a chosen restaurant, let alone daily changing menus.

Discussing the subject with chefs who already work with the small food supply chains and have the consciousness when buying goods has unveiled sensitive issues on the food system, and the need to improve it. This food purchasing and delivery network can aid the day-by-day life.

There are simple yet transforming actions to be taken. Chefs have to put themselves in the role of food managers, with the authority to choose and change. Mostly, they are starting to realize how much power they've got, be it in the media, be it in the tag they carry along themselves, be it by just doing what they think is right for all of the involved.

## 5 CONCLUSIONS

Although the timeframe of this study wouldn't allow for the Prototyping phase, it was just enough to accomplish the main objectives. Notable professionals are aiming at better practices, and that can only lead to a better future for the environment and society as a whole, besides enriching the gastronomic panorama.

After mapping a range of initiatives, deterrents and, successful ideas, a local background scenario can be pictured, so as to, from there, take a step forward in systematizing and multiplying the thriving cases. Along with that, some preliminary steps have already been given towards the undertaking of the most promising of the ideas: an initial talk with the owner of a strategically positioned local produce market and the creators of an online website offering goods from local and small farms and artisans. All of them foresee the services working hand to hand to empower and facilitate access. Furthermore, a number of farmers and artisans already belong to both business' networks, making it even easier to test and implement.

The use of this tool, along with feedback, can result in a solid way of surpassing the constraints identified in this work. On the route to shortening the food supply chain, the link between the chef and the final consumer is key to unite both ends. The chef has a variety of tools to explore and become the connection, merging farm and city, promoting the consciousness in buying and consuming food goods.

## REFERENCES

Adrià, F.; Roca, J. *The world's 50 Best Restaurants 2017.* www.theworlds50best.com. Access in February 2019.

Ballantyne-Brodie, E., Wrigley, C.; Ramsey, R. *Evolution of the Docklands Food Hub: A Design-Led Innovation Approach to Food Sovereignty Through Local Food Systems,* Journal of Design, Business & Society 1: 1. 2015.

Ballantyne-Brodie, E.; Ramsey, R. et al. *Design-led innovation to rejuvenate local food systems and healthy communities: An emerging research agenda.* 323–330. 0.1109/TIDMS.2013.6981254. 2013.

Barber, Dann. *The third plate.* Penguin Books, 2014.

Borges, C.D.; Santos, M.A. *Aplicações metodológicas da técnica de grupo focal: fundamentos metodológicos, potencialidades e limites.* Rev. SPAGESP, v.6, n.1. 2005.

Brown, Tim. *Design Thinking.* Harvard Business Review América Latina, Alta Books, 2008.

Brown, Tim; Wyatt, J. *Design thinking for social innovation.* Stanford Social Innovation Review, 8(1), 31–35. 2010.

Creswell, John W. *Projeto de pesquisa: métodos qualitativo, quantitativo e misto.* Porto Alegre: Artmed, 2007.

Deakin, Lynda. *IDEO's Approach to Designing a Better Food System.* Podcast under: Creative Confidence Series, design for Food. Access in June 2019.

EAT-Lancet Commission (https://eatforum.org/eat-lancet-commission/). Access in May 2019.

Fernald, Anya et al. *A World of Presidia: Food, Culture and Community,* Slow Food Editore, 2004.

Food and Agriculture Organization of the United Nations (http://www.fao.org). Access in May 2019.

Goodman, D., Dupuis, E. *Knowing food and growing food: beyond the production-consumption debate in the sociology of agriculture.* Sociologia Ruralis Volume 42, Issue 1, pp. 5–22, 2002.

https://nacoesunidas.org/pos2015/agenda2030/ Access in July 2018.

IDEO, *The Field Guide to Human-Centered Design.* Canada, IDEO.org, 2015.

Manzini, E. *Context-based wellbeing and the concept of regenerative solution. A conceptual framework for scenario building and sustainable solutions development.* The Journal of Sustainable Product Design, 2(3), 141–148. 2002.

Manzini, E. *Design, when everybody designs: an introduction to design for social innovation.* The MIT Press, 2015.

Nature Hub, Conscious consumer (https://medium.com/naturehub/what-is-a-conscious-consumer-and-why-does-it-matter-4b7a14ca08fc). Access in May 2019.

Nestlé, Marion. *Unsavory Truth.* Strand Books, 2018.

Petrini, Carlo. *Slow Food.* Columbia, Columbia University Press. 2001.

Pocketbook 2018, Preparations and outcomes of the 2012 United Nations Conference on Sustainable Development (Rio +20) (http://www.fao.org). Access in April 2019.

Pollan, Michael. *The Omnivore's Dilemma.* Penguin Books. 2006.

Roep, D.; Wiskerke, H. *Nourishing networks: Fourteen lessons about creating sustainable food supply chains.* Reeds Business Information, 2006.

Silva; Veloso, A. *Focus Group: Considerações Teóricas e Metodológicas.* Portugal. Revista Lusófona de Educação, n.26, p. 175–190. 2014.

Steel, Carolyn. *Hungry Cities.* Vintage Books, 2013.

Steel, Carolyn. Sitopia*: How Food can save the world.* Chatto & Windu, 2019.

Stewart, D.; Shamdasani, P. *Focus Groups: Theory and Practice*. Thousand Oaks, California. Sage. 2007.

Stickdorn, Marc.; Schneider, Jakob. *Isto é Design Thinking de Serviços*. Bookman, 2014.

The Fair Trade Foundation (https://www.fairtrade.org.uk/). Access in March 2019.

The Small Footprint Family (https://www.smallfootprint family.com/can-organic-farming-feed-the-world). Access in April 2019.

UN Agenda for Sustainable Development Goals, Food and Agriculture Organization of the United Nations, World Food and Agriculture Statistical, Access in May 2018.

UN Paris Agreement (https://unfccc.int/process-and-meetings/the-Paris-agreement/d2hhdC1pcy). Access in June 2019.

Vianna, M et al. *Design Thinking: Business Innovation*. Gráfica Cruzado. 2018.

Wiskerke, Johannes S.C.; Viljoen, André. *Sustainable food planning: evolving theory and practice.* E-book, 2016.

World Design Organization https://wdo.org/ Access in July 2018.

Zampollo, F. *The four Food Design pillars.* Online School of Food Design – onlineschooloffooddesign.org. published on academia.edu on December 15, 2017.

Zampollo, F. *The wonderful world of Food Design: A conversation with Marije Vogelzang.* International Journal of Food Design, 2015, Volume 1, Number 1, p. 65–71.

Zampollo, F. *Welcome to Food Design.* International Journal of Food Design, 2015, Volume 1, Number 1, p. 3–9.

*Experiencing Food: Designing Sustainable and Social Practices – Bonacho, Pires & Lamy (Eds)*
© *2021 Taylor & Francis Group, London, ISBN 978-0-367-49414-8*

# From Asia to Portugal – fermentation, probiotics and waste management in restaurants

F. Abreu & N. Félix
*ESHTE, Estoril Higher Institute of Hotel and Tourism Studies, Estoril, Portugal*

M.J. Pires
*ESHTE, Estoril Higher Institute of Hotel and Tourism Studies, Estoril, Portugal*
*CEAUL, Universidade de Lisboa, Lisboa, Portugal*

ABSTRACT: After visiting Asia, on a journey about the fermentation process, the aim was to study the work of probiotics which enhance parts of foods prepared to be discarded, creating new products. Accordingly, a Waste Reduction System through Fermentation with 10 phases was created to implement a system in the restaurant or at home to reduce waste. After this process, food becomes a vehicle for a complex experiment that represents the development of thousands of living microorganisms and by completing it with one more phase – from turning a waste into a new product through fermentation, including the positive health effects – we increase profits in a restaurant.

## 1 INTRODUCTION

The tour to the Asian continent, a reference in terms of the history of fermentation and the diversity of fermented products, included Hong Kong, Macao, Vietnam, Cambodia, Bangkok, Laos and Singapore (Jan–March 2018). Several forms of fermentation are here briefly presented, as well as their uses and, mainly, their benefits.

Some types of fermentation have been described as being more suitable for the development of bacteria beneficial to humans, thus making us particularly interested in the synergy that these living microorganisms exert after their consumption. In fact, we cannot ignore the fact that fermentation can be seen, and used, as a way of reducing food waste and of food preservation, or how this can generate profits in the food industry area.

In addition, apart from the research and its analysis, there was the opportunity to test some of the fermentations in Fome Restaurant (literally translated as Hunger) in Lisbon. Such an empirical experience was essential and what was then appropriately named "Fermenting through Asia" soon became "Fermenting in Lisbon".

### 1.1 *The focus*

It was because of our focus on improving health through food intake that we came across probiotics – "Microbes that after ingestion confer some benefits to the body" (Katz, 2012: 26)[1]. The research was on these and on how to introduce them in food; therefore,

fermentation, an ancestral technique that uses the microorganisms present in the food itself, or not, in order to create a new product with a much richer biota, aims at the development of the microorganisms of our intestine.

Following Dr. Emeran Mayer[2] in *The Mind-Gut Connection*, among others, we need to highlight how the intestines and all of their flora are closely related to the brain. Food is a source of information that upon reaching our body will influence it and our trillions of microbes which degrade food; all this is reflected in our health and well-being and so in our life. What we eat is really who we are. It is at this stage that fermentation allows the inoculation/development of microorganisms in foods, thus enhancing the diversity of intestinal flora. A rich and healthy flora generates a healthy organism.

Fermentation can, and should be used in any food, not only for the preservation of a particular food, but also as a resource of the benefits from the consumption of bacteria and yeasts produced by this technique, namely probiotics, further enhancing its use in order to promote better management and reduction of food waste, in order to obtain profit in the restaurant industry.

According to FAO, "33% of everything produced annually in the world goes to waste" (FAO, Issue No. 711/2015)[3], raising political and governmental issues, given the need to solve this problem. Accordingly, we have verified the introduction and implementation of food waste reduction policies, such as the Urban Waste Prevention Program (UWPP/PRU), which is based on "the promotion of individual composting (mixed, rural and collective areas, as schools and green spaces), the concept of 'right dose', and support for food banks and also in stimulating responsible consumption" (Lima, 2017)[4]. However, in spite of various awareness-raising policies, promotion of food banks and increased composting, food waste remained at around 30%.

FAO also estimates that about 1.3 billion tons of food, which accounts for approximately one-third by weight of all food produced for human consumption in the world, are lost or wasted every year (European, 2017)[5]. When reflecting on knowledge, training and experience, an alternative has emerged, an alternative that is already practiced in some restaurants: fermentation, which is used by some of the most famous restaurants in the world, such as NOMA, Geranium and AMASS, all of which are based in northern Europe and have chosen fermentation processes with Asian inspirations.

In the Portuguese case, despite the use of fermentations in the favorite national products, such as bread, cheese, wine and sausage, the state of the art lies asleep. The application of similar techniques in day-to-day products, such as greens, fruits and vegetables in order to increase their longevity, for example, or to obtain much more interesting nutritional values, is just not performed. Such scarcity (fermentation techniques) results, in part, from the lack of knowledge of the general public about fermentation processes, what they originate and the probiotic effect they may have on everyone's health.

Fermentation is a technique that involves the development of microorganisms and the growth of certain bacteria, molds and yeasts. Due to the fact that the fermentation involves the handling of living microorganisms, it is necessary to take extra care to develop and keep alive those we want, namely the probiotics, that we address here. In addition to the interaction of these microorganisms (probiotics) with the host organism (via consumption), this technique also increases the shelf life of the products, thus reducing or avoiding food waste, as well as developing new flavors; these last uses create the possibility of increasing profits in the restaurant area.

Given the concept of probiotic – microbes that are provided with life forms, favoring them, as these are mostly bacteria – we were able to notice that the species most heavily used as probiotics, approved by the World Organization of Gastroenterology (GMO), are particularly "*Lactobacillus, Bifidobacteria, Saccharomyces cerevisiae* and some species of *E. coli* and *Bacillus*" (Kaufmann et al., 2011: 4)[6]. In this way, there are similarities with the same species used to work in various fermentations, such as yogurt, beer, sourdough, kefir, among others. Thus, with the probiotic(s) present in a large quantity in fermented foods and having a given food associated probiotic, it is possible to admit that the consumption of a certain fermented food will have a beneficial effect on the organism, favoring its consumption, instead of the introduction of probiotics by

synthesized route. This factor is accompanied by a greater bioavailability to the natural factor vs synthetic factor. In addition to the bioavailability, there is also the symbiosis between the respective microorganisms that create synergies between them to create a better environment to coexist.

This leaves us one last question to close the circuit: is it possible to elaborate the fermentations, full of probiotics, through products that were initially considered waste in order to increase profit? After confirming and understanding the relationship between fermentation and probiotics, and vice versa, we proceeded to use this knowledge to create new products loaded with probiotics, hence relating this practice to the use of food, in order to avoid and reduce the waste in the restaurant industry, and as a cause-effect situation, to increase the resulting profits in a restaurant. To perform these tests it was first necessary to understand what can be fermented, as well as how best to use the product resulting from the fermentation. As an example the banana peel was fermented using *Lactobacillus bulgaricus* and *Streptococcus thermophilus*; in this way two new products were obtained: the serum, now with a slightly acidified banana palate, and the peel, now less fibrous, completely black, and with intensified flavored banana and sour notes. Through these two new products, many more have been made. The serum was used in milkshakes, pancakes and juices, enriching these by-products with probiotics and a higher nutritional value. The peel has been chopped finely and incorporated into a guacamole, which now together with the peppers, onion, lime, tomato, avocado and coriander, awaken us to new flavors – the fruity notes and the acidity of the guacamole itself. It is possible, from this concrete example, to discover that not only it is possible to transform waste into new food, but it is also quite feasible to develop a fermented product through the use of what would be a waste, which can lead to complete polyvalences of uses in the area of gastronomy taking advantage of both their consumption and the sale itself (profit).

## 1.2 *Fermentation*

Fermentation is the transformative action of microorganisms. This action can be triggered by various bacteria and fungi, and therefore also by their respective enzymes. In order for fermentation to occur, the following two factors are required: bacteria/fungus and substrate. In each food we want to ferment, regardless of its origin, vegetables, fruit, dairy products, meat, fish, shellfish, eggs, legumes, seeds, oilseeds and tubers, among others. There is never only one type of microorganisms present, but a lot of different microorganisms and this community is called microbiota.

In this microbiota all the microorganisms contribute with genetic code or with metabolic products, so that they can thus reproduce on favorable conditions and the efficiency of the microbiota is maintained in the best possible conditions. It is through these basic principles of community management that the fermentation is governed and it is also through fermentative processes the lactic acid bacteria is released into their medium antimicrobial properties which include "organic acids, hydrogen peroxide, antibiotics and bacteriocins" (A.R. Sarika, 2010: 291)[7]. They are consequently fighting the external aggressions through the production of internal compounds, which are permanently alive and adapt to the aggressors.

Lactic acid bacteria (BAL/LAB) – part of the genera "*Lactobacillus, Leuconostoc, Pediococcus, Streptococcus, Lactococcus, Enterococcus, Carnobacterium e Vagococcus* (Fernandes, 2011: 2)[8]" – produce lactic acid, which can be homolactic (homofermentative) type with the highest amount of this component (lactic acid), having a "minimum content of 85%" (Katz, 2012: 96) in relation to the other formed products, such as diacetyl, ethanol and $CO_2$, or heterolactic (heterofermentative), when the proportions of these products are practically the same (Franco & Landgarf, 1996: 10)[9]. Heterofermentative bacteria can produce, in addition to lactic acid, also acetic acid (Franco & Landgarf, 1996: 10).

According to Katz (2012)[10] the fruit is fermented primarily in alcohol and acetic acid if exposed to oxygen, while the vegetables ferment primarily in lactic acid. Consequently, some actions are necessary in order to perform a lactic fermentation in the fruit: the activity of the endogenous yeasts of the fruit, responsible for the transformation of the sugars into alcohol, can be inhibited through a brine process or through the addition of a culture of LAB such as whey.

Concerning the fermentation process of sugars, it is characterized by the action of yeasts, such as the genus "*Saccharomyces, Kloeckera, Candida, Hansenula, Hanseniospora, Pichia, Zigossacharomyces*", (Mamede & Pastore, 2004: 453)[11] among others, in the transformation of sugars into alcohol. This is a process of spontaneous fermentation, so it is not necessary the action of man for the appearance of alcohol – it "happens in fruits too ripe, split, happens in honey that is diluted with water, [it] happens in plants that expel juices out of the plant" (Katz, 2012: 69).

By reading Katz (2012), it is possible to perceive that yeasts, responsible for the transformation of sugars into alcohol, can act in two ways and they are able to perform: (1) anaerobic fermentation, (2) and/or oxidative respiration. In the oxidative mode they grow and reproduce faster, but do not produce alcohol, since the alcohol is only accumulated in the anaerobic mode (absence of oxygen).

The most well-known and used yeast is *Saccharomyces cerevisiae*, which is predominantly used in alcoholic fermentation and in the bakery; however, there are numerous others capable of performing alcoholic fermentation, such as *Kloeckera apiculata*, which dominates the initial stages of the spontaneous fermentation of fruit juices and grapes. To these

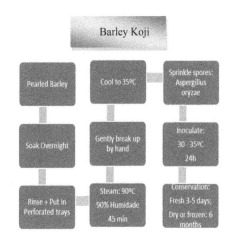

Figure 1. Demonstration of Barley Koji production; Source: Johnson & Williams (2016: 54–55)[23].

fermented fruit drinks based on simple sugars we call country wines.

As for beer, Katz (2012: 247) defines it as "a fermented beverage in which alcohol derives essentially from complex carbohydrates of cereals or tubers with starch." For alcohol production cereals require the conversion of complex hydrates into simple sugars and this conversion takes place through enzymatic activity. According to McGee (2004)[12] the enzymes responsible for this conversion arise due to the malting process; in this process the germ within the grain activates a mechanism to restart all the biochemical activity of the cereal itself and thus produces several enzymes, performing actions of breaking the starch and proteins within the cells of the endosperm.

In the conversion of complex sugars into simple ones, there are more ways to work with. The oldest form is the use of mastication of cereals, a technique called "insalivation, enzymes present in saliva (amylases)" (Gastoni & Filho, 2016: 30)[10] perform actions of breaking the complex carbohydrates into simple ones. Gastoni & Filho (2016) focus on how the technique widely used in Asia derives from the production of fungi and on how the growth of molds outside the grain, usually of the genus *Aspergillus, Rhizopus* and/or *Neurosopora*, is induced – in this case high amiolytic activities degrade the starch.

According to Katz (2012), mold growth is extremely simple to perform. Since molds as aerobic beings require oxygen to survive and reproduce, in addition to oxygen they also need moisture and heat. These are the three basic factors for the development of molds: oxygen, temperature (between 27°C and 32°C) and humidity (80%). Figure 1 shows the *Aspergillus oryzae* mold, and its effect on barley in order to produce Koji. Koji is a product transformed through the action of *Aspergillus oryzae* and the substrate to be used in the production of Koji can vary immensely essentially between cereals and leguminous. Koji is also the basis of all Asian cuisine, it is through this that saké, miso, soy sauce, amazaké, rice vinegar, mirin and even pickles with vegetables are made – that is, all the seasonings of the Asian gastronomy.

## 1.3 *Asia*

Fermentation is a millennial process, used essentially as a way to extend the shelf life of the foods, which often maintain the fermentation process for more than a year. In its origin, in addition to increasing the life span of food, fermentation is a technique used as a natural remedy.

All cultures have a bit of fermentation: "the miso of Japan, the Kombucha of China, the kimchi of Korea, the labneh of the Middle East and the lassi of India, through the fermented pickles of cabbage, cucumbers and carrots, from Eastern countries and Northern Europe, from Bulgaria to Scandinavia" (Pike, 2016: 6)[13]. In addition to these, "most fermented milk products, which are very familiar these days, were developed by Asian nomads, breeders of cattle" (Lambert, 2016: 14)[14]. Also, as mentioned, "most of the tradition of fermented beans, essentially soybeans originate and are most commonly found in China, Japan, Korea, Indonesia and other parts of Asia" (Katz, 2012: 316).

Miso, the basis of traditional Japanese cuisine, corresponds precisely to a mixture of well-cooked and crushed grains, to which koji, salt and other ingredients are added, and after the second fermentation ends, it is ready to be consumed. The use of miso knows no limits, this is used as a paste that acquires flavor and high nutritional value regardless of where it is placed.

In Japan, soybeans are fermented by the action of a bacterium (*Bacillus subtilis* var. *natto*) that produces a viscous network in its own grain similar to the gum of okra. This fermented product is called natto – "Ferments very similar to natto are found in China (tan-shih), Thailand (thua-no), Korea (joenkuk-jang and damsue-jang), Nepal (kinema), and in several more East Asian sites" (Katz, 2012: 329). According to Katz (2012) and Cook (2015)[15] it should be noted that natto has a unique compound, nattokinase, produced by bacteria found in bean gum. This compound has a strong fibrinolytic activity, which means that it is able to break blood clots, and is also effective in breaking the amyloid plaque, characteristic of Alzheimer's disease. For Lambert (2016: 28) "the medicinal use of the Japanese fermented plum umeboshi can be found 1,000 years ago [and] umeboshi continues to be used on Japan's days, as a remedy that heals everything"

Having the first records of production and consumption in China, Kombucha is a fermented beverage which uses the leaves of *Camellia sinensis*, popularly called the tea plant: "Tea has been consumed in Asia for thousands of years" (Katz, 2018: 46)[16]. Kombucha is thus a sweet tea fermented through a community of bacteria and yeast – SCOBY. It is widely consumed and made in many different ways – "Kombucha contains

glucuronic acid, a compound produced in our liver, which aggregates itself with various toxins in order to eliminate them" (Katz, 2012: 168).

These are some of the fermented foods used in the Asian cuisine, but there are numerous other varieties and the diversity of each of them is endless, just as in India each different house has its curry, in Asia each house has its own miso.

## 1.4 *The probiotic world*

The concept of probiotic was delineated between 1965 and 1989 as a factor of microbiological origin that stimulated the growth of other microorganisms. However, the definition of probiotic was only complete in 1989, after Roy Fuller added that, in addition to stimulating resistance to the acidic environment of the stomach, to the bile and to the enzymes of the pancreas, it promoted a good adhesion to intestinal mucosal cells; a good colonization capacity; the production of antimicrobial substances that aim to act against pathogenic bacteria and the absence of translocation, so that, after setting in the mucosa, they do not migrate to another site.

Probiotics that are often used are divided into two large microbial domains, bacteria and yeast. Bacteria in turn are divided into two groups: acid-lactic bacteria (BAL/LAB) where we find the genus *Lactobacillus, Lactococcus* and *Streptococcus* and its various species; and the genus *Bifidobacterium*, which is not lactic acid bacteria because it does not produce lactic acid when fermenting the food, is also taxonomically different (Kaufmann, et al., 2011). In relation to yeasts, the genus *Saccharomyces* stands out, but only two of this species are used: *Saccharomyces boulardii* and *Saccharomyces cerevisiae*.

*Lactobacillus* are gram-positive, non-sporulated, facultative anaerobic bacteria, without flagella, which are *bacillus* or *cocobacillus* forms. There are 56 species recognized (Stefe, Alves & Ribeiro, 2008)[17] and the most commonly used are *Lactobacillus acidophilus, Lactobacillus brevis, Lactobacillus bulgaricus, Lactobacillus gureri, Lactobacillus gasseri, Lactobacillus paracasei, Lactobacillus plantarum, Lactobacillus reuteri, Lactobacillus salivarius and Lactobacillus rhamnosus* (Cook, 2015).

The genus *Bifidobacterium* is characterized by the following: Gram-positive, non-sporulated bacteria, without flagella, without the presence of the enzyme that degrades hydrogen peroxide (catalysis) and anaerobes. This genus has a variety of 30 species, the most known being *Bifidobacterium bifidum, Bifidobacterium breve, Bifidobacterium infantis, Bifidobacterium lactis* and *Bifidobacterium longum* (Cook, 2015). Bifidobacteria are capable of using galactose, lactose and fructose as sources of energy (Stefe, Alves & Ribeiro, 2008).

*Saccharomyces*, among which the *S. boulardii* stands out, tolerate high temperatures and are not pathogenic. When *S. boulardii* is ingested it has the particularity of becoming insensitive to the action of gastric and antibacterial acids, an important factor to consider in the use of antibacterial to combat stomach infections (Stefe, Alves & Ribeiro, 2008).

Concerning bacteria, "it is estimated that the microorganisms in our body weigh about one kilogram" and "there are more than one billion bacteria in our intestines, it is estimated that they are composed of a thousand different species" (Cook, 2015: 34). As Shinya (2011)[18] points out in her book *The Microbe Factor: Your Innate Immunity and the Coming Health Revolution*, there are 3 types of intestinal bacteria – beneficial, harmful and intermediate – and the proportion of bacteria in our intestines is approximately twenty (20) percent of beneficial bacteria, 30 (thirty) percent of harmful bacteria and the remaining 50 (fifty) percent are composed of intermediate bacteria. According to Cook (2015), the key bacteria that contribute to the control of the intestinal environment are the intermediate bacteria, since they act as a neutral intestinal element; when less healthy meals are eaten, part of the intermediary goes to the harmful ones, the opposite is true. In this way we succeed.

Oelschalaeger (2009)[19] said that the effects of probiotics on health, can be classified into three groups: (a) ability to articulate the defense of their host to which the probiotic provides a synergistic relationship; (b) application of a direct action on other foreign microorganisms, for example pathogenic, in this way probiotics play a pivotal role in the prevention and treatment of infections in the intestinal mucosa, as well as a recovery of the microbial balance; and (c) cleansing the intestine by eliminating residues resulting from microbial metabolism such as toxins.

Through Ng, Hart, Kamm, Stagg, & Knight (2008)[20], it is possible to realize that all these effects are performed by mechanisms of action that are exerted by probiotics. These mechanisms of action are divided into three phases, the antimicrobial phase, the reinforcement phase of the barrier function and the immunomodulation phase. In this way these mechanisms consist of: (I) – Antimicrobial phase – competition for nutrients, local of adhesion and production of antimicrobial metabolites; (II) – Strengthening phase of the barrier function – changes in environmental conditions; (III) – Immunomodulation phase – modulation of the immune response of the host.

It is through these stages that probiotics improve our health, and subsequently our quality of life. Probiotics also have several anticancer effects. These occur, it is known, due to three actions carried out by probiotics, namely:

(a) Firstly by the inhibition of polycyclic aromatic hydrocarbons and nitrosamines, in other words, compounds prior to the formation of carcinogenic compounds – pre-carcinogenic.
(b) Secondly, when the cells responsible for tumor formation are formed, an inhibitory action is applied.
(c) Thirdly, because of the high binding capacity of probiotics to carcinogenic substances, which are

formed by tumor cells, preventing them from forming and thus inactivating the carcinogenic substances which would result therefrom.

Probiotics act on carcinogenic compounds to the extent that they "produce antitumorigenic or antimutagenic compounds in the colon (such as butyrate), alter the metabolic activity of the intestinal microbiota, leading to a change in the physicochemical conditions of the colon with decreased pH and effects on the physiology of the host" (Costa, Balthazar, Moreira, Cruz, & Júnior, 2013: 1394)[21].

Another characteristic of probiotics is the production of bacteriocins, "which are proteins or protein complexes with bactericidal or bacteriostatic activity, directly against species that are usually related to the bacterial producer" (Klaenhammer, 1987: 337)[22]. KVR Reddy (2004) has shown that the peptides are produced by bacteria, and thus have a spectrum of action against a wide variety of microorganisms, including Gram-positive and Gram-negative bacteria, protozoa, fungi and virus, which are called bacteriocins.

It is in this context that Cook concludes that "studies show that probiotic bacteria are far more intelligent than we have ever thought. They can recognize the molecular patterns of harmful microbes that cause disease and respond by secreting proteins that destroy these harmful microbes" (Cook, 2015: 34).

## 2 FERMENTATION AND SUSTAINABILITY

### 2.1 *WRSF/SRDF*

Due to the amount of waste that exists in the world, and the amount of waste that exists in the area of the restaurant industry, it is urgent to create a system capable of reducing this waste. Consequently, we have created the WRSF/SRDF system – Waste Reduction System through Fermentation.

This system works in an extremely simple way so that it can be applied in the restaurant industry. At the moment it is being applied by us, partially, in the restaurant "FOME". Some of these policies have been in place since July to reduce waste and boost profits and will soon be running at a 100 percent.

WRSF works in tandem with seasonality, respecting the ingredient, while working on a product in its fullness. It also implies more work on each ingredient and rethinking the menu daily according to the seasonality and the products transformed by the fermentation that we already have.

Thus, the WRSF presents 10 phases, as follows:

- 1st Phase – Seasonality database of products;
  - Software that demonstrates the ideal fruit and vegetable season.
  - Software is also used to view the closed fish season (fish breeding season, so they cannot be fished at that time);

- 2nd Phase – Contact with small suppliers;
  - They will supply the products of the season, very fresh;
  - Small suppliers of meat and fish, including game, this way we can vary our menu, having offers that few have.
- 3rd Phase – According to the seasonality acquire more quantity;
  - It will enable a greater quantity of a product at a more affordable price.
- 4th Phase – Decide the menu according to the products that are bought, of the season and, therefore, cheaper, and not the opposite;
- 5th Phase – Use a product in a variety of ways;
  - It will allow a greater variety of by-products to be presented in the menu. For example, when buying extra quantity of carrots, make carrot and cardamom jelly, carrot and mango foam and carrot bread. This allows us to add more variety to the menu, using a single ingredient, this way we are boosting profits.
- 6th Phase – Prolong the life of the ingredients, acquiring a new product through the fermentation;
  - At this stage it is necessary to make ferments that fit well with any dish in the menu;
  - For example: with the carrot left over from our purchase, make a Sauerkraut of carrot which can last for more than a year, and serve as a complement or side-dish of several dishes.
- 7th Phase – Reuse what seems to be untapped through fermentation;
  - An example of fermenting: use the banana peel to make guacamole; grind carrot peel, potato peel, cabbage/broccoli stalks, beetroot …to do miso; remove the peel of the orange and the lemon that would go in the trash and ferment the zests along with the Sauerkraut, the white part can be dehydrated and crushed, to be used to thicken jams; use the skin of the peeled tomatoes that would also go in the trash mixed with a SCOBY so as to obtain a tomato kombucha; use the peach kernel to make brandy or even grate the core of an avocado in order to make a mature butter.
- 8th Phase – Reuse the by-products of fermentation;
  - We have as an example water of Kefir that can be used with sourdough for faster acidification of the dough.
- 9th Phase – Development of a compound waste, made with the leftovers from the living room and the kitchen;
- 10th Phase – Rethink the menu daily to get the best out of the system.

## 3 EXPERIMENTATION AND RESULTS

By exploring the theme of fermentation and all the concepts and theory inherent to it, adding to the concerns and known info about food waste and the claim to profit in the area of the restaurant industry, we have been identifying the possibilities of performing and developing this process, practicing some of the fermentation techniques approached. For this, the availability of the "Fome" restaurant in Arroios/Lisbon was essential, which emphasized the importance of reducing waste, and thus left it to us to transform it. There, it was possible to carry out for example the following fermentation, obtaining the result shown below.

### 3.1 *Mead*

Mead production started on the 1st of August 2018, and finished on the 28th of February 2019.

For the production of mead, the endogenous yeast of ripe fruits was first incubated in a mixture of 80% water to 20% honey, this mixture had to be vigorously wrapped every day for 2 weeks, then strained and transferred to the bottle shown in Figure 2. Then the bottle was sealed and the second fermentation occurred.

Food Resources: Fruit and stone, excess of the mackerel prime plate, which would normally be a waste. Results: Fruit (destined for trash) was turned into a tasty alcoholic drink, and one-shot (sold in a shot) so a profit was created out of waste. It is also a differentiating factor in the restaurant, as there are few places that have mead. Figure 2 demonstrates the respective mead, that was made from waste.

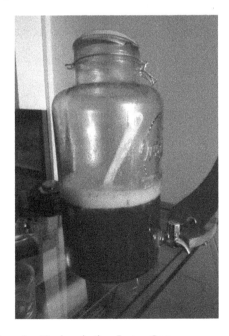

Figure 2. Mead production; Source: Own.

As a result, we have verified and achieved a waste reduction in the identified restaurant, which led to a better management of the resources acquired and the investment made for this purpose.

## 4 CONCLUSION

Fermentation is a technique that through bacteria, molds and yeast transforms food. Despite its ancestral origin and being associated with various physical and chemical processes, it is relatively simple to elaborate if its basic principles are taken into account – that is, inhibition of pathogens through minor actions of salinity control, substrate control as well as temperature control, and surrounding conditions.

In this path, and as a result of the Asia trip, we were able to gain visual and taste knowledge and also open our horizons to the point of realizing that there are ways to make edible even an avocado seed.

Although we were unable to further demarcate the theme "Fermenting through Asia" (given the language barrier that did not allow us to report a more traditional process) our presence on that continent had a great influence on the way we see and think about food and people, even enhancing it.

The benefits of fermentation know no boundaries, particularly with regard to health, as new probiotics are constantly being discovered, which are associated with the improvement of certain diseases.

## REFERENCES

[1] Katz, S. E. (2012). *The Art of Fermentation.* United States: Chelsea Green.

[2] Mayer, E. (2016). *The Mind-Gut Connection: How the Hidden Conversation within Our Bodies Impacts Our Mood, Our Choices, and Our Overall Health.* United States: HarperCollins Publisher. https://www.amazon.com/Mind-Gut-Connection-Conversation-Impacts-Choices/dp/0062376551#reader_0062376551.

[3] FAO. (2015). *The State of Agricultural Comodity Markets IN DEPHT.* United States: http://www.fao.org/3/a-i5225e.pdf

[4] Lima, S. http://www.fao.org/3/a-i5225e.pdf (2017). *Redução do Desperdício Alimentar.* https://www.apambiente.pt/index.php?ref=16&subref=84&sub2ref=106&sub3ref=273

[5] Europeu, P. (16 May 2017). *Utilização mais eficiente dos recursos: reduzir os resíduos alimentares.* http://www. gpp.pt/images/MaisGPP/Iniciativas/CNCDA/Resolucao_PE-INI_desperdicio_20170516.pdf

[6] Kaufmann, P., Paula, J., Fedorak, R., Shanahan, F., Sanders, M., Szajewska, H., ...Kim, N. (2011). *probióticos e prebióticos.* World Gastroenterology Organization. http://www.worldgastroenterology.org/UserFiles/file/guidelines/probiotics-portuguese-2011.pdf

[7] A.R. Sarika, A. L. (2010). *Bacteriocin Production by a New Isolate of Lactobacillus rhamnosus GP1 under Different Culture Conditions* (Vol. 2). Vizhinjam – 695521, Kerala, India: Maxwell Scientific Organization. http://maxwellsci.com/print/ajfst/v2-291-297.pdf.

[8] Fernandes, S. d. (2011). *Monitoramento da Microbiota de Iogurtes Comerciais.* Rio de Janeiro. https://tede.ufrrj.br/bitstream/jspui/1240/2/2011%20-%20Simone%20de%20Souza%20Fernandes.pdf.

[9] Franco, B. D., & Landgarf, M. (1996). *Microbiologia dos Alimentos.* Brazil: Atheneu. https://drive.google.com/file/d/0ByedtynnbmhGQVRqRXdjcUNNS0U/view.

[10] Gastoni, W., & Filho, V. (2016). *Bebidas alcoólicas: ciência e tecnologia.* (2º). São Paulo: Blucher. https://books.google.pt/books?id=4ytdDwAAQBAJ&pg=PA30&lpg=PA30&dq=mastiga%C3%A7ao+dos+cereais+na+produ%C3%A7ao+de+cerveja&source=bl&ots=dtR2ZZa4Br&sig=wjpLa3Q8VAUK0cKlmKySbNXeEWI&hl=ptPT&sa=X&ved=2ahUKEwjM3fKw8vbdAhUHdcAKHTxcDKoQ6AEwBnoECAAQAQ#v=onepage&

[11] Mamede, M. E., & Pastore, G. M. (2004). *Avaliação da produção dos compostos majoritários da fermentação de mosto de uva por leveduras isoladas da região da "Serra Gaúcha" (RS).* Campinas, São Paulo. de http://www. scielo.br/pdf/%0D/cta/v24n3/21942.pdf.

[12] McGee, H. (2004). *On Food And Cooking: The Science and Lore of the Kitchen.* (Scribner, Ed.) New York. http://wtf.tw/ref/mcgee.pdf.

[13] Pike, C. (2016). *A arte da fermentação.* Estarreja: MEL Editores.

[14] Lambert, D. (2016). *Fermenting Recipes & Preparation.* United Kingdom: Flame Tree Publishing Ltd.

[15] Cook, D. M. (2015). *Probióticos – A Solução: A chave para uma vida saudável.* Amadora: Agir, Camarate.

[16] Katz, S. E. (2018). *Os segredos da fermentação.* Alfragide: Lua de papel. Agosto de 2018.

[17] Stefe, C., Alves, M., & Ribeiro, R. (2008). *Probióticos, Prebióticos e Simbioticos – Artigo de revisão* (Vol. 3). http://www.educadores.diaadia.pr.gov.br/arquivos/File/2010/artigos_teses/Biologia/Artigos/alimentos.pdf.

[18] Shinya, H. (2011). *The Microbe Factor: Your Innate Immunity and the Coming Health Revolution.* United States: Millichap Books, LLC.

[19] Oelschalaeger, T. (2009). *Mechanisms of probiotic actions – A review.* (PubMed, Ed.) Würzburg, Alemanha. doi:10.1016/j.ijmm.

[20] Ng, S., Hart, A., Kamm, M., Stagg, A., & Knight, S. (7 May 2008). *Mechanisms of Action of Probioticos: Recent Advances.* Middlesex, London: Crohhn's & Colitis Foundation of America. doi:10.1002/ibd.20602.

[21] Costa, M., Balthazar, C., Moreira, R., Cruz, A., & Júnior, C. (2013). *Leite fermentado: Potencial Alimento Funcional.* Rio de Janeiro, Brazil. http://www.conhecer.org.br/enciclop/2013a/agrarias/LEITE%20FERMENTADO.pdf.

[22] Klaenhammer, T. R. (14 August 1987). *Bacteriocins of lactic acid bacteria.* North Carolina: Societe de Chimie biologique/Elsevier, Paris. doi:10.1016/0300-9084(88)90206-4

[23] Johnson, A., & Williams, L. (2016). *A Field Guide to Fermentation.* Copenhaga: Dystan & Rosenberg.

# The experience of the natural world in a moment of fine dining – interwoven approaches to sustainability

R. Bonacho, A. Gerardo & M.J. Pires
*Estoril Higher Institute for Tourism and Hotel Studies, Estoril, Portugal*

ABSTRACT: Our study begins with a pedagogical and transdisciplinary approach of the Master in Innovation in Culinary Arts (ESHTE, Portugal), commonly used in the development of gastronomic experiences from a creative process in Design adapted to Gastronomy. Students created four gastronomic moments with different approaches to food, environment and social sustainability, presenting diners with a holistic gastronomic experience, product and process – *Do Prado to Prato* (From farm to plate) in order to understand how the experience of the natural world can be reflected in a moment of fine dining. In this edition the association *Planting a Tree* joined students in the development of a commemorative dinner for the association's 10th anniversary that would become mediatic, sensory and sustainable and would present guests with a full gastronomic experience for all the senses – *Momentum: From Forest to the Plate*. Accordingly, the students made several visits to the Portuguese forest in order to analyze, together with experts from the association, the native plant and animal species that could be used for culinary purposes. To study the results of our experience, a questionnaire was conducted on the experiments carried out and we have adopted the ethnographic design methodology to better understand how the guests experienced these fine dining moments.

## 1 INTRODUCTION

In the Master in Innovation in Culinary Arts (MIAC) at the Estoril Higher Institute for Tourism and Hotel Studies (ESHTE, Portugal) students are encouraged to develop their project activity under current themes of the food system based on a creative process in design (Bonacho, 2019) and in an interdisciplinary manner. Based on the theme of the 6th edition of the master's degree *Do Prado ao Prato* (From farm to plate), students and the coordination of MIAC were challenged to create a gastronomic experience that reflected the guiding principles of the non-governmental association *Planting a Tree* on the celebration of its 10th anniversary as a non-profit movement that preserves the Portuguese forest, since it "develops and implements voluntary programs, (…) for the recovery of ecologically degraded areas through the restoration of native forests and species" (Associação Plantar uma Árvore, 2019).

Food, according to Hegarty (2005), encompasses more than its production, consumption and nutrition, it reflects a socio-cultural interaction with symbolic meanings. Schösler & De Boer (2018) even mention that in the last decades we have seen a growing interest in the theme of food sustainability that promotes the adoption of new diets. According to the authors, this idea of sustainability of the food system can only be achieved if consumers themselves adopt and develop a set of changes in their diet, such as reducing protein consumption, for which they are not yet prepared (Schösler & De Boer, 2018, 2013). In a globalized world where food is available or scarce, where there is diversity and abundance, gastronomy is increasingly revised into two essential concepts: creativity and experience. We understand that more and more chefs are "rescuing traditions, using local ingredients and transforming them into authentic experiences with an innovative touch, while respecting flavors and products" (Bonacho, 2018).

In this sense, MIAC seeks to instill a pedagogical model in which students work on the idea that food consumption reflects a much boarder dimension, especially with regard to gastronomic experiences. The challenge we propose to students is to imagine that haute cuisine surpasses the physical and mental barrier of what a restaurant is, to cook something that is not recognizable as "food" when using disruptive codes (de Albeniz, 2018).

Such a concept of experience is what Gómez-Corona & Valentin (2019) refer to as hyper-consumerism that circulates between the accumulation of objects and experiences. The consumer is moving from a culture of mass production (standardized and inauthentic) to an aesthetic culture, a unique one where artisanal products are valued.; s/he is moving from a material collector to an experience collector, *Homo experientialis* – "Today, consumers want to be immersed in a world in which they are free to express themselves through products, and experience them with all their senses. The products in the hyper-consumption market that can generate these experiences will have what Lee et al. (2018) have called, an experiential advantage" (Gómez-Corona & Valentin, 2019).

The consumer wants more than the delivery of a product or service, he seeks consumption that meets products and services which create unique and memorable experiences – "Through the experience, the consumer no longer 'destroys', but becomes the builder of emotions and moments." Successful products must offer "experiences" (Pecoraro & Uusitalo, 2014), "memorable experiences" (Pine & Gilmore, 1998) or "extraordinary experiences" (Linberg & Ostergaard, 2015).

In Gómez-Corona & Valentin (2019) we can see a brief literary review of the concept of experience, what the authors tell us is that experience contains two contradictory phenomena that are important to connect. In the first case, experience is a way of feeling, as being invaded by an emotional state, which the authors refer to as an aesthetic or loving experience, but this is juxtaposed with another that has to do with cognitive activity, the way we build the real world, how we receive and experience it. Then we have to be aware of the fact that there are different types of experience, see for example "product experience" (Desmet & Hekkerts, 2007), "consumer experience" (Darpy, 2012), "user experience" (Warell, 2008) or "drinking experience" (Schifferstein, 2009). However, what interests us in the context of our study is the concept of "food experience" that can also be used as "dining experience" or "gastronomic experience", terms that are mostly used to describe the experience in a restaurant or a complete meal.

Moreover, Kauppinen-Raisanen, Gummerus & Lehtola (2013) break down the food experience into five dimensions, in which the intrinsic characteristics of food are just a single component. The other components are: the dinner, the place, the food, the context and the time. Another aspect that usually influences the eating experience is the act of cooking, as well as the culture that is not always taken into account but that has a close relationship between food and regional culture, especially when we talk about gastronomic experiences. As such, in order to better bring students closer to this idea of culture and the relevance that "the kitchen" and actually "cooking" have in the construction of gastronomic identities, students visit diverse producers and have the opportunity of attending "Food Talks", open access masterclasses organised by MIAC.

Through these opportunities, it becomes easier to understand how food is divided into being edible for pleasure (eatable) and edible without bringing any possible danger (edible); the first, although it can be natural and/or artificial, circulates in both worlds (culture and nature), but only with the discovery of fire was the human being allowed to act in order to process food, making it into something artificial – to cook as a home practical task and cooking at a restaurant for others (Montarani, 2004). This was the context in which the project *Momentum: From the Forest to the Plate*, a sensory experience, was developed. Starting from the challenge suggested by the association *Planting a Tree* made to MIAC students, the latter created a menu whose concept reflected not only the association's concerns, but also the values of the Portuguese gastronomy from a sensory and sustainable point of view, appealing to the consumption of indigenous raw materials.

*Momentum: From Forest to the Plate* was constituted as an interdisciplinary, creative and differentiating project, seeking to create synergies by using environmental sustainability applied to teaching-learning practices, contributing to the visibility of all the institutions involved. The menu was inspired and aligned with the principles of the association: the recovery of biodiversity and the strengthening of ecosystems. A menu that reflected the production cycle and respected the identities of the territories, the proximity of the products to their origin and the way they are treated in the kitchens. The menu embodied the tree's life cycle; basically, taking care of environmental and food sustainability, valuing Portuguese forests. The staging moment created for the menu was accompanied by the performance of the cultural association Byfurcação, which created characters related to the imaginary world of the forest, seeking to combine theatrical activity in the search for an awakening of the consciousness of the guests for the mission of the Association, which on a daily basis passes is based on the individual and collective action.

## 2 METHODOLOGY

Our study was based mainly on a mixed methodology that used mostly qualitative methods. In a first phase, we are presenting a brief review of the literature on the concepts that are fundamental to our study: "experience"; "fine dining" [1] and "sustainability" in the food context and their direct relationship with the process of creating a gastronomic experience that seeks to follow the principles of the association *Planting a Tree*. The second part describes the process by which students responded to the challenge proposed by the association and the theme proposed in the context of the master's program based on Bonacho's research (2018; 2019). Finally, we are presenting the experience in four different contexts, where, with the help of questionnaires (moments II & III), it was possible to measure results that also complete a perspective adopted by an ethnographic method in design – immersion of the researcher in all the experiences during a certain period time (usually the preparation period and the experience itself), where observations were also made on the behavior of the clients/guests through informal conversations and short interviews on issues that are not directly observable but which could respond to the stated hypotheses. The ethnographic dimension is important in this context because the sensory evaluation under controlled conditions, such as laboratories, has numerous limitations for a better understanding of the dinner preferences of the diner – "Ethnographic observation can be a form of engagement and can be a part of transitional practices (…). Involving ethnography within processes of designing is not detached observation, rather practices unfold, are concerned with working *with* people and closing the gap between observation and understanding" (Gunn & Donovan, 2012). Most of the food we eat depends on the way we eat and the context of the food situation (García-Segovia et al., 2015; Schifferstein, 2009). That is why sensory studies have gone beyond the properties of the food itself, see for example the studies by Spence (2014; 2017) and Mouritsen & Styrbaek (2018) and the experiences already developed by the authors (Bonacho et al., 2018a,b). "Observations of the world is natural and essential to design. But ultimately, what matters is less what you look at, and more what you see and what you make of it. From designers we ask for a designed world that has meaning beyond the resolution of purely functional needs. We ask for poetry and subtlety that make sense – not just by fitting in with the culture and environment, but by adding a new dimension to it" (Suri, 2018).

In such a context, our hypotheses are: (a) a gastronomic experience may reflect the principles of biodiversity recovery and the strengthening of the Portuguese forest ecosystems; (b) can this experience be transposed to different geographies and maintain the same guiding principles; (c) can the raw materials used reflect the idea of seasonal and local consumption; (d) the previous hypotheses can be transferred to a fine dining gastronomic experience; and (e) the processes used from a technical and hedonic point of view can maintain the sensory integrity of the raw materials used.

## 3 THE PROCESS

The challenge proposed to students was based on the pedagogical model adopted in the MIAC, considering that in every edition of the MSc course students are encouraged to develop two projects based on a common theme. In the 2018/2019 edition, the theme *From Farm to Plate* was projected in order to instill in students a greater awareness of the sustainability of the Portuguese food system, encouraging them to have greater contact with the product in order to integrate the entire production cycle in the final result of the proposed projects. Students are asked to carry out a project across all disciplines, where they must design a food product and/or service based on the proposed theme to be developed in groups of two and create a gastronomic experience based on the same theme, but in this latter

case it is planned to be developed jointly by the group of 10 students who attend the MSc annually. Based on this theme, the *Planting a Tree* association launched the challenge of reconfiguring this experience at their 10th anniversary celebration dinner. Accordingly, after several visits to the Sintra forest accompanied by biologists and experts on matters of seasonality and the local flora, for instance, from the association, students chose elements not commonly used in the Portuguese gastronomy, like borage, elderberry, myrtle, pine and chamomile, creating then the appropriated narrative to the forest cycle of life.

## 4 THE MENU

The menu concept created by the students starts with the ROS (Figure 1, 1M1) (dew) moment, when the guests are received by the forest beings (guardians and goddess) who, in a performative moment, create the purification of the guests entering the forest with the ritual of washing their hands. This ROS reflects the dew of the plants and a citronella and elderberry kombucha is served – it makes sense for being a probiotic, which through fermentation becames a sustainable technique for food waste. The kombucha is served outside or away from the place where the gastronomic experience takes place, as a moment of conviviality among diners. In the first experience guests enjoyed this moment under an American sequoia, since it is already planted as an ornamental tree in several parks and gardens in Portugal, where the species finds exceptional conditions for its culture. In all the four experiences, the beings of the forest received the guests and purified them for the next moments.

The second moment, CYNTHIA (Figure 1, 1M2) (named after Sintra, the town where the first gastronomic experience took place) is a four-piece moment in a specific order of consumption, because each of the elements reflects the stages of the concept of the menu itself (seed, sapling, leaf and flower): a salted choux pastry served with nettles and crunchy topping with seeds; a liver pate with mint from the river, coriander, citronella, lemon and lime and sprouts; a shiso leaf filled with raspberry, cherry, mint and elderberry gel and a sphere filled with river prawn tartar with pollen vinaigrette. The third moment, EXITIUM (Figure 1, 1M3), expresses the idea of destruction in an allusion to the devasting fires which have been destroying the Portuguese forests over the years. Accordingly, for the guests to have a better perception of everyone's responsibility they are asked to cook river crayfish at the table over a controlled fire and dip it in hollandaise sauce with lavender and flavoured with the crayfish shells. The new cycle comes with the idea of ashes and ruin, entitled CINIS (Figure 1, 1M4), by presenting a piece of apparent charcoal sorrel flavored with a liquid. The fifth moment, SEMEN (Figure 1, 1M5), a bed of bar inside ley, fermented vegetables and broth (again to emphasize the sustainable principle), and other crunchy seeds with activated charcoal earth is then finalized with a broth served running down the dish reminiscent of the course of the river in the forest. Then REPENTARE (Figure 1, 1M6) brings the sprouts moment with mushroom brulé with edible soil (beet, malt flour) topped with some sprouts and mushrooms where the guest has to "dig" to eat while sensing the smell of wet earth. As for the seventh moment, FOLIA I (Figure 1, 1M7), it is a green leaf dish with a mix from microgreens, snail caviar, fake snail stuffed with snail, roasted tomato gel and caper gel, fig leaf sorbet and huakatai vinaigrette, flowed by FOLIA II (Figure 1, 1M8) with tubers, pine crust, hay, juniper, egg yolk, wild boar, crispy tubers styled/shaped as paper-thin leaves and FOLIA III (Figure 1, 1M9) of phisalis leaves, flower petals, elderberry and chamomile gel all placed in wood crafted physalis petal shaped wood. The tenth and eleventh moments, FLOS I (Figure 1, 1M10) with Koji crumble, wild berry gel, myrtle sorbet and meringue with blackberry and raspberry and FLOS II (Figure 1, 1M11) with honey, brandymel, orange, ginger and almond symbolized flower pollination presented as a honeycomb. Finally, the FRUCTUS (Figure 1, 1M12) moment, petit-fours shaped as fruits for guests to pick from a tree (flavors: passion fruit, pear and lemon). These are hanging from the tree being just held by a suspended leaf with the name of the diner who has previously stated his/her preference. As a last note on the menu, several breads are served throughout the dinner: Fire (activated charcoal and smoked grissini; three-seed bread with beet; dried leaves; flat bread flavored with lemon balm). These are harmonized to better complement the experience, along with the selected wines.

## 5 THE EXPERIENCES

According to Hekkert & Schifferstein (2015) food must engage experiences to seduce the consumer and define the product experience as an awareness of the psychological effects that the interaction with the diner produces, including also the way the senses are stimulated, the meaning and the value that people add to the product and the emotions and feelings that are aroused in its consumption. It is important, in addition, to the sensory component, to understand the aesthetic response of the product: "Because food experiences are not determined solely by the physical product, the development of new food products should take the usage situation and the consumption context into account." (2015:27).

### 5.1 Momentum: from forest to the plate – part I (Sintra, June 2019)

The issue of sustainability was also reflected in terms of resources, creating dialogues between institutions, students and study areas. An example was the partnership with a Design School which brought about all the challenges of creating an interchange between those who cook and design a sustainable menu and those

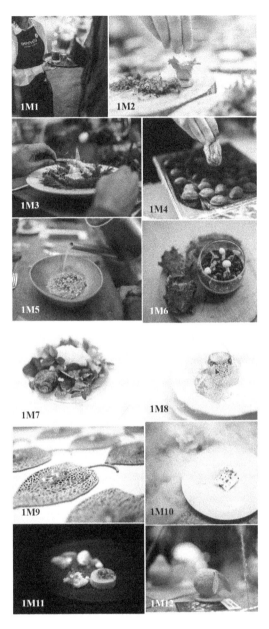

Figure 1. Menu momentum: from the forest to the plate (Photography: Gabriell Vieira, 2019).

who create the dishware and the tableware in harmony with the forest; the participation of the Social Communication School (ESCS-IPL), which was equally valued with the creation of a video mapping experience for the event; and some of the moments were accompanied by the performance of the cultural association Byfurcaçao, who helped to portray the immersive spirit of this detailed project in the special environment of the about to be under renovation Quinta da Riba Fria (Sintra). Meiselman et al. (1988) *apud* García-Segovia et al. (2015) define the context as "the numerous variables in our eating environments which make it easier or harder for us to begin, continue, or complete a meal." (2015:1) This has been another challenge when creating the settings in the diverse regions, as clearly the diverse partnerships helped reaching beyond the boundaries of academia to include these other cities (moments II, III & IV).

The partner association protects Portuguese forests and helped to better understand and explore our food region – its seasonality, the invading plants, the national heritage and the place to present an experience to policymakers, the media, the catering industry and those responsible for diverse levels of education to test this concept. We believe in the culinary experience as a way of living to apprehend, i.e. creating in order to transfer/transmit the experience – "Powerful stories can transport consumers into imaginary worlds" (Mossberg & Eide, 2017).

### 5.2 Momentum: from forest to the plate – part II and III (Lagoa and São Brás de Alportel, November 2019)

Following the first experience developed in Sintra and which served as a milestone for the 10th anniversary of the *Planting a Tree* association, students were invited to join the program of the *Forgotten Food Festival* that took place in the Algarve in different locations (Lagoa and São Brás de Alportel). The festival aimed to "revive recipes and ingredients lost in memory" or bring to our knowledge moments/recipes which somehow faced extinction of its kind, either through an association with poverty or rurality, or because they are not species of agricultural interest. With different logistic and raw materials, the menu was adapted according to the festival's needs, maintaining its initial concept. A survey was made of the homegrown products from the locations where the dinners took place and the recipes were changed only with respect to the raw materials used. Unlike the invited guests of the Sintra moment, these applied for the experience in each location and they comprised both Portuguese and international guests, which created a more challenging task, even if the menu was reduced in terms of the numbers of courses. The references to the local and seasonality would vary much more, we assumed. A final note on the quite different and challenging logistics in terms of preparation facilities, but also on the choice of having guests sitting in long benches to bring everyone together, as well as showcasing the forest elements in the table decoration – although different during each of the four moments, these choices were essential for the experience.

### 5.3 Momentum: from forest to the plate – part IV (Lisbon, November 2019)

The challenge to create an experience of the natural world in a moment of fine dining changed in the fourth setting; not only in terms of the logistic, since the kitchen now included members from the catering company who had also supported us in the first event and the setting defied us in a diverse way (Teatro Thália, a recently restored building), but also because some of the guests returned from the first experience. In fact, the objective was to invite diners who have "cultivated their (gustatory) taste and are open to and even looking for its further refinement" and surprising moments (Lane, 2014). Bearing in mind that the "location contributes significantly to food acceptance, both to the appreciation of particular food attributes, as well as to overall acceptability" (Edwards et al., 2003), the fourth experience proved to bring together an even greater acknowledgement of the message conveyed. Such considerations do not subsume the notion that food products must engage experiences to seduce the consumer; as Hekkert & Schifferstein (2009) portray, the experience of the product, as an awareness of the psychological effects that the interaction between the product and the consumer produces, includes also the way the senses are stimulated, the meaning and value that people add to the product and the emotions and feelings that are aroused in its consumption. In this case, in addition to the sensory components, it is important to understand the aesthetic response of the product, since; as we also concluded "experiences may change over the different stages of the user-product interaction and can be affected by items consumed previously" (2015: 27) [2].

## 6 RESULTS AND CONCLUSIONS

Our main questions were on how we can create a gastronomic experience that reflects the principles of biodiversity recovery and the strengthening of Portuguese forest ecosystems; how this experience can be transferred to different geographies following the same guiding principles; which of the raw materials used can reinforce its concept of seasonal and local products; on its liability to be transposed to a gastronomic experience and which processes can be used from a technical and sensory point of view to maintain their sensory integrity.

During our gastronomic experiences (moments II & III) in the Algarve we surveyed and interviewed the diners. The direct questions came to: "Regarding the food products used in this experience, how do you rate them from the perspective of Sustainability, Seasonality and Local". All the diners answered that the food products were local and sustainable according to their knowledge. This was because we changed most of the products according to the geography in which the experience happened.

Other comments, during interviews, were that the food was challenging sometimes, something not "experienced before", "the atmosphere was a bit strange, with the smells and the sounds", "it was definitely an unusual experience" and "I think the Algarve should be opened every day of the year", saluting the 365Algarve project that brings together several associations [3].

Our "gastronomic experience could be defined as a result of the interaction of all the processes that are activated in gastronomy, especially in haute cuisine, when it is realized that the kitchen contains a complexity that exceeds the functional fact of feeding. The traditional boundaries of cuisine are surpassed when it becomes part of an economy of experience in which processes (*the how*) have a greater weight than the product (*the what*). The gastronomic experience thus has a high sublimation component that goes beyond the limits of a functional or subsistence cooking." Accordingly, this comes to showcase that considering how "food experiences are not determined solely by the physical food product, the development of new food products should take the usage situation and the consumption context into account" (Kauppinen-Räisänen et al., 2013) as we believe to have been the case with the *Momentum | From Forest to the Plate* detailed gastronomic experiences.

## REFERENCES AND NOTES

[1] The term is a contentious one commonly used for those who value high quality food and service – a more elaborate food preparation as a "result of very skillful and imaginative cooking, and together with attentive service and a pleasing ambience, turns a meal in to an inspiring 'special occasion'" – and are open to surprising and creative interpretations" (Lane, 2014).

[2] https://www.facebook.com/fa.ulisboa/videos/962526697479154/

[3] https://youtu.be/B2D8iPi4pP4

Bonacho, R. (2019). *Design Bites: A prática do Design nas Artes Culinárias*. Lisbon: Faculdade de Arquitetura da Universidade de Lisboa. Tese de Doutoramento não publicada.

Bonacho, R.; Pires, M.J.; Viegas, C. (2018a). "A Saudade Portuguesa: Designing a dialogical food narrative." In. Bonacho, et al (2018) (Ed.) *Experiencing Food, Designing Dialogues. Proceedings of the 1st International Conference on Food Design and Food Studies* (EFOOD2017). London: Taylor & Francis – CRC Press.

Bonacho, R.; Coelho, A.; Pinheiro Sousa, A.; Pires, M.J. (2018b). "Angela Carter: Receiving Literature through food & design". In. Bonacho, et al (2018) (Ed.) *Experiencing Food, Designing Dialogues. Proceedings of the 1st International Conference on Food Design and Food Studies* (EFOOD2017). London: Taylor & Francis – CRC Press.

Darpy, D. (2012). *Comportements du consommateur*. Paris: DUNOD.

De Albeniz, I. M. (2018). Foundations for an analysis of the gastronomic experience: From product to process. *International Journal of Gastronomy and Food Science*, 13, 108–116.

Desmet, P., & Hekkert, P. (2007). Framework of product experience. *International Journal of Design*, 1(1), 57–66.

Edwards, J. S. A., Meiselman, H., Edwards, A. & Lesher, L. (2003). The influence of eating location on the acceptability of identically prepared foods. *Food Quality Preference*, Vol. 14, 647–652.

Gómez-Corona, C.; Valentin, D. (2019). An experiential culture: a review on user, product, drinking and eating experiences in consumer research. *Food Research International*, Vol. 115, 328–337.

Hegarty, J. A. (2005). Developing "Subjects Fields" in Culinary Arts, Science, and Gastronomy. *Journal of Culinary Science and Techonology*, 4:1, 5–13.

Hekkert, P., & Schifferstein, H. N. J. (2008). Introducing product experience. In H. N. J. Schifferstein, & P. Hekkert (Eds.). Product Experience. UK: Elsevier.

Kauppinen-Räisänen, H., Gummerus, J., & Lehtola, K. (2013). Remembered eating experiences described by the self, place, food, context and time. *British Food Journal*, 115(5), 666–685.

Lane, C. (2014). *The Cultivation of Taste: Chefs and the Organization of Fine Dining*. Oxford University Press.

Lee, J. C., Hall, D. L., & Wood, W. (2018). Experiential or Material Purchases? Social Class Determines Purchase Hapiness. *Psychological Science*, 1–9.

Linberg, F., & Ostergaard, P. (2015). Extraordinary consumer experiences: Why immersion and transformation cause trouble. *Journal of Consumer Behaviour*, 14, 248–260.

Meiselman, H. L., Hirsh, E. S., & Popper, R. D. (1988). Sensory hedonic and situational factors in food acceptance and consumption. In D. M. H. Thomson (Ed.), *Food Acceptability*, 77–87. London: Elsevier.

Montarani, M. (2004). *La Comida como Cultura*. Gijón: Ediciones Trea.

Mossberg, L. & Eide, D. (2017). Storytelling and meal experience concepts. *European Planning Studies*, 25:7, 1184–1199.

Mouritsen, O. G. & Styrbaek (2018). *Mouthfeel: How texture makes taste*. New York: Columbia University Press.

Pecoraro, M., & Uusitalo, O. (2014). Exploring the everyday retail experience: The discourses of style and design. *Journal of Consumer Behaviour*, 13, 429–441.

Pine, B. J., & Gilmore, J. H. (1998). Welcome to the experience economy. *Harvard Business Review*, 76, 97–105.

Schösler, H.; De Boer, J. (2018). Towards more sustainable diets: insights from "gourmets" and their relevance for policy strategies. *Appetite*, Vol. 127, 59–68.

Schifferstein, H. N. J. (2009). The Drinking experience: cup or content? *Food Quality and Preference*, 20(3), 268–276.

Spence, C. (2017). *Gastrophysics: The new science of eating*. UK: Penguin Random House.

Spence, C. & Piqueras-Fiszman, B. (2014). The Perfect Meal: The multisensory science of food and dining. UK: John Wiley Blackwell.

Suri, J. F. (2018). Poetic Observation: What Designers Make of What They See. In: Clarke, A. (Ed.) *Design Antrophology: Object Culture in Transition*. London: Bloomsbury.

Warell, A. (2008). Multi-modal Visual experience of Brand-specific Automobile Design. *The TQM Journal*, 20(4), 356–371.

*Experiencing Food: Designing Sustainable and Social Practices – Bonacho, Pires & Lamy (Eds)*
*© 2021 Taylor & Francis Group, London, ISBN 978-0-367-49414-8*

# Floating dish, a sustainable, interactive and fine dining concept

R. Mota & P. Mata
*LAQV, REQUIMTE, Departamento de Química, Faculdade de Ciências e Tecnologia/Universidade Nova de Lisboa, Caparica, Portugal*

R. Bonacho
*Centro de Investigação em Arquitetura, Urbanismo e Design, Faculdade de Arquitetura da Universidade de Lisboa, Lisbon, Portugal*

ABSTRACT: A floating plate composed by an organic fig's leaf, which levitates by the application of magnets, was used to serve an *amuse-bouche* called Mooning Walk, developed in the context of a multisensory designed menu. The design process was built up around an interactive plate and sustainable conscious ingredients. Its presentation under ultraviolet (UV) black-light results in different visualizations and perceptions of the dish that triggers emotions and influences taster's perceptions imparting also playful characteristics.

*Keywords:* Food-Design, Food Sustainability, Gastrophysics, Ergonomics

## 1 INTRODUCTION

Design and Food are universes with common characteristics, both involving a conception and an execution of an idea (Catterall, 1999). Human creativity and Design have always sought to improve the feeding process, providing tools to obtain food, to eat and to cook (Capella, 2015). This new emerging territory of Design, known as Food Design, intends in this research to serve our senses and be sustainable by using the Design Thinking Process (Schön, 1992; Zampollo, 2013).

Food has many features: pleasure, disease, medicine or fuel, since the live beings empirically visualize and evaluate food (externally) before placing it in the mouth (Garner, 1974; Rozin, 1982). The first contact with food is through vision, and it contributes not only to its perception, but also to its acceptance, with color, shape, exterior texture, brightness, clarity and transparency being the most relevant characteristics for this. Color is the characteristic that most contributes to the creation of food related expectations (Spence, 2015).

For most chefs, the plating of food is approached in an intuitive manner, the understanding of the influence of the visual characteristics of the food on a plate on the diner's expectations, and their subsequent experience of the food, is still far from understood, but a great amount of research is being undertaken about this subject (Capella, 2015). The influence of the glassware and plateware on the perception of food is also an important aspect to consider (Deroy & Spence, 2016).

Research conducted at the Alicía Foundation in Spain, found out that exactly the same frozen strawberry mousse was rated as tasting 10% sweeter and 15% more flavourful, and was liked significantly more, when eaten from a white plate instead of from a black plate (Spence, 2017). The visual shape or format also influence taster perception, as sweet tastes have been found to be associated with roundedness, and bitterness is associated with angularity (Spenceand Ngo, 2012), the latter is unpleasant (Bar & Neta, 2006; Spence, 2017b; Spence & Piqueras-Fiszman, 2014).

Diners can also find difficulty to distinguish between flavours in the absence of visual cues. Commonly sighted individuals have a great deal of stored knowledge concerning the appearance properties of foods and beverages. These multisensory mental images might define the cognitive aspects of the eating process (Delwiche, 2012; Shankar et al., 2010).

Furthermore, it is important to consider the colour of the lighting in the restaurant. Indeed, the temperature, intensity and type of illumination can all be expected to exert some influence on the perceived colour of the plate, the food placed on it, and on the atmosphere, and hence on the flavour of the food itself, not to mention on the mood of the guests (Spence et al., 2014).

An increasing number of chefs, artists, and designers are currently interested in utilizing different materials and/or textures in their food, plateware, cutlery, and even the texture of the restaurant seats (Watz, 2008). Movement and technology are becoming a trend at fine

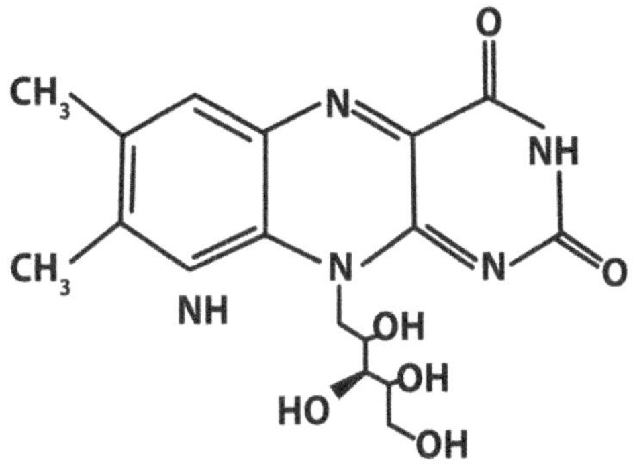

Figure 1. Riboflavin structure, Johnson, 1955.

dining restaurants, to enhance the taste/flavour of food, to provide entertainment and/or to deliver memorable experiences around food and beverages, and to provide healthier eating (Spence & Piqueras-fiszman, 2013). For example, through the use of interactive containers that react on contact with the food, emitting sounds and vibrations and generating luminescence and moving images. Other examples of this approach are the edible luminescence work of Pastry Chef Janice Wong (Wong, 2017), The El Somni project by El Celler de Can Roca (Aleu, 2014), Sublimotion by Paco Roncero and The Fat Duck by Heston Blumenthal (Aleu, 2014).

Magnetic levitation or magnetic suspension is a method by which an object is suspended with no support other than magnetic fields (Halliday et al., 2004; Powell & Danby, 2003; Simon et al., 2001). This technology was already used in restaurants, for example at Sublimotion and The Fat Duck (Spence & Piqueras-fiszman, 2013).

Luminescence is the emission of light by any substance that has absorbed light or other electromagnetic radiation. The energy of the emission is typically less than that of absorption. Fluorescent materials, exhibit a particular type of luminescence, and cease to glow immediately when the radiation source is turned off (Lakowicz, 2006). The most striking example of fluorescence occurs when the absorbed radiation is in the UV region of the spectrum (e.g. black light), and thus invisible to the human eye, while the emitted light is in the visible region, which gives the fluorescent substance a distinct colour that can be seen only when exposed to UV light (Berlman, 1965; Sauer et al., 2011; Wong, 2017).

Examples of fluorescence molecules are: quinine, which is present in tonic water (Berlman, 1965; Johnson, 1955; Schmillen, 1967), Riboflavin (Glow by SOSA) a compound best known as vitamin B2 (see Figure 1), and Curcumin, a bright yellow chemical produced by some plants as for example Curcuma longa known as turmeric (Johnson, 1955).

These concepts and products were applied under the lens of design process in order to develop a Floating, Sustainable, Interactive and Fine Dining Dish.

## 2 MATERIALS AND METHODS

### 2.1 *Food stimulus*

The dish here described, called Mooning Walk, is a component of a multisensory designed menu (Mota, 2018). It is an amuse bouche, served in bite-sized pieces. Composed by eight elements. The main ingredients used are wild pigeon, katsuobushi, tonic water, figs and their leaves (as an organic plate) and white grapefruit essential oil.

**Wild pigeon** – the breast was cleaned, blanched, deboned, browned, simmered, thinly shredded, deep fried, strained and plated. It's texture reminds a straw bale with an aerated texture.

**Tonic water fluid gel** was made by adding 8,5 g gellan gum, 0,4 g salt, 0,3 ml white grapefruit essential oil and 100 g sugar to 500 g tonic water. The mixture was boiled until complete dissolution and cooled to set. Finally, it was blended in a thermomix equipment and sieved. After plated when under blacklight it glows and when under sunlight it becomes transparent.

**Katsuobushi flakes** – Flakes of dried, fermented, and smoked skipjack tuna, having distinct umami taste due to its high inosine acid content. Upon being placed on hot food, the heat waves cause the thin and light katsuobushi flakes to move upwards, giving it a special aesthetic look, contributing for an additional visual component

**Riboflavin sauce** – The glowing mixture, used for holding and making katsuobushi flakes move, was done using 500 ml of hot water, 5 g Glow by SOSA (E101) and 2 g xanthan gum which were blended together.

**Tagete petals** – contribute to colour contrast and provide dry and acid vegetal flavour to the dish, under blacklight turn bordeaux. Provided by Microgreens® under organic and certified production.

**Pea sprouts** – freshly picked, washed and plated. Apart from the interesting spirals shapes, this sprout tastes as dry cereals. Also provided by Microgreens® under organic and certified production.

**Fig's jam** – contributing for a sweet taste on the dish, matches the pigeon flavour well plus works as a base for stability. Another reason for applying this fruit, was to match the fig leaf used as plate.

It was prepared using 400 g figs, 300 g sugar, 150 g water, 150 g lemon juice, 2 g salt, 1 vanilla bean and 1 cinnamon stick cooked at low heat for about 45 minutes.

**Curcuma powder** – A spice with yellowish pigments, that also glows in the dark. This Indian spice, after being toasted, was sprinkled on the pigeon.

### 2.2 *Container*

All the elements above referred were placed on top of a fig's leaf (see Figure 2). The leaf floats due to a magnetic levitation system (Figure 3). The top magnet disk was concealed between two leafs and glued, while the bottom base magnet (Figure 4) was craved below

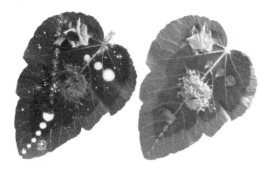

Figure 2. Mooning walk plating 1, under blacklight (left) under sunlight (right), 2018.

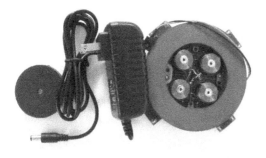

Figure 3. Magnetic levitation equipment (Thompson, 2000).

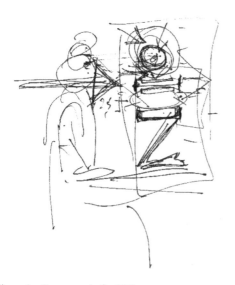

Figure 4. Ergonomy drafts, 2018.

the dining table. The plate rotates as a consequence of the placing impulse by the waiter.

In order to allow a direct contact with the levitation system and food, no cutlery is provided with this dish, fingers are intended to be used when tasting it.

## 2.3 *Procedure*

The plating options on the figs leaf were guided by general principles of visual harmony, which were selected to include movement, unity, variety, balance, rhythm, emphasis, contrast, proportion and pattern (Cross et al., 1993; Hutchings, 2017; Stummerer, 2010; Swann, 2002; Stummerer & Hablesreiter, 2013; defining a completely natural form with organic edges and colours. Movement, rhythm and optical illusion were enhanced by the levitation system.

As light changes, from blacklight to normal LED light, while the dish is served, different visual compositions will come up which allow different readings, produces new expectations and an innovative sensory perception. The dish was photographed by an analogic digital camera in two moments, under 18 watts blacklight and normal LED light (Figure 2), revealing different identities and perspectives.

## 2.4 *Design process*

This dish was developed in 4 phases, applying the Double Diamond design process (Design Council, 2017): **1st Phase** – Identify sight cues that can be used in the dish to influence sensory perception. **2nd Phase** – Define and select the relevant sight cues to achieve the intended objectives. **3rd Phase** – Develop prototypes, test elements and recipes. Check the whole ergonomy of the system, confirm colours and light set, define plating. **4th Phase** – Delivery of the final version of the dish.

## 3 DISCUSSION

Visual receptors are the first to be stimulated prior to the consumption of food. Apart from increasing the production of saliva and gastric juices, vision insights trigger emotions, interest and expectations related to the taste, flavour, and enjoyment of a given dish (Michel et al., 2015). One of the main objectives in the development of this dish was to create illusion, bluff, mystery, darkness, surprises, arouse curiosity and introduce cues to some elements common in a forest at night. Constant feeling of surprise, based on the delivery of unusual sensory experiences, can contribute to make this dining experiences unusual, intriguing and memorable for the customers (Spence, 2017). The various aspects of the visual composition included, for instance, the colour of the food or elements of the dish, the visual texture of the components and their combination, the shape of the individual components, and the higher-order spatial arrangement of the various elements. One relevant aspect of this dish is the double reading, with blacklight and normal LED light creating different perspectives of food elements. The elements of the dish were selected and tested in order to create two distinct visual perception moments during consumption of this dish. These represent the night and day light perception of a forest,

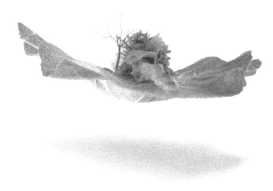

Figure 5. Mooning walk plating 2, under sunlight.

including the fauna and flora elements characterizing them. Changes of colours from dark blue, brown, black, grey and neon bright lights (yellow, white, light blue) to green, orange, yellow, brown and even transparent, contribute to arouse interest and interrogation and mark the memory of the taster (Hutchings, 2017; Stummerer, 2010).

The technology, namely the use of the magnetic levitation system and the fluorescence, in this dish, was used to make the building of a multisensory dining experience possible. The risk of this becoming more important than the food itself should be considered. The use of technology already present in the work of several chefs, can only be justified if it constitutes a benefit in terms of enhancing the diner's multisensory experience. H. Blumenthal's dish 'The sound of the sea' is an example in which digital technology was used to deliver a genuinely different kind of multisensory dining experience, in these cases, it is also expected that the diner ends up by getting to pay more attention to dish which results in an increased perception (Spence and Piqueras-Fiszman, 2014). Some restaurants also use the possibilities associated with projecting images directly onto the food sitting on the dinner table. For example, at El Celler de Can Roca in Spain (Aleu, 2014), a variety of projections over the food dishes give the impression of bringing the food very much to life (Spence & Piqueras-fiszman, 2013). In summary, the range of scientific insights that are now available concerning the effects of the multisensory atmosphere on the pleasantness and enjoyment of food can be used, potentially giving it a purpose in terms of enhancing the diner's experience, rather than just serving to offer the diner an entertaining distraction (Spence & Piqueras-fiszman, 2013). No studies were encountered regarding the effect of the use of these technologies in the perception of the dishes (Figure 5). Although this aspect is not in the scope of the present work, it should be mentioned that it is a relevant area of research.

Concerning the plate's visual characteristics, mostly food is eaten from round white plates, as the plate used in the dish described is a triangular green leaf, this could be the first detail to focus on. Plating does not stop with the choice of plate, but extends to the complexity of the overall arrangement on the plate and the interactions between the various visual attributes of plateware (Spence et al., 2014). Apart from the organic edges, a leaf inserts its own lines on the plan, symmetry and perspective to the composition.

As Deroy & Spence (2016) quoted, in triangle-like shapes (as that of the fig's leaf), orientation appears to matter, with downward pointing triangles being associated with a threat, Michel et al. (2015) also demonstrate that orientation matters and say that optimally orienting the plate translates into an increased willingness to pay for the food. In the case of the dish developed, however, the fig's leaf was in constant rotation provided by the magnetic levitation, so no upward or downward orientation was defined. In fact, this fact can also provide different reading moments of the dish.

The non-existing cutlery when tasting this dish, also introduces different perception components. Many people around the world eat without the aid of cutlery, and claim their food to be much tastier when consumed in this way (Biggs et al., 2016).

Ingredients were chosen considering not only its organoleptic and visual relevant characteristics, but also sustainability and symbolism. The pigeon meat was chosen due to its distinctive flavours and leanness but also due to the fact that pigeons, in terms of threat status at European level, are considered as "Unthreatened" (BirdLife International, 2004). Wild pigeons are also guided by the magnetic fields of the planet. For these reasons this bird was chosen as the main ingredient in this dish in which magnetic effects are used. Due to the chosen cooking process its consistency and lightness remind a bundle of crispy straws.

Tonic water has quinine that glows under blacklights, and is transparent under normal light, allowing to provide different visual readings. It also gives a bitter taste to the dish. White grapefruit essential oil was chosen to pair the flavours of the pigeon, contributing to its citrus profile. Due to the increasing attention to natural additives, essential oils from several plants have been more widely used and are processing aids in green technologies (Adelakun et al., 2015; Espina et al., 2014; Hyldgaard et al., 2012).

Under normal light is yellow and under blacklight becomes fluorescent. Represents the fireflies and all the mysterious night animals. Riboflavin is used as an additive to soft drinks and yogurt (Buehler, 2011).

## 4 CONCLUSION

The use of technology in food service certainly holds the potential to enhance the diner/drinker's experience, and/or to allow a restaurant to differentiate itself in the challenging world of fine dining. This can also be effective in contributing to a deeper and more informed appreciations, reducing unconscious consumption, and promoting education, and food sustainability consciousness. Moonlight Walk, the dish described in this paper, was designed to produce a multisensory and innovative perception.

The dish uses technology, such as magnetic levitation and UV light (blacklight), and a designed visual composition to create effects that intend to improve the experience of the diners when eating it.

There is a growing public interest in the topic of food aesthetics. The science of plating, or rather the scientific approach to aesthetic plating, will continue to grow in the years to come (Velasco et al., 2016). Digital technologies will constitute an increasingly common feature of the dining table of the future (Spence & Piqueras-fiszman, 2013), contributing to allow people to control/modify their eating behaviours and perception, in order to improve it.

Studying food presentations under the lens of psychology and sensory science could give precious insights to the so far empirical, art of plating (Michel et al., 2014). This is an important area of research to allow chefs to do a more grounded work and to promote the teaching of food design at culinary arts school.

## ACKNOWLEDGEMENT

The work described is a component of a research project developed for a MSc dissertation which consists on the development of a menu inspired by a forest and composed by five dishes, each one focused in stimulating a particular human sense – Sight, Smell, Hearing, Taste and Touch (Mota, 2018). Each dish involves different contents and techniques and is based in different hypothesis and research results in the literature.

## REFERENCES

Adelakun, E., Oyelade, J. and Olanipekun, F. (2015) 'Use of essential oils in food preservation', *Essential Oils in Food Preservation, Flavor and Safety* (November), pp. 71–84. doi: 10.1016/B978-0-12-416641-7.00007-9.

Aleu, F. (2014) *El Somni del Celler de Can Roca*. Barcelona, Spain.

Bar, M. and Neta, M. (2006) 'Humans prefer curved visual objects', *Psychological Science*, 17(8), pp. 645–648. doi: 10.1111/j.1467-9280.2006.01759.x.

Berlman, L. (1965) *Handbook of fluorescence spectra in aromatic molecules*. Vol. 1. New York: Academic Press.

Biggs, L., Juravle, G. and Spence, C. (2016) 'Haptic exploration of plateware alters the perceived texture and taste of food', *Food Quality and Preference*. Elsevier Ltd, 50, pp. 129–134. doi: 10.1016/j.foodqual.2016.02.007.

BirdLife International (2004) *Abundance of bird species*.

Buehler, B. (2011) 'Vitamin B 2: Riboflavin', *Complementary Health Practice Review*, 16(2), pp. 88–90. doi: 10.1177/1533210110392943.

Capella, J. (2015) *Tapas – Spanish design for food*. Barcelona: Sociedad Esatal de Accion cultura, SA.

Catterall, C. (1999) *Food: Design and Culture*. London, UK: Laurence King.

Cross, N., Vries, M. and Grant, D. (1993) 'A history of design methodology', in *Design Methodology and Relationships with Science*. Dordrecht: Kluwer Academic Press, pp. 15–26.

Delwiche, J. (2012) 'You eat with your eyes first', *Physiology and Behavior*, 107(4), pp. 502–504. doi: 10.1016/j.physbeh.2012.07.007.

Deroy, O. and Spence, C. (2016) 'Crossmodal correspondences: Four challenges', *Multisensory Research*, 29(1–3), pp. 29–48. doi: 10.1163/22134808-00002488.

Design Council (2017) *The Double Diamond*. Available at: https://www.designcouncil.org.uk/ (Accessed: 16 January 2018).

Espina, L., Garc, D. and Pag, R. (2014) 'Impact of Essential Oils on the Taste Acceptance of Tomato Juice, Vegetable Soup, or Poultry Burgers', *Journal of Food Science*, 79(8), pp. 1575–1583. doi: 10.1111/1750-3841.12529.

Garner, W. (1974) *The processing of information and structure*. 6th edn. New York: Potomac, L. Erlbaum Associates.

Halliday, D., Resnick, R. and Walker, J. (2004) *Fundamentals of Physics*. Edited by David Halliday. EUA: John Wiley & Sons, Ltd.

Hutchings, J. (2017) *Colour in food, Colour Design: Theories and Applications: Second Edition*. doi: 10.1016/B978-0-08-101270-3.00006-0.

Hyldgaard, M., Mygind, T. and Meyer, R. (2012) 'Essential oils in food preservation: Mode of action, synergies, and interactions with food matrix components', *Frontiers in Microbiology*, 3(JAN), pp. 1–24. doi: 10.3389/fmicb.2012.00012.

Johnson, F. (1955) *The luminescence of biological systems*. Washington, D.C: Amer. Assoc, Adv. Sci.

Lakowicz, J. (2006) *Principles of fluorescence spectroscopy, Principles of Fluorescence Spectroscopy*. Baltimore, Maryland, USA: Springer. doi: 10.1007/978-0-387-46312-4.

Michel, C. et al. (2014) 'A taste of Kandinsky: assessing the influence of the artistic visual presentation of food on the dining experience', *Flavour*, 3(1), p. 7. doi: 10.1186/2044-7248-3-7.

Michel, C. et al. (2015) 'Rotating plates: Online study demonstrates the importance of orientation in the plating of food', *Food Quality and Preference*. Elsevier Ltd, 44, pp. 194–202. doi: 10.1016/j.foodqual.2015.04.015.

Mota, R. (2018) *Designing for the senses through food design and psychophysiology*. Universidade de Lisboa.

Powell, J. and Danby, G. (2003) 'Maglev: The New Mode of Transport for the 21st Century', *21St Century Science and Technology*, pp. 43–57.

Rozin, P. (1982) '"Taste-smell confusions" and the duality of the olfactory sense', 31(4), pp. 397–401.

Sauer, M., Hofkens, J. and Enderlein, J. (2011) *Fluorescence: Handbook of fluorescence imaging*. Weinheim: Wiley & Co.

Schmillen, A., *et al.* (1967) *Luminescence of organic substances*. Berlin: Hellwege Verlag.

Schön, D. (1992) 'Teaching and Learning as a Design Transaction', in Cross, D. & R. (ed.) *Research into Design Thinking*. Delft: University Press.

Shankar, M., Levitan, C. and Spence, C. (2010) 'Grape expectations: the role of cognitive influences in color–flavor interactions', *Consciousness and Cognition*, 19(1), pp. 380–390. doi: https://doi.org/10.1016/j.concog.2009.08.008.

Simon, M. et al. (2001) 'Diamagnetically stabilized magnet levitation', *American Journal of Physics*, 69(6), pp. 702–713. doi: 10.1119/1.1375157.

Spence, C. (2015) 'On the psychological impact of food colour', *Flavour*. doi: 10.1186/s13411-015-0031-3.

Spence, C. (2017a) 'Enhancing the experience of food and drink via neuroscience-inspired olfactory design', *Senses and Society*. Routledge, 12(2), pp. 209–221. doi: 10.1080/17458927.2017.1270800.

Spence, C. (2017b) *Gastrophysics – The new science of eating*. Edited by P. M. Classics. Oxford, England: Viking.

Spence, C. and Ngo, M. (2012) 'Assessing the shape symbolism of the taste, flavour, and texture of foods and beverages', *Flavour*, 1, p. 12.

Spence, C. and Piqueras-fiszman, B. (2013) 'Technology at the dining table', *Flavour*, 2(16), pp. 1–13.

Spence, C. and Piqueras-Fiszman, B. (2014) *The Perfect Meal: The multisensory science of food and dinning*. First edit. Oxford, England: John Wiley & Sons, Ltd.

Spence, C. et al. (2014) 'Plating manifesto ( II ): the art and science of plating', *Flavou*, 3(Ii), pp. 1–12.

Stummerer, S. (2010) *Food Design XL*. New York: Springer Wien.

Stummerer, S. and Hablesreiter, M. (2013) *Eat Design*. Berlin: Metro Verlag Wien.

Swann, C. (2002) 'Research and the Practice of Design', *Design Issues*, 18(1), pp. 49–61.

Velasco, C. et al. (2016) 'On the importance of balance to aesthetic plating', *International Journal of Gastronomy and Food Science*. Elsevier, 5–6, pp. 10–16. doi: 10.1016/j.ijgfs.2016.08.001.

Watz, B. (2008) 'The entirety of the meal: a designer's perspective', *Journal of Foodservice*, 19, pp. 96–104.

Wong, J. (2017) *Janice Wong*. Available at: https://www.janicewong.com.sg/ (Accessed: 10 March 2018).

Zampollo, F. (2013) *Meaningful eating: a new method for food design*. Edited by M. and D. Sir John Cass Department of Art. London, UK: London Metropolitan University.

# Author index